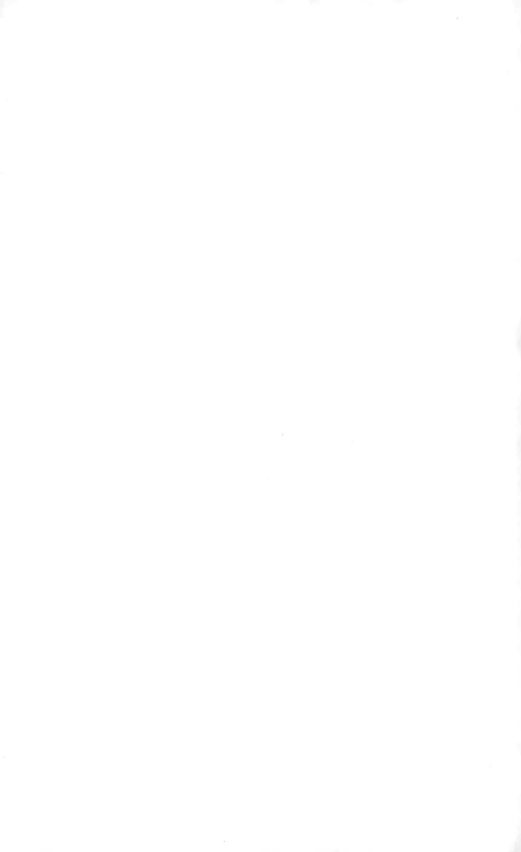

SEXUALLY TRANSMITTED DISEASES

A JOHNS HOPKINS PRESS HEALTH BOOK

SEXUALLY TRANSMITTED DISEASES

A PHYSICIAN TELLS YOU WHAT YOU NEED TO KNOW

Second Edition

LISA MARR, M.D.

THE JOHNS HOPKINS UNIVERSITY PRESS
BALTIMORE

Note to the Reader: This book is not meant to substitute for medical care of people with sexually transmitted infections, and diagnosis and treatment should not be based solely on its contents. Instead, treatment must be developed in a dialogue between the individual and his or her health care provider. This book has been written to help with that dialogue.

Drug dosage: The author and publisher have made reasonable efforts to determine that the selection and dosage of drugs discussed in this text conform to the practices of the general medical community. In some sections, while the medications that are generally used to treat infections are listed, dosages are not.

Remember, this book does not substitute for a visit to a health care provider. It is important not to try to treat yourself, since the decision about which medications to use is a complicated one, and self-treatment often makes it more difficult in the long run to identify the problem and ensure proper treatment.

The medications described do not necessarily have specific approval by the U.S. Food and Drug Administration for use in the diseases and dosages for which they are recommended. In view of ongoing research, changes in governmental regulations, and the constant flow of information relating to drug therapy and drug reactions, the reader is urged to check the package insert of each drug for any change in indications and dosage and for warnings and precautions. This is particularly important when the recommended agent is a new and/or infrequently used drug.

© 1998, 2007 Lisa Marr
All rights reserved. Published 2007
Printed in the United States of America on acid-free paper
2 4 6 8 9 7 5 3 1

The Johns Hopkins University Press
2715 North Charles Street
Baltimore, Maryland 21218-4363
www.press.jhu.edu

Library of Congress Cataloging-in-Publication Data

Marr, Lisa.
Sexually transmitted diseases : a physician tells you what you need
to know / Lisa Marr. — 2nd. ed.
p. cm.
Includes bibliographical references and index.
ISBN-13: 978-0-8018-8658-4 (hardcover : alk. paper)
ISBN-13: 978-0-8018-8659-1 (pbk. : alk. paper)
ISBN-10: 0-8018-8658-9 (hardcover : alk. paper)
ISBN-10: 0-8018-8659-7 (pbk. : alk. paper)
1. Sexually transmitted diseases—Popular works. I. Title.
RC200.2 M27 2007
616.95′1—dc22   2006100443

A catalog record for this book is available from the British Library.

Illustrations by Jacqueline Schaffer

To my husband, Joe, for his love and support

C O N T E N T S

P R E F A C E

Sexually transmitted diseases used to be known as *venereal diseases* (a term derived from *Venus*, the name of the goddess of love) or simply *VD*. The term *VD* was mostly used to describe gonorrhea and syphilis—the "dynamic duo" up until the 1940s. When penicillin was introduced in 1945, there was a euphoric period during which it was hoped that all sexually transmitted diseases would soon be wiped out.

Unfortunately that euphoria was short-lived. There are now more than twenty sexually transmitted infections that we know about (and these days they are known as *sexually transmitted diseases*, or *STDs*, *and sexually transmitted infections*, or STIs, rather than *venereal diseases*), with viral infections such as that caused by the human immunodeficiency virus (HIV) often of greatest concern. The HIV epidemic, understandably, has opened up discussions about sex and STDs, but many people are still in the dark about STDs in general, and attention is seldom given to other, more common, sexually transmitted infections, such as chlamydia and herpes.

Sexually transmitted infections are very common. The fact is that more than half of sexually active adults acquire one or more STDs at some point in their lives, and over twelve million persons are infected with an STD every year in the United States. Although more than half of new infections occur in adolescents and young adults, people of any age, socioeconomic background, and education can be infected. Because so many people are infected, it is very important to understand what STDs are and how they are transmitted. Such knowledge allows people to take steps to protect themselves and helps to keep fear from controlling their lives. People who have information about STDs can lead richer sexual lives because they do not have to live in fear—they know how to lower their risk of acquiring infection.

Sexually transmitted infections have been around for a long time—probably as long as people have been having sex. Throughout history, the discussion of these infections has been colored by their social context and the beliefs and prejudices particular to a certain place and time. From references to gonorrhea in the Old Testament, to the first descriptions of syphilis at the time of Columbus, to warnings to soldiers against getting "VD" from "loose" women in World War II, people have been scared, and misinformed, about STDs. The main reason for that fear is probably the stigma associated with these infections. Many associate them with prostitutes, or with people who "sleep around," and most people do not think that they themselves could be at risk. This is not true. Sexually transmitted infections cut across all boundaries. Furthermore, although we are to this day bombarded with sexual imagery in the media and sex is a favorite topic of conversation, people are still generally misinformed about their risk, do not have accurate information about sexually transmitted infections, and are too scared to ask for the information they need.

Think about it: Where did most of us get our information about these infections? From classes in school? From parents? From peers? From the media? From health care providers? Discussing issues of sexuality in a serious way is difficult in our society, and because of this the information delivered is often incomplete or completely wrong. Usually the people who talk the most about infections know the least, and our friends are as much in the dark as we are. Most school-age children, adolescents, and young adults are too embarrassed to ask questions in school. Besides, school health classes often have moralistic overtones that turn off students.

While growing up, some people are fortunate to have a knowledgeable parent or other adult with whom to discuss issues of sexuality, but most do not. Very often, information obtained through the media is inaccurate, although this situation is improving. Sometimes health care providers, if they are not specialists in sexually transmitted infections, may not be up to date on this topic, and many of the volumes on bookstore and library shelves perpetuate inaccuracies or convey out-of-date information.

The consequences of *not* having accurate information can be devastating: although some STDs are no more than a minor nuisance, others can cause significant pain and discomfort and can become chronic—that is, last a lifetime. Some are curable; others are not. Some can increase the risk of cancer. Some can result in death. Some can lead to difficulty having children in the future, for both men and women. All of these consequences can be avoided if you have accurate information about sexually transmitted infections. It is important to know that most of the STDs that are discussed in this book can be present in people and transmitted without their even knowing it. I find that most people think that if they do not have symptoms, then they could not possibly have an infection. This is why we are seeing epidemic numbers of new infections each year, and this is one reason it is important to have all the facts when you are making decisions about having sex. Your life could depend on it.

Here are some of the most common statements made about sexually transmitted infections. These and others are discussed thoroughly in this book. See how many of these statements you believe are true:

1. "If I don't have any symptoms, I can't have an STD."
2. "If my partner and I get HIV tests and we're negative, that means we don't have to worry about using condoms."
3. "When I got my yearly Pap smear, my doctor would have told me if anything were wrong."
4. "If I use a condom, I can't get an STD."
5. "Oral sex is safe. I can't get an infection with oral sex so I don't need to use a condom."
6. "Only promiscuous people get STDs."
7. "I had chlamydia before, and I had symptoms. Since I don't have any symptoms now, that means I don't have an STD."
8. "Douching after sex will help protect me from getting an STD."
9. "People with herpes always have symptoms."
10. "I can't transmit herpes if I don't have an outbreak."

If you assumed these are true statements, you are not alone. Contrary to what you may have heard, however, all these statements are *false.* One of the purposes of this book is to dispel myths such as these.

In this book I tell you the facts about what sexually transmitted infections are, how they are transmitted, how to recognize them, and how you can protect yourself from getting them. The book is not meant to substitute for a visit to a health care provider; however, as a better-informed person, you are more likely to be a better consumer of health care—you will understand why it is important to take medications as they are prescribed and why it is important to keep follow-up appointments, and you will know what questions to ask. If you do acquire an infection, this book describes standard-of-care treatment. It gives you the knowledge to make well-informed decisions about your sexual health. It provides information for persons of all ages, racial/ethnic backgrounds, and sexual orientations. Its audience is anyone who is sexually active and anyone who is not active but is thinking about becoming active. I hope this book will bring you the information you may have been afraid to ask for and replace some of the misinformation you were given in the past.

In this book, the term *health care provider* is an all-inclusive one used to describe a person who provides you with care on health matters. Physicians, nurses, nurse practitioners, and physician assistants, to name a few, are all health care providers.

There are also infectious disease specialists, and even specialists who are expert in diagnosing and treating specific STDs. Someone who has an infection that seems to be resistant to standard treatments (i.e., is not improving with these treatments) may benefit from consulting with a specialist. This is especially true for people infected with HIV, because the new drugs for controlling that infection must be prescribed very carefully to be effective.

In choosing a health care provider, you should find someone you feel comfortable talking with, someone who listens to you and takes your concerns seriously. You should also feel comfortable about the medical care you're getting and feel confident that the advice and treatments you're being offered are what you need to ensure your good health. Most health care providers are competent and caring and do a good job. If you have doubts, however, try to get a second opinion. You do not need to feel guilty about this, because health care providers are used to patients getting a second opinion. One of the primary themes of this book is that you must do what's right for you. That goes for medical care as well as personal relationships.

As you read this book, I hope you will become armed with knowledge to make smart decisions about sex. The following pages contain the latest, most accurate information about sexually transmitted infections. You should keep in mind, however, that intense medical research on STDs is in progress and recommendations may change over time, so this book does not replace an up-to-date and knowledgeable health care provider. Part I provides general information about the diseases: what symptoms they cause, how they are spread, and how they are diagnosed in a medical examination. It also explains how you can protect yourself from disease through communication and safer sex. Part II, which is in the form of an encyclopedia, provides detailed information about each infection. By providing the most up-to-date information, this book will, I hope, help dispel your fears with knowledge, help you protect yourself and others, and help you get the medical treatment you need to ensure your own good health.

Thanks to Myriam Coppens, ANP, and Terri Warren, ANP, for reviewing selected portions of the original manuscript, and to the staff and practitioners at Westover Heights Clinic in Portland, Oregon, who continue to provide excellent patient care and expand the knowledge of STDs through their research programs.

P A R T I

WHAT YOU NEED TO KNOW

GENITAL
ANATOMY

n this chapter I review normal male and female genital anatomy. A complete understanding of this anatomy will help in understanding how sexually transmitted diseases occur and where the symptoms may be noticed. (Symptoms are discussed in detail in Chapter 2 and throughout Part II.)

Both men and women have urinary tracts and lymph nodes, and these parts of the anatomy can be affected by STDs. I begin by describing these structures and then move on to the genital area, where men and women look very different from each other.

The bladder is where urine is stored. Urine is made in the kidneys and travels to the bladder through the ureters. Because in women the opening of the urethra is so close to the openings of the vagina and the anus, bladder infections are not uncommon in women. Men, on the other hand, rarely get bladder infections, because there is a large distance between the urethra and the anal area. (As discussed in Chapter 2, however, some underlying structural problems and some sexual acts may make a man more likely to develop a urinary tract infection.) Symptoms usually associated with a bladder infection, such as burning with urination, may also be caused by sexually transmitted infections such as chlamydia or herpes.

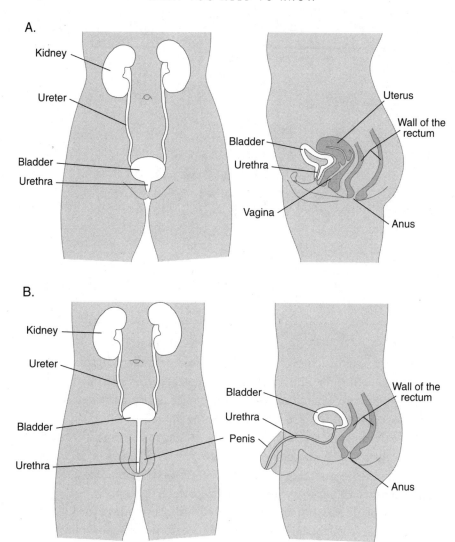

FIGURE 1. The urinary tract in (A) a woman and (B) a man.

The lymph nodes are part of the immune system and are found throughout the body. The immune system is the body's defense against foreign invasions of bacteria, viruses, and protozoa, as well as cancer cells, and the lymph nodes are where the cells of the immune system congregate as they flow throughout the body. People have lymph nodes in the neck, under the arms, and in the groin, among other places. The lymph nodes usually cannot be felt with the fingers (in medical language, they are "not palpable"), or else they are palpable but are very small. They can become swollen in response to infection or sometimes from invasion with cancer cells. The lymph nodes that swell with a genital infection are located in the groin. Lymph node swelling in the groin may be the only indication that a person has a genital infection.

MALE ANATOMY
PENIS

The penis is the organ through which men both urinate and produce semen. There are no muscles or bones in the penis, which is composed of three tubes of tissue. The top two tubes are called the corpora cavernosa (singular: corpus cavernosum). These tubes are composed of spongy tissue and blood vessels that, during sexual excitement, become full of blood and thus cause an erection. When not erect, the penis is soft and limp (flaccid). The bottom tube of tissue is called the corpus spongiosum, and through it runs the urethra, the hollow tube that carries both urine and semen.

At the end of the penis is the glans or head. The corpus spongiosum is connected to the glans, and the urethra opens at the tip of it. The glans of the penis has more nerve endings than any other part of the penis, which is why it is so sensitive. Stimulation of the glans is important in sexual arousal and orgasm: it is analogous to the clitoris in women. All men are born with a retractable layer of skin, called the foreskin, that covers the head of the penis. Many males have the foreskin surgically removed at birth in a procedure called circumcision. In some men, small, shiny, painless bumps called pearly penile papules are present around the edge of the head of the penis. Although they are sometimes confused with warts by both patients and health care providers, they are a normal part of male anatomy.

> James was sick with worry that he had contracted a sexually transmitted disease. When he noticed small, painless bumps along the ridge of the head of his penis, he did some research in the library, and now he was convinced that he had genital warts.
>
> After several weeks of worrying, James finally went to a local STD clinic, where he was relieved to learn that the bumps weren't warts after all, but *pearly penile papules*, a normal part of male anatomy. While he was there, he and the physician discussed safer sex prac-

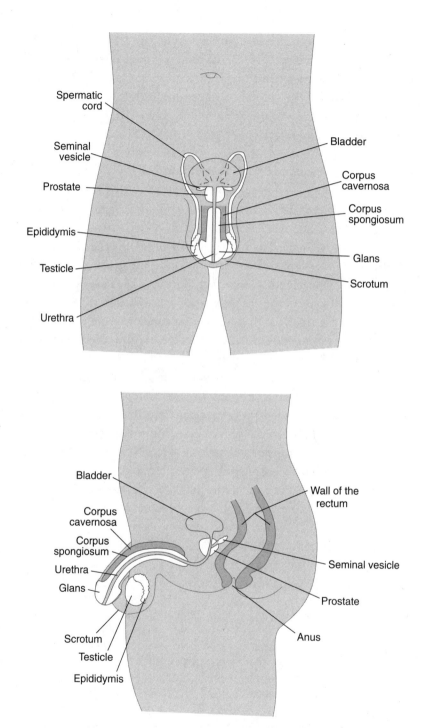

FIGURE 2. The internal and external sex organs of a man.

tices and how to prevent becoming infected with an STD in the future. James learned so much and wished he had gone earlier to be checked out.

SCROTUM

The scrotum is the bag of skin that sits below the penis and contains the testicles and, for each testicle, the epididymis and the vas deferens (spermatic cord), and blood vessels that lead to the testicles. The skin is normally loose and wrinkled, and sparsely covered with hair.

Testicles

The two testicles, which are located inside the scrotum, are the structures that make sperm and testosterone. (Testosterone is the hormone primarily responsible for the development of male physical characteristics.) The testicles sit away from the body to keep them below body temperature (the lower temperature is required for the production of sperm). The testicles should feel smooth to the touch and have the consistency of a hard-boiled egg. They vary in size, from the size of a large grape to the size of an egg. Normally, most men have one testicle that hangs lower than the other.

When a male infant is in the womb, the testicles start out in the pelvic area and descend into the scrotal sac. Sometimes one or both testicles do not descend; they remain in the pelvis and are not visible from the outside. This condition must be surgically corrected, since an undescended testicle is a risk for developing testicular cancer.

Every month all men should do a self-examination of the testicles, feeling for any bumps or irregularities on them, which can be a sign of testicular cancer. The testicles can be a site of infection, called orchitis, which can be caused by mumps in men who were not adequately immunized or (rarely) by sexually transmitted infections or other viruses.

The area above the testicles feels like cords of string. This area contains the epididymis, which stores sperm; the vas deferens, which carry sperm into the urethra during ejaculation; and blood vessels going to and from the testicles.

Epididymis

The epididymis is a collection of coiled tubes, the main purpose of which is storing sperm and providing a place for the sperm to mature.

The tubes also carry sperm from each testicle to its vas deferens, which carries the sperm into the urethra. Sperm move slowly and mature as they travel through the epididymis. The epididymis can become infected with sexually transmitted bacteria (such as those causing gonorrhea and chlamydia) or nonsexually transmitted bacteria. Infection of the epididymis is called epididymitis.

Vas Deferens
The vas deferens is a straight, hollow tube that carries the sperm from the epididymis on each side to the urethra as it travels through the prostate. These are the tubes that are cut in the sterilization procedure for men called vasectomy.

URETHRA
The urethra is a hollow tube that leads from the bladder, through the prostate gland, and through the penis to open at the tip of the glans. It carries urine to the outside of the body to empty the bladder. The vas deferens leads sperm from the testicles into the urethra during ejaculation. In addition, there are glands called the seminal vesicles that empty fluid into the urethra during ejaculation. The ejaculate, called semen, contains a mixture of sperm and secretions from each vas deferens, the seminal vesicles, and the prostate. Pre-ejaculate, the small amount of fluid released before ejaculation, may contain sperm and cause pregnancy, and it may transmit infection as well. The urethra should not burn or itch, and normally there should not be any discharge from it. The urethra can become infected with bacteria (such as those that cause gonorrhea, chlamydia, and nongonoccal urethritis), viruses (herpes, genital warts), and protozoa (trichomoniasis) through sexual contact.

PROSTATE
The prostate is a gland that sits at the base of the bladder and secretes fluids that are one component of semen. Because the urethra (the tube that carries urine from the bladder) runs through the prostate into the center of the penis, any swelling of the prostate caused by infection, inflammation, or cancer can disrupt the flow of urine. The prostate can be examined during a rectal examination, when it is palpated (felt) for enlargement, irregularity, or tenderness by the health care pro-

vider. It is usually about the size of a walnut and is firm. The prostate can become infected with sexually transmitted bacteria, occasionally after a urethral infection, but this is uncommon when treatment with antibiotics is started early in response to these infections. Men can also acquire infections of the prostate that are not sexually transmitted (this is much more common). Cancer of the prostate occurs more commonly in men over the age of fifty, and a noncancerous swelling of the prostate, called benign prostatic hyperplasia (BPH), occurs more often in this age group, as well.

FEMALE ANATOMY
VULVA

Vulva is the term used to describe the outside, visible parts of the female genital anatomy. This includes the labia (lips), the clitoris, and the urethral and vaginal openings.

Labia

There are two sets of labia: the labia majora, or outer lips, and the labia minora, or inner lips. The outer lips extend from the clitoris to the bottom of the vaginal opening. They are covered with hair and are composed of fatty tissue. The labia minora sit inside the labia majora and are not visible until a woman reaches puberty. The labia minora have little or no hair and extend from the clitoris, covering the urethra and the vaginal opening. Several STDs can cause visible symptoms in this area, including herpes, genital warts, and syphilis.

Clitoris

The clitoris is a small (about 2–3 cm) structure that sits at the top of the vulva. It is very sensitive and is analogous to the glans of the penis in men. It is partially covered by the labia minora. Stimulation of the clitoris is important in sexual arousal and orgasm.

Urethra

The urethra is the tube that carries urine from the bladder to the outside. The opening of the urethra is located below the clitoris, and it can sometimes be difficult to see when a woman examines herself. The urethra can be the site of sexually transmitted infections, such as chlamydia and gonorrhea, which can cause burning with urination.

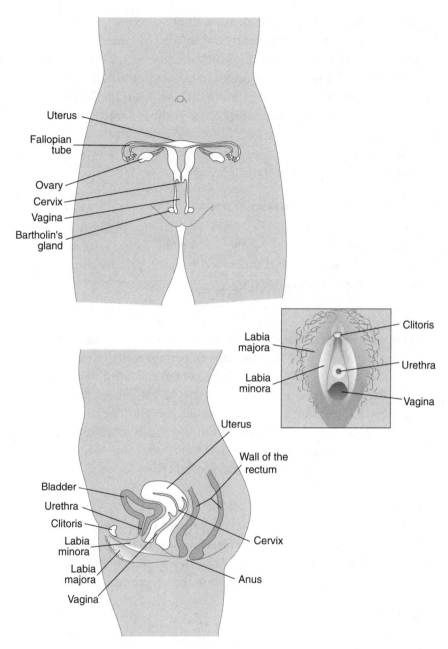

FIGURE 3. The internal and external sex organs of a woman.

Bladder infections (which, unlike in men, are very common in women) can also cause irritation of the urethra.

Glands on each side of the urethra, called Skene's glands, supply lubricating fluid to the vaginal area during sexual stimulation. These can sometimes become the site of sexually transmitted bacterial infections.

Vagina

The vagina is a muscular canal that is visible when the labia minora are spread open. From the time of birth, a membrane of tissue called the hymen covers the opening of the vagina; this membrane is usually torn with first sexual intercourse, though it can be torn before. The vagina is usually only 3–4 inches in length, but it can expand during childbirth and slightly during sexual intercourse in women who are past the age of puberty. There are normally bacteria in the vagina, the most common type being *Lactobacillus*. Some common infections of the vagina (which are discussed in detail later in the book) are fungal (yeast) infections, bacterial vaginosis, and trichomonas infections. The vagina should not hurt or itch. A clear, odorless discharge from the vagina is normal for some women, especially during ovulation (the production of an egg from the ovaries), which occurs in the middle of the menstrual cycle. The cells of the vagina are shed constantly. This process, and the vaginal secretions that are normally produced, keep the vagina clean. Douching is not necessary.

Women whose mothers took the medication diethylstilbestrol (DES) during pregnancy in the 1960s have a higher risk for an unusual cancer of the vagina called vaginal adenocarcinoma. It is important to tell your health care provider if you fall into this category, since special tests must be done during your yearly Pap smear to screen for this type of cancer.

BARTHOLIN'S GLANDS

Bartholin's glands sit on each side of the lower part of the vaginal opening and secrete lubricating fluids during sexual stimulation. They can also become infected (in particular with gonorrhea and chlamydia), and this would make them enlarged and painful. They are not usually noticeable.

CERVIX

The cervix is a round structure that sits at the end of the vaginal canal. The cervix is visible during a gynecological examination, and a woman can sometimes feel the cervix herself by inserting one or two fingers into the vagina. It looks like a small doughnut. The cervix has an opening, called the os, through which menstrual blood flows during a period. The opening in the cervix leads to the uterus (womb), which sits above the vagina. For fertilization to occur, sperm must pass through the os and into the uterus and Fallopian tubes, to reach the egg released by the ovary during ovulation (which normally happens once a month).

Two types of cells are found on the cervix. The columnar cells are on the inside of the cervix, and they are also found inside the uterus. Sometimes these cells are seen on the outside of the cervix (a condition called ectopy), especially in younger women and women who are taking birth control pills. As women age, these cells move into the cervix and can only be reached with an instrument such as the brush used to collect cells for a Pap smear. These cells may become inflamed and move to the outside again when a woman has an infection of the cervix (called cervicitis).

The second type of cell is the squamous cell. These cells are located on the outside of the cervix and are also found in the vagina. The place on the cervix where the columnar cells and the squamous cells come together is called the transformation zone or squamocolumnar junction. It is here that precancerous or cancerous changes can occur, and cells for a Pap smear are taken from the transformation zone during screening for cervical cancer.

The cervix can become infected with STDs. Cancer of the cervix can also occur; it is caused by certain strains of the human papillomavirus, which also causes genital warts. Pap smears are an excellent screen for cervical cancer and are part of the yearly examination recommended for all sexually active women. During the Pap smear, cells that are removed with a brush from the cervix are sent to a laboratory for examination under a microscope.

UTERUS (WOMB)

The uterus is shaped like a small pear that sits upside down in the pelvic cavity, with the cervix as the "stem." It is where a fertilized egg implants itself at the beginning of a pregnancy. (An ectopic pregnancy occurs when the fertilized egg implants itself somewhere outside the uterus, such as in the Fallopian tubes.) The uterus has a very rich blood supply and provides nourishment for the developing embryo. The uterus is very muscular and can grow to a very large size during pregnancy, but it shrinks back to just a little bit bigger than its prepregnancy size afterward. The lining of the uterus (called the endometrium) builds up each month in preparation for a pregnancy, and the lining is shed during menstruation (the period) if the woman does not become pregnant.

The lining of the uterus can also undergo cancerous changes, called endometrial cancer or uterine cancer. This is more common among older women. Fibroids are noncancerous growths in the muscle layer of the uterus that can cause pelvic pain and increased bleeding during and between periods.

FALLOPIAN TUBES

The Fallopian tubes are two thin, muscular tubes located between the upper (wider) part of the uterus and the ovaries. They transport the egg from the ovaries to the uterus, where it can be fertilized. The Fallopian tubes can become infected in pelvic inflammatory disease. Sometimes a fertilized egg can stop here instead of traveling to the uterus to implant. This type of ectopic pregnancy, called a tubal pregnancy, is a medical emergency, since such a pregnancy can lead to rupture of the tube and cause internal bleeding. This condition is more common in women who have had an infection in the Fallopian tubes as a result of pelvic inflammatory disease, which often leads to scarring in the tubes.

OVARIES

Every woman has two ovaries, one on each side of the pelvic cavity. The ovaries are located at the ends of the Fallopian tubes. In addition to containing ova (eggs), the ovaries are vital in the production of the hormones estrogen and progesterone; ovaries are analogous to the testicles in men. Each ovary is normally 3–4 cm across. Each month before a woman reaches menopause (the cessation of menstrual cycles, usually at about the age of fifty for most women), one of the ovaries releases an egg at the middle of the menstrual cycle. If the egg is not fertilized by sperm, then it does not implant in the uterus and menstruation occurs. The ovaries, too, can be infected in pelvic inflammatory disease.

IN THIS CHAPTER I mentioned briefly the kinds of things that can go wrong in the genital area. In the next chapter I tell you about the symptoms caused by these problems.

A KEY TO
SYMPTOMS

People are always asking themselves and their health care providers what is normal and what is abnormal when it comes to symptoms in the genital area. When to worry and when not to worry—that is the question. This chapter describes common symptoms in the genital area as well as some possible causes of those symptoms; it will help you to decide when a symptom could be the result of a sexually transmitted infection. Many different infections have similar symptoms, however, so examination and testing are usually the only way to know for certain what is causing the symptoms. See your health care provider any time you have a concern, and also for regular checkups. (Chapter 3 describes what's involved in examination and testing for a sexually transmitted disease and explains what goes on during the examination.)

Many sexually transmitted infections may never produce symptoms, or may take a long time—sometimes months or years—to produce symptoms. *So, as you read this chapter, remember that just because you don't have the symptoms listed here this doesn't necessarily mean you are free of the infection.* Testing is the only way to find out. (Part II of this book

> **You can have a sexually transmitted disease without having any symptoms.**

lists all of the STDs and describes each one in detail, including symptoms, diagnostic tests, and treatments.)

The first part of this chapter describes common genital symptoms in women, the second part describes common genital symptoms in men, and the third part describes symptoms that can occur in women and men. Within the section describing each symptom, possible causes of these symptoms are listed in alphabetical order. The most common causes of the symptoms are listed, but a symptom could be from a cause not included in this list. It is also possible that your symptoms may seem to have a nonsexually transmitted cause, which may prevent you from seeking treatment. That is not the intent of this section. *If you are having any of these symptoms, it is a good idea to stop having sex and see your health care provider,* because only a health care provider can know for sure what the cause of the symptoms is. And ask your partner to be evaluated. It is also a good idea to be evaluated *while you are having the symptom.* Some conditions may cause symptoms at first, but after a while the symptoms go away. After the symptoms have disappeared, it may be more difficult or even impossible to diagnose what caused them. For more information on each topic listed, please refer to the relevant sections in Part II of the book.

SYMPTOMS IN WOMEN
DISCHARGE FROM THE VAGINA

As mentioned in Chapter 1, most women have a clear, odorless discharge from the vagina that is perfectly normal. The amount of discharge varies from woman to woman, and it varies for most women over the course of the monthly cycle. The discharge is the normal fluid or lubrication produced by the vagina and the cervix. It can be especially noticeable during ovulation (when an egg is released from an ovary), which occurs during the middle of the menstrual cycle (halfway between the periods). *Normal discharge is usually clear to white, and it is not accompanied by odor, itching, or pain in the genital area.* As a woman ages, the amount of normal discharge may change.

Discharge from the vagina may be a sign of infection, however, so if there is any question about whether the discharge is normal, it is a good idea to see a health care provider for evaluation. The most common infections that can cause a vaginal discharge are described below.

Bacterial vaginosis (BV). The discharge of bacterial vaginosis is usually *white to slightly gray in color* and is usually not accompanied by significant irritation of the labia or vagina, although there may be mild itching. There is often a strong odor from the vagina, often described as a *fishy odor, which can be more prominent after sexual intercourse or during menstruation.* The symptoms may sometimes resolve on their own, only to recur again later.

> Barbara had not had sex in over a year, so she was surprised when she noticed a discharge from her vagina. The discharge had a fishy odor and was grayish in color. There was a little bit of itching on her labia, but not as bad as when she had had yeast infections in the past. She tried douching, but the odor persisted—if anything, it got worse. She went to see her nurse practitioner, who did a careful pelvic examination and found evidence of bacterial vaginosis, after examining vaginal secretions under the microscope. The nurse practitioner explained that bacterial vaginosis is not an STD, although it is more common in women who have been sexually active at some time in their lives. Barbara was screened for STDs—the first time in her life. She was relieved that the test results were negative.
>
> Barbara was given samples of metronidazole cream to use for five days, and her symptoms went away. She was advised not to douche, because although douching may lessen some of the symptoms, it doesn't cure vaginal infections. In fact, it may obscure evidence of the problem on examination, making diagnosis more difficult.

Cervix infection (mucopurulent cervicitis, or MPC). Mucopurulent cervicitis is an infection of the cervix that may be caused by several types of bacteria, including chlamydia and gonorrhea. Other infections, such as herpes and trichomoniasis, may also cause irritation of the cervix. The most common symptom of MPC is a discharge, which can range in color from *clear-white to yellow-green.* Occasionally, there may also be *spotting of blood between periods, or after sexual intercourse,* because the cervix is inflamed and bleeds very easily.

Herpes. Although the typical symptoms of herpes is sores or breaks in the skin, discharge may be the only symptom if there is an outbreak on the cervix that is causing irritation. The discharge is usually *white to yellow in color, and it may be accompanied by external sores or irritated areas on the skin.* Occasionally lymph nodes in the groin may become swollen, the woman may have pain in the back of the legs, and flu-like symptoms may occur, especially with a first infection.

Pelvic inflammatory disease (PID). The most common symptom of PID, or infection of the pelvic organs, is *pelvic or lower abdominal pain.* There may also be *discharge, spotting of blood between periods or after sex, pain with intercourse, and heavier than usual periods.* The color of the discharge can range from *clear-white to yellow-green, and it may be thin or thick.* Other symptoms may include fever, chills, and nausea.

Trichomoniasis. A *thin, yellow-green discharge* is common with trichomonas infection. Trichomonas often causes *irritation and itching of the labia and vagina,* and there can be fishy odor as well. There may also be *pain with intercourse* because of the significant irritation that can occur.

Yeast. The discharge caused by a vaginal yeast infection is often *thick, white, and clumpy,* and it is sometimes described as looking like *cottage cheese;* however, it may be thinner in consistency. Usually the *labia and vagina are irritated and itchy.* The irritation can become severe and can cause *breaks in the skin.*

ITCHING IN THE GENITAL AREA

Contrary to common misperceptions, not all itching in the female genital area is caused by yeast infections. Because of the availability of over-the-counter yeast treatments, however, many women self-treat for genital itching with these medications and never receive professional evaluation of their symptoms. For this reason, some women never receive an accurate diagnosis of what's really causing their symptoms. For instance, a herpes outbreak may cause genital itching, which a woman may think is caused by a yeast infection; she may start treating herself with an over-the-counter cream. Her symptoms resolve, and she believes she has successfully treated the yeast infection, when in fact the herpes outbreak merely resolved on its own, which it will do without treatment. So even if you think your symptoms are "typical yeast" symptoms, it is a good idea to be evaluated by a health care provider while you are having symptoms (especially the first time you have these symptoms), or if the symptoms recur. There are many possible causes of genital itching.

Allergic reactions. Many women have allergic reactions or increased sensitivity to certain products used in safer sex practices, such as latex condoms. About one-third of people have allergic reactions to spermicides such as nonoxynol-9 and other lubricants, which can range from mild to severe. Allergic reactions most often occur *immediately or shortly after intercourse* and may consist of *redness, itching, and breaks in the skin.*

Bacterial vaginosis. Although BV usually doesn't cause significant irritation of the labia and vagina, sometimes there can be *mild itching.* More common is a *white to gray discharge, which has a strong, fishy odor,* usually most prominent after sex or during menstruation.

Herpes. Herpes outbreaks often itch, and in fact this may be the only sign of an outbreak. There may be *tingling, redness, a bump, or a break in the skin, such as a blister, ulcer, or slit.* Lymph nodes in the groin may be swollen, and a woman may also experience leg pain and flu-like symptoms.

Jock itch. Also caused by a fungus, but by a different fungus than *Candida* (see the section on fungal infections in Part II), this condition is very common in both men and women. It is caused by the fungus *Tinea cruris* and most commonly causes an itchy, scaly red rash on the genitals and the upper thighs.

Lice. Pubic lice, also known as "crabs," are tiny parasites that infect the pubic hair and sometimes the hair under the armpits and the eyelashes. They can but do not always cause *itching.* A person with lice may also notice *tiny blood spots on the underwear,* resulting from the openings in the skin where the lice have bitten.

Scabies. Scabies causes *itchy bumps and small lines* (which are the burrows of the mites that cause the infection) on the body in a characteristic pattern. Most often, these are seen in the genital area, around the belt line, in the armpits, and in the webs between the fingers. The *itching is usually worse at night and after a shower.*

Trichomoniasis. The itching resulting from a trichomonas infection can range from mild to severe. The discharge is usually *thin and yellow-green in color.* There may also be a strong, *fishy odor.*

Warts. Warts are usually *small, hard, flesh-colored bumps* that can occur anywhere in the genital or anal area. They may also be *cauliflower-like* in appearance. Although warts usually don't produce any accompanying symptoms, about 20 percent of people with warts experience itching, which is usually mild.

Yeast. Yeast infections—usually caused by the fungus *Candida albicans*—can occur at any time of the year, but they occur more often in the warmer months. Often there is *itching, which can range from mild to severe,* as well as a *thick, white, clumpy discharge.* If the inflammation is severe or if a woman scratches in the genital area, there may be *breaks in the skin* as well. A woman who has recently taken an antibiotic is more likely to develop a yeast infection, since antibiotics temporarily diminish the quantity of the normal vaginal bacteria and allow yeast to overgrow.

BLEEDING BETWEEN PERIODS

Bleeding between periods (called *irregular bleeding*) is not unusual and may be related to a sexually transmitted infection, but it can be from other causes as well. (Sometimes irregular bleeding is the *only* symptom of a sexually transmitted infection.) Some of the common causes of bleeding between periods are listed in this chapter. An examination is necessary to explore all of the possibilities and rule out infection as a cause.

Anovulation. The occurrence of a menstrual period, or uterine bleeding, each month is the result of a complex interplay between signals from the brain and the pelvic organs. The lining of the uterus (the endometrium) builds up each month in anticipation of the implantation of a fertilized egg. If a fertilized egg is not implanted, the lining is shed during the woman's period. Many women, at some point in their lives, experience irregularity in their cycles. Certain women have irregular periods from the time they start menstruating. Others normally have regular periods and then occasionally miss a period. The most common cause of the latter event is *anovulation,* when the signals between the brain and the ovaries "misfire" and an egg is not released from the ovary in the middle of the cycle. If an egg is not produced, there may also be gradual shedding of the lining of the uterus throughout the cycle, rather than a full shedding at the end of the cycle. Usually, the cycle picks up the next month where it would have if an actual period had occurred. But if the periods do not resume, an evaluation is necessary to determine the underlying cause and to check for pregnancy.

Bleeding disorders. Blood clots as the result of a complex interplay between cells in the blood and components called *clotting factors.* Any underlying medical problem that disrupts this relationship may cause unusual bleeding from any place in the body, including the vagina. Often, but not always, there will be unusual bleeding from other areas as well.

Cervical problems. A cervix infection (mucopurulent cervicitis) can be caused by bacteria (such as gonorrhea and chlamydia), viruses (such as herpes), and protozoan infections (such as trichomonas). *Unusual bleeding, including bleeding between periods and after intercourse,* can occur from a cervix that is irritated for any reason. Other cervix conditions, such as cancer or a polyp (a small, noncancerous growth on the cervix), may sometimes also cause bleeding. A Pap smear is used to detect cervical cancer.

> Anne, 36, had had regular periods all her life, "like clockwork, every 28 days." After two pregnancies, she had a tubal ligation about three years ago. She and her husband recently divorced, and Anne was once again in the dating game.
>
> Anne began seeing Brian about two months ago, and they had sex on their third date. They discussed STDs and condom use before becoming intimate and decided that since neither of them had had many sexual partners in their lifetimes, and they both "looked clean," they didn't need to use condoms. Anne wouldn't become pregnant because her tubes had been tied.
>
> Soon Anne began experiencing burning and itching on her labia, and intercourse was painful. She also noticed a fishy odor every now and then, and blood on the toilet tissue after she urinated. She talked it over with Brian, who had no symptoms and suggested that she see her gynecologist.
>
> After a thorough examination, Anne's gynecologist diagnosed trichomoniasis. Tests were performed for gonorrhea and chlamydia, and both were negative. Both Anne and Brian were surprised that Brian could have had the infection without symptoms. They were treated with antibiotics, and both of them decided to have tests for other STDs before having sex again.

Hypothyroidism. People with hypothyroidism have a lower than usual level of hormones produced by the thyroid gland. There are several possible causes for this condition. These hormones are important in the body's metabolism, so someone with hypothyroidism *may experience low energy, may gain weight, and may have irregular periods.* A simple blood test can screen for hypothyroidism.

Pregnancy. Sometimes spotting occurs early in pregnancy. Usually there will also be signs of pregnancy, such as a missed period, breast tenderness, or morning nausea. Spotting may occur *even if the pregnancy is proceeding without complications,* but it can also signal a problem with the pregnancy, either a "threatened abortion" (meaning that a *miscarriage* may occur) or an actual miscarriage (spontaneous abortion), or a condition called an *ectopic pregnancy,* in which the pregnancy is occurring outside the uterus. Any pregnant woman who is experiencing bleeding should consult her health care provider.

Starting a hormonal method of birth control (birth control pills, progesterone shots or implant). Many women have spotting between periods when they begin using a new hormonal method of birth control, sometimes for *several months after starting the new contraceptive,* until the body adjusts to it. Remember that birth control pills or shots do not protect against STDs. If you and your partner have been using a barrier method (condom) and stop using it when starting to use the pill, infection may be a cause of the spotting. Talk with your health care provider about this. If the spotting persists after a few months, or is accompanied by other symptoms that may indicate infection (discharge, pain, and so on), evaluation is important to make sure the bleeding is the result of the hormones and not an infection.

Uterine problems. There are several possible causes of abnormal bleeding from the uterus. PID may cause *spotting between periods, and heavier than usual periods, as well as pelvic pain and discharge.* *Fibroids,* which are noncancerous growths in the muscle wall of the uterus, may also cause spotting and heavier periods. Spotting after menopause (when periods stop) may be a sign of *uterine cancer* and should be evaluated immediately. Your doctor may perform a procedure called an *endometrial biopsy.* This can be done in the doctor's office and consists of removing a sample of uterine lining and examining it under the microscope. Uterine cancer is more common in women over age fifty.

Vaginal infections. Some vaginal infections, such as *yeast or trichomonas,* may cause severe irritation of the vaginal tissue, which can in turn cause spotting, especially after intercourse.

BURNING WITH URINATION

Not all burning with urination (called *dysuria*) signals a bacterial urinary tract infection, as is often assumed by both the public and health care providers. Several common sexually transmitted infections, such as herpes and chlamydia, can also cause burning with urination. Dysuria can occur if there is infection inside the urethra (*internal dysuria*), or when there are sores or breaks in the skin around the urethra (*external dysuria*). A medical evaluation is necessary to sort out these possibilities.

Chlamydia and gonorrhea. These common sexually transmitted bacteria can cause infection of the urethra as well as the cervix. Sometimes, the only symptom a woman may notice with gonorrhea or chlamydia is *burning with urination.* Some of the other symptoms of these infections—such as *discharge, spotting between periods, or pelvic pain*—may or may not be present. (Sometimes these infections cause no symptoms at all.) A urine sample may show white blood cells indicating an infection, as with a routine bladder infection, but a culture of the urine for the bacteria commonly associated with urinary tract infections will be negative. Special tests must be done for gonorrhea and chlamydia.

Herpes. Herpes outbreaks may occur in the urethra and cause burning with urination. If the herpes outbreaks are on the vulva, the woman may experience burning when urine hits the lesions. Thus, herpes can cause both internal and external dysuria. Other symptoms of herpes outbreaks are *itching or tingling in the genitals, a discharge, swollen lymph nodes in the groin, pain in the back of the legs, and flu-like symptoms.*

Urinary tract infection (UTI). Because in women the openings of the urethra, the vagina, and the anus are so close together, infection of the urethra by bacteria that are commonly present in these other areas occurs fairly easily. Other symptoms of a UTI are *increased frequency of urination and lower back pain.* Wiping back to front instead of front to back after urinating or defecating can cause an infection of the urethra and bladder; sexual intercourse may also move bacteria from the anal area to the urethra. About one-third of women will get a bacterial UTI in their lifetime. The best way to test for a UTI is to evaluate the urine for white blood cells and culture the urine for bacteria. A UTI may progress and cause infection of the kidneys, called *pyelonephritis*. Symptoms of this infection include *fever, chills, nausea, vomiting, and upper back pain.*

Vulvar and vaginal irritation. Anything that causes vaginal and vulvar irritation—such as yeast and trichomonas infections, or allergic reactions to latex or spermicide—may cause burning when urine hits these areas.

ODOR FROM THE GENITAL AREA

Sometimes a stronger than usual odor from the genital area indicates infection. Occasionally a woman inserts something into the vagina, such as a tampon, and forgets that it is there, which can cause a strong odor. It is not uncommon for a woman to think that an abnormal genital odor is her normal genital odor, especially if the odor has been there for a long time. Any unusual odor should be checked out by a health care provider. A woman should never douche in an effort to get rid of the strong odor. Douching will not cure the infection and will increase the risk of developing pelvic infection.

Bacterial vaginosis. BV may cause a *fishy odor* in the genital area, often more pronounced after sexual intercourse and during menstruation. A fishy smell is not a normal smell from the genitals. Some women with BV may also experience a *scant discharge and mild itching*, but usually not significant irritation or inflammation. BV can sometimes be a sign that there is other infection in the genital area, such as chlamydia, but it may also be present exclusive of other infections.

Gonorrhea and chlamydia. Although it is not the most common symptom, strong genital odor may occur with bacterial infections of the cervix and pelvic organs. Other symptoms of these infections are *discharge, spotting between periods, and pelvic pain.*

Trichomoniasis. This protozoan infection can also produce a *fishy odor* from the genital area. There is usually much more *discharge, itching, and irritation* from the genitals than with BV.

Yeast. Although *genital itching and inflammation and a thick white discharge* are the most common symptoms of a yeast infection, there may be a *strong bread-like odor* from the genital area as well.

PAIN WITH INTERCOURSE

There are many reasons that a woman may experience pain with intercourse, only some of which are related to sexually transmitted infections. Pain can originate from sores on the outside of the genitals (herpes) or from vaginal infections (yeast or trichomonas), which often cause pain with initial penetration. Infection of the cervix or pelvic organs (gonorrhea, chlamydia, MPC, and PID) usually causes pain with deeper penetration. Causes of pain with intercourse that are not related to infection include atrophy (thinning) of the tissue as a result of estrogen loss in postmenopausal women, endometriosis, and spasm of muscles in the vaginal opening, called vaginismus. Pain with intercourse should be evaluated by a health care provider.

Endometriosis. This condition occurs when the tissue lining the uterus (the endometrium) dislodges from the uterus and becomes implanted in other areas of the pelvis or other areas of the body. Even though this tissue is no longer part of the uterus, it continues to respond to hormonal changes just like the endometrium, and it bleeds monthly. This bleeding irritates the structures where the tissue has become implanted, causing pain, usually with the menstrual cycle. Because of this irritation, intercourse, especially with deep penetration, may be painful. The best way to diagnose endometriosis is through a procedure called a *laparoscopy,* during which a special tool called a *laparoscope* is inserted through a small incision into the abdomen so the surgeon can view these pieces of implanted tissue. The typical treatments for endometriosis involve medications or surgery.

Estrogen deficiency. Women who are going through or who have gone through menopause and who do not receive estrogen replacement therapy (ERT) may develop *thinning of the vaginal tissues (atrophy) and therefore increased susceptibility to tearing with intercourse.* This is true whether a woman's menopause is natural (brought about by a decline in the amount of estrogen produced by the ovaries, which occurs for most women around the age of fifty) or due to surgical removal of the ovaries (such as with a total hysterectomy, which may be performed for various reasons). ERT after menopause will help to prevent these changes and can reverse atrophy when it has occurred. However, ERT is not for everyone, and the decision to start ERT is an individual one. Discuss the pros and cons with your health care provider.

Herpes. Herpes causes pain with intercourse only during an outbreak. Therefore *episodic* pain with intercourse could be the result of herpes, since herpes symptoms are themselves episodic (meaning they come and go). Any *sores in the genital area* may cause pain when rubbed. The pain is from contact with the sores and is not usually associated with deep penetration. Other common symptoms of herpes outbreaks are *itching or tingling in the genitals, lymph node swelling in the groin, pain in the back of the legs, and flu-like symptoms.*

Pelvic inflammatory disease. Infection of the pelvic structures, caused by bacteria such as gonorrhea and chlamydia, can cause pain with intercourse. The pain is usually associated with *deep penetration,* as the penis or sex toys strike the inflamed cervix and pelvic organs. There may also be *pelvic and lower abdominal pain without intercourse, discharge, spotting between periods and heavier than usual periods, fever, chills, and nausea.*

Trichomoniasis. Trichomonas may cause irritation and *inflammation of the vulva or vagina or both,* so intercourse (both initial and deep penetration) may be painful.

Vaginismus. Sometimes pain with intercourse may occur because of a condition called *vaginismus,* which is the tensing or spasm of vaginal muscles with intercourse or when inserting a tampon or undergoing a pelvic examination. This may occur if a woman has an underlying genital problem, such as those listed previously, and she anticipates that intercourse will be painful. Vaginismus may sometimes occur in women who have been sexually abused. Vaginismus is best managed with the help of a gynecologist and a therapist with expertise in this field.

Yeast. If a yeast infection causes *inflammation and irritation of the genital area,* then intercourse may be painful. If the vulva and vagina are inflamed, both initial and deep penetration may be painful. Yeast infections also commonly cause a thick white discharge.

PELVIC PAIN

Pain in the pelvic area can originate from the pelvic structures themselves, or what may feel like pelvic pain may in fact originate from other structures, such as the intestines. There are various causes of pain in this area. Of these, pelvic inflammatory disease, ectopic pregnancy, and appendicitis are medical emergencies and require immediate attention. Pelvic pain must be assessed by a health care provider as soon as possible.

Appendicitis. The appendix is a small out-pouching of the colon in the right lower abdomen that can become infected and inflamed and cause pain in this area. Although the appendix is not in the pelvis, sometimes pain from an inflamed appendix may be difficult to distinguish from other types of pelvic pain. *Usually the pain begins around the navel and then migrates down to the right lower abdomen.* There may also be *fever.* Appendicitis (an inflamed appendix) can usually be distinguished from other causes of pelvic pain by a physical examination and appropriate testing such as a CT (computerized axial tomography) scan.

Endometriosis. Endometriosis is the condition in which the lining of the uterus (the endometrium) dislodges and becomes implanted in other areas of the pelvis or intestinal tract. The tissue is still responsive to the changes in hormones that cause a period and therefore bleeds, and this can cause pain, usually during a menstrual period. Endometriosis is diagnosed through a procedure called a *laparoscopy,* in which the internal structures are examined through a small incision using a *laparoscope.*

Irritable bowel syndrome (IBS). IBS is a very common problem among young women. It may cause pain that is experienced in the pelvis by most women, but the source of the pain is in fact the bowel. IBS causes *abdominal and/or pelvic pain, bloating, and constipation and/or diarrhea.* Sometimes the diarrhea and constipation alternate. Usually no structural abnormality is seen on examination of the colon, and no abnormalities are evident with laboratory tests. IBS is a diagnosis of exclusion, meaning that all other possibilities should be ruled out first. Although it is a chronic problem, IBS can be managed with diet, exercise, and medications in most people, and it does not cause more severe problems, such as cancer.

Ovarian cyst. In the normal menstrual cycle, each month one ovary releases an egg to be fertilized. If ovulation (the release of an egg) does not occur, a cyst, called a *follicular cyst,* may form. When an egg is released from an ovary, another kind of cyst, called a *corpus luteum cyst,* may form. These two kinds of cysts may grow quite large and may cause pain either if they remain intact or if they rupture. An *ultrasound* device, which bounces sound waves off internal structures to visualize them, is used to diagnose an ovarian cyst. Most cysts go away on their own, or they can be reduced through hormone suppression with birth control pills or drained through a laparoscopy. Ovarian cysts must be differentiated from ovarian cancer, which usually has a different appearance from a cyst on ultrasound and does not shrink with hormone suppression.

Pelvic inflammatory disease. PID is an infection of the uterus, Fallopian tubes, ovaries, or all of these structures, and it is usually caused by sexually transmitted bacteria such as gonorrhea and chlamydia. These bacteria cause inflammation of the cervix, and then they, as well as vaginal bacteria, may move through the cervix up into the pelvic organs. Pelvic infection may also be caused by a complication of pregnancy such as incomplete abortion or by bacteria introduced during gynecological surgery. The consequences of PID can be severe; for example, scarring can lead to *chronic pelvic pain or infertility, or can increase the chance of a tubal pregnancy.* There may be other symptoms of infection—such as *discharge, spotting between periods or heavier than usual periods, fever, chills, and nausea*—or pain may be the only symptom.

Pregnancy in a Fallopian tube (ectopic, or tubal, pregnancy). When a fertilized egg becomes implanted in a Fallopian tube instead of in the lining of the uterus, there will be pain, and the tube may rupture, causing significant bleeding and possibly even death. Any sexually active woman with pelvic pain should promptly seek medical care to rule out or treat this medical emergency.

Trichomoniasis. Although trichomoniasis, a vaginal infection, does not usually cause symptoms higher up in the genital tract, occasionally pelvic pain occurs with trichomoniasis for unclear reasons. The other, more common, symptoms of trichomonas infection—such as *inflammation and itching of the vulva, discharge, and a fishy odor*—may also be present.

SYMPTOMS IN MEN
DISCHARGE FROM THE PENIS

Discharge from the penis is never a normal occurrence, and any man experiencing this symptom should be examined by a health care provider while he is having the symptom. The most common causes are sexually transmitted infections, such as gonorrhea, chlamydia, and nongonoccal urethritis. Some men think this symptom is caused by not drinking enough fluids, drinking too much caffeine, or having too much or too little sex, but there is no evidence that any of these can cause discharge from the penis.

Chlamydia and nongonococcal urethritis (NGU). NGU is a sexually transmitted infection in the urethra (*urethritis*) that is not caused by gonorrhea. The most common cause is chlamydia, but other bacteria, as well as herpes and trichomonas, can also be responsible. The discharge caused by this infection is *usually clear, and there is not much of it.* There also may be *redness at the top of the penis.* Symptoms typically start a week or two, or up to a couple of months, after infection. Most men, however, experience no symptoms with this infection.

Epididymitis. Characterized by *swelling and pain in the epididymis,* epididymitis may be accompanied by a *discharge and burning with urination.* The swelling and pain usually occur on *only one side.*

Gonorrhea. The discharge from gonorrhea is usually *thick, copious, and yellow.* It usually starts within a *day to a week or two after infection.* There may be *burning with urination* and *redness at the tip of the penis.* However, some men experience no symptoms with gonorrhea.

Herpes. Herpes can cause discharge, with outbreaks occurring in the urethra or on the skin of the genitals. The discharge is usually *clear.* Outbreaks inside the urethra usually cause *extreme pain with urination,* with men typically reporting "I feel like I'm peeing ground glass."

Prostate infection. Infection of the prostate (called *prostatitis*) can be either bacterial or nonbacterial in origin. Bacterial prostate infection can be acute or chronic, and it may cause a *discharge from the urethra.* There may also be *pain between the scrotum and the anal area, frequent urination, pain with urination and ejaculation, and blood in the semen.* Prostate infections may be caused by sexually transmitted bacteria or, more often, by other bacteria. Rarely, a sexually transmitted urethral infection that is not promptly treated may progress to infection of the prostate.

Reiter's syndrome. Reiter's syndrome is a condition that can result after chlamydial infection or NGU or after certain intestinal infections. Men with Reiter's syndrome complain of an *inflamed urethra, discharge, and burning with urination,* as well as *joint pain and inflammation of the conjunctiva of the eyes.* Symptoms usually start one to four weeks after the infection that triggered the advent of Reiter's syndrome, whether or not the infection was treated.

BURNING WITH URINATION AND PAIN, ITCHING,
OR IRRITATION INSIDE THE PENIS

Burning with urination and experiencing pain, itching, or irritation inside the penis are not normal. When these symptoms are experienced, they may be constant or may come and go. They may be subtle or severe, and there may or may not be discharge. Men sometimes incorrectly attribute these symptoms to being dehydrated, to consuming too much caffeine or alcohol, to allergic reactions, or to other causes. Any man with pain, itching, or irritation inside the penis must visit a health care provider.

Chlamydia and nongonococcal urethritis. Although half of the time these infections are symptom free, there may be *pain, itching, or burning in the urethra and burning with urination, as well as a small amount of discharge,* which is usually clear. There may also be *redness at the tip of the penis.*

Epididymitis. The epididymis, which sits above each testicle, can become infected with bacteria, which may or may not be sexually transmitted. Half of the scrotum is usually *swollen, hot, red, and painful,* and there may be urethral irritation and discharge, particularly if the infection was caused by sexually transmitted bacteria.

Gonorrhea. This bacterium can cause infection in the urethra and result in *pain, itching, or burning in the urethra and burning with urination,* as well as a *thick yellow discharge.* There may also be *redness at the tip of the penis.* The intensity of the symptoms can range from mild to very strong, although some men do not experience any symptoms at all with gonorrhea. Symptoms usually start within a day to a week or two after infection.

Herpes. A man with a herpes outbreak in the genital or anal area may report *pain, burning, or itching in the urethra and burning with urination.* Even without visible skin lesions, a man may have a herpes lesion inside the urethra; this usually causes severe burning with urination.

Prostate infection. Infection of the prostate (called *prostatitis*) can be either bacterial or nonbacterial in origin. Bacterial prostate infection can be acute or chronic, and it usually causes *pain in the area of the prostate (between the scrotum and anal area), increased frequency of urination, and interruption in the flow of urine,* as well as other symptoms, such as fever and chills. There may also be *irritation inside the urethra, as well as discharge.*

Urinary tract infection. Although UTIs are not very common in men, they can occur. The symptoms include *burning with urination and an increased frequency of urination.* If the kidneys are infected as well (a condition called *pyelonephritis*), there may be fever, chills, and back pain in the area of the kidneys. When a man does develop a UTI, an assessment is usually made to determine whether there is an anatomical problem that is making it more likely for him to develop infection; the presence of kidney stones is another possible promoting factor. Men who perform unprotected anal intercourse on a partner may also get a UTI from the bacteria that are in stool. *The most common cause of burning with urination in men, however, is not a UTI but a urethral infection from a sexually transmitted infection.*

Warts in the urethra. Warts are one of the most common STDs, if not the most common. They usually appear as *flesh-colored bumps on the skin that are harder than the surrounding skin,* but sometimes they occur *inside the urethra and may cause irritation, discharge, and a disruption in the flow of urine.* A thin scope is inserted into the urethra so that the doctor (usually a urologist) can see the warts and treat them.

PAIN IN THE TESTICLES

There are many possible reasons that a man may develop pain in the testicles. This symptom should be evaluated as soon as possible, since both infection and more worrisome possibilities, such as torsion or testicular cancer, require prompt treatment.

Epididymitis. Infection of the epididymis usually affects only one side of the scrotum. The most common symptom is a *swollen, hot, red, and very painful half of the scrotum.* There may be *discharge from the penis,* if the infection that is causing epididymitis is also causing urethral infection—a common combination. The onset of pain is usually more gradual than that experienced with testicular torsion (see below).

Orchitis. Orchitis is an infection of the testicle that is usually caused by the mumps virus. Other causes are infection with *bacteria (gonorrhea, tuberculosis, syphilis) or with a virus other than mumps.*

If orchitis occurs in an adult man, permanent testicular scarring and failure may result. There is usually *severe pain and swelling in one or both testicles;* other symptoms associated with mumps (such as parotid gland enlargement) and bacterial or viral infections may also be present.

Testicular cancer. More common among young men, this is a completely treatable cancer if detected early. To make early detection more likely, men must perform monthly testicular self-examinations, just as women do monthly breast self-examinations. Testicular cancer produces a *swelling or bump on the testicle itself,* not above the testicle in the epididymis or spermatic cord (vas deferens). It may cause testicular discomfort as well. A health care provider can distinguish this disease from benign causes of swelling in the scrotum, such as spermatoceles (which are temporary swellings in the spermatic cord) or cysts in the epididymis. An ultrasound study (in which sound waves are bounced off an internal structure to allow that structure to be visualized) may be ordered to help with the diagnosis.

Torsion of the testicle. Torsion of the testicle is a medical emergency. It is a twisting of the spermatic cord and the blood vessels to the testicle, which can kill the testicle unless it is repaired quickly by surgery. The primary symptom is *severe pain and swelling on one side of the scrotum that often comes on rapidly.* It is more common among *adolescent men.*

BLOOD IN THE SEMEN

Although surprisingly common, the presence of blood in the semen can be very frightening. It usually occurs without warning, and even a tiny bit of blood in the semen can look like much more. The most common cause is a ruptured blood vessel in the urethra. However, infection and malignancy must be ruled out.

Infection in the prostate. Prostatitis, or prostate infection, may cause blood in the semen. Prostate infection can be *acute, with severe pain in the area of the prostate (between the scrotum and the anal area), fever, chills, and difficulty urinating,* or chronic, with subtler symptoms.

Infection in the urethra. Any of the possible causes of infection in the urethra (*chlamydia or the other NGU bacteria, gonorrhea, trichomonas, or the intestinal bacteria for men who perform anal sex*) can cause inflammation producing blood in the semen, although this is not common. However, urethral infection must be eliminated as a possibility in a man with blood in his semen. There may or may not be other symptoms of infection, such as *discharge from the penis, burning with urination, and irritation inside the penis.*

Prostate cancer. More common among older men, usually those over the age of fifty, prostate cancer usually does not cause symptoms, but there may be *blood in the semen or, if the enlarged prostate obstructs the urethra, difficulty urinating.* A prostate examination and blood and imaging tests are used to make a diagnosis.

Ruptured blood vessel. The rupture of a blood vessel is very common and harmless. It usually occurs *after masturbation or ejaculation during sex.* There is usually *no pain* and no other symptoms consistent with infection. The rupture resolves on its own after a few days to a week in most cases. This is a diagnosis of exclusion; the other possible causes of blood in the semen listed above must be ruled out first.

SYMPTOMS IN BOTH MEN AND WOMEN
RECTAL PAIN AND DISCHARGE

In both men and women who engage in unprotected anal sex, there is a risk of infection with STDs. In women who contract an infection of the cervix or urethra through unprotected genital sex, anal infections can occur as well, probably because infected secretions are spread to that area from the genitals. Someone with infection in the anal and rectal area may be completely symptom free or may have severe symptoms of pain and discharge.

Chancroid. Chancroid is not an infection commonly seen in the United States, but it is common in other areas of the world. The symptoms—*painful genital or anal ulcers,* depending on where the infection took place—are similar to those of genital herpes. Like herpes, chancroid can cause *pain in the rectal area, discharge, and bleeding.* The lymph nodes may also become extremely swollen and painful; they may spontaneously rupture and drain infected fluid.

Donovanosis (granuloma inguinale). Donovanosis is a very uncommon infection in the United States. The typical lesions are *heaped up, beefy-red ulcers in the genital or anal area* that slowly enlarge over time and can cause significant *scarring.* If the scarring is in the anal area, the flow of stool may be impaired.

Gonorrhea, chlamydia, and NGU bacteria. Gonorrhea, chlamydia, and NGU bacteria may cause inflammation in the rectal area after anal sex is received from an infected partner. Women may also have simultaneous infection in the cervix and anal area when secretions carry infection from the genitals to the anal area. There is usually *rectal pain, discharge, difficulty having a bowel movement because of the pain, and rectal bleeding.*

Hemorrhoids. Hemorrhoids are very common inflammations of the blood vessels in the anal area that occur with straining to have a bowel movement. They are not caused by a sexually transmitted infection. There is usually *rectal pain,* and there may also be *bleeding from the anal area.* The symptoms may disappear on their own, and they may recur.

Herpes. A person can become infected with herpes in the rectal area through unprotected sex—often, but not always, anal sex. In addition, a person may experience recurrences of genital herpes in the anal area or on the buttocks, whether or not he or she has ever received anal sex. This does not mean that the virus has spread; rather, it is just recurring in a different area that the nerve that has been infected supplies. There may be *sores* (they often look like slits in the skin), *rectal pain, difficulty having a bowel movement, rectal discharge, and bleeding.*

Intestinal infections. There are many intestinal infections—such as those caused by giardia, salmonella, and shigella—that can be transmitted through unprotected anal sex with an infected partner. These infections can also be spread through actions unrelated to sex, such as ingesting contaminated food or water. Where the infection occurs—in the small intestine (*enteritis*), the rectum (*proctitis*), or a combination of the rectum and colon (*proctocolitis*)—determines what symptoms will develop. There may be *rectal pain, bleeding and discharge from the anal area, diarrhea (which may be bloody), and abdominal pain.*

Lymphogranuloma venereum (LGV). Often confused with herpes, LGV begins as a painful ulcer at the site of the initial infection. If it occurs in the anal area, there may be *rectal pain and discharge and bleeding from the rectal area.* There may also be *lymph node swelling in the groin* (this usually occurs in the second stage). The ulcer will go away, but the infection remains until it has been treated. The infection can spread from the genital area to the anal area even if a person has never received anal sex. LGV is not common in the United States.

Syphilis. Through unprotected anal sex, a person may acquire syphilis in the rectal area. Usually the first symptom of syphilis is a *chancre,* a *painless sore* that may not be noticed, especially if it is in the rectal area. However, it may cause *bleeding or discharge from the rectal area,* which may warn the person that the infection has occurred. The chancre will disappear on its own, but the infection remains unless treated.

Ulcerative colitis and Crohn's disease. Not STDs (and indeed not caused by infections of any sort), ulcerative colitis and Crohn's disease are inflammatory diseases of the bowel and rectum that can cause *diarrhea, bloody stools, and rectal and abdominal pain.*

Warts. Warts may occur in the anal area of those who receive anal sex, but they can also occur there even if a person has never received anal sex. Warts higher up in the rectum are usually acquired through anal sex. Anal warts are usually *painless, skin-colored growths* that can become very large and *sometimes obstruct the flow of stool.* If they are large and if they tear, they can become irritated and painful.

BODY RASH

Many conditions, such as allergic reactions and viral illnesses, can cause body rashes. In addition, certain STDs can cause skin changes in parts of the body other than the genital area. The most common rashes caused by sexually transmitted infections are described below.

Gonorrhea. In a small percentage of cases, genital gonorrhea infection spreads throughout the blood stream and causes *skin lesions and joint infection* in addition to the more common symptoms of *pain with urination and discharge from the penis or the vagina.* The skin lesions usually occur on the arms and legs and look like *small blood- or pus-filled sores with redness surrounding them.*

Human immunodeficiency virus (HIV) infection. Many skin conditions can occur with HIV infection. Within *two to six weeks after infection,* about a third of people experience a *severe flu-like illness with a diffuse rash, sore throat, and lymph node swelling throughout the body.* This occurs when the body is mounting an immune response to the virus and is producing proteins called antibodies. These symptoms go away after about a week. After this illness, most people will show a positive blood test for HIV, although some may take up to six months to test positive after infection. There are many skin infections that can occur when HIV infection has progressed to AIDS (acquired immunodeficiency syndrome); these infections are beyond the scope of this book.

Lice. There are three types of lice: head lice, pubic lice, and body lice. The variety that can be sexually transmitted is pubic lice. The lice usually cause *itching and irritation in the genital area where they occur.* As the lice attach to the skin, there may also be a small amount of bleeding, which can look like *rust-colored stains on the underwear.* The lice may also infest the eyelashes and the hair in the armpits and on the lower abdomen.

Scabies. This common infection can be sexually transmitted by body contact with an infected person or through infected bedding or clothing. Scabies causes *itchy red bumps and lines on the skin (the burrows of the mites that cause the disease),* with the itching usually *worse at night and after a shower.* The rash most commonly develops on the genitals, in the webs between the fingers, at the belt line, under the armpits, behind the knees, and at the ankles.

Syphilis. A person who has second-stage syphilis may develop a *rash all over the body, including on the palms and soles.* The rash usually does not itch and is not painful. Other symptoms of second-stage syphilis are *hair loss, lymph node swelling (not only in the groin but in other areas of the body, such as under the arms and in the neck), fever, and bumps in the genital area that look like warts but are not.*

GENITAL SORES, RASHES, ABRASIONS, OR BUMPS

Many of the sexually transmitted infections, and other nonsexually transmitted skin conditions, can cause bumps or sores in the genitals. When a person notices a rash, sores, or lesions, he or she should see a health care provider as soon as possible after the symptoms start, since the appearance of the rash may change over time and seeing the rash as soon as possible helps the health care provider make the correct diagnosis. Certain of the most common causes of genital skin changes are listed in this section; many other, nonsexually transmitted, infections can also cause genital rashes (as well as rashes in other areas of the body), but they are beyond the scope of this book.

Note: Some men may have pearly penile papules, which are painless, tiny bumps around the head of the penis. Although often mistaken for warts, they are a normal part of male anatomy.

Allergic reaction. Usually the symptoms from an allergic reaction—to a condom or spermicide, for example—occur immediately after a person comes into contact with it and recur whenever there is further exposure to it. The symptoms generally include a *red, itchy rash in the genitals,* where contact took place.

Behçet's disease. Behçet's disease is an autoimmune disease that causes *mouth and genital ulcers.* (Some other autoimmune diseases are lupus and rheumatoid arthritis.) Behçet's disease is more common in women, and its cause is not known. The ulcers are *very painful; there are usually many of them and they tend to recur.* People with Behçet's disease are sometimes mistakenly diagnosed as having herpes, because the ulcers may look like herpes lesions and recur.

Chancroid. Chancroid is another cause of genital ulcers, although in the United States it is much less common than herpes or syphilis. There can be *one or several ulcers,* with several being the more common condition. They are usually *painful.* The *lymph nodes in the groin* usually swell and also become very painful. They may spontaneously rupture and drain thick yellow fluid. If not treated, the lesions may persist for one to three months and then spontaneously vanish, although the underlying infection remains, and the lesions may recur over time.

Donovanosis (granuloma inguinale). Even rarer in the United States than chancroid, donovanosis also causes genital ulcers, which can *persist for a very long time* if left untreated. Usually the lesions continue to enlarge over time and can form *large, beefy-red heaped-up sores* in the genital area. Without a biopsy these lesions may be difficult to distinguish from those of skin cancer.

Epidermoid cysts. Epidermoid cysts are yellow bumps that can occur anywhere on the skin, but the genital area, particularly on the scrotum, is a common location. These cysts do not hurt or itch, but they can become larger and painful if infected with bacteria.

Herpes. The classic herpes lesions are *painful blisters or ulcers* in the genital area. However, there are many exceptions to this rule. The reactivation of the herpes virus may cause a *recurrent red, itchy, or tingling area on the genital skin or buttocks;* a *small slit in the skin;* or *a typical blister or ulcer.* There may be a *discharge* from the vagina and *diffuse or localized itching or tingling* in the genitals. There may be *pain down the back of the legs* or *lymph node swelling* in the groin. There are many variations from person to person, and sometimes from outbreak to outbreak in the same person. Herpes lesions usually spontaneously resolve whether or not they are treated, but the infection is not gone and may *recur* with time.

Infected hair follicles (folliculitis). Hair follicles anywhere on the body can become infected with staphylococcus, a bacterium that is normally present on the skin. Folliculitis tends to occur most often where the skin is rubbed with clothing, such as the thighs, pubic area, belt line, and buttocks. It is not a sexually transmitted disease. The infection may involve one hair follicle or many, and it is revealed by the presence of *tiny pimples on a small red area of skin, each with a hair follicle in the center.* Sometimes the infection can spread and cause infection of the surrounding skin, called cellulitis. Although cleansing the area with a mild soap generally clears up the infection, sometimes topical or oral antibiotics are necessary as well.

Molluscum contagiosum. Often confused with warts, molluscum skin lesions are usually *white, waxy, painless bumps with a dimple in the center.* In the center of the lesion is a hard white core, which contains the virus. There are usually many lesions at a time, and they can continue to appear long after the initial infection (sometimes for months to years). The lesions will *clear up without treatment,* but treating them usually speeds up the healing process. Molluscum lesions can become infected with skin bacteria and take on a pimple-like appearance, which may resemble that of herpes lesions.

Psoriasis. Psoriasis is a usually benign skin rash that is not sexually transmitted; its cause is not known. It can occur anywhere on the skin, but the genitals are a common site. The typical rash is characterized by *red splotches, often with silvery or white scales on top.* It can look very similar to fungal rashes in the genital area, and it is often suspected when the usual antifungal creams do not work. The rash usually does not hurt or itch. Several topical treatments, including steroid creams, are effective. Treatment is usually best coordinated with a dermatologist.

Scabies. Scabies usually forms *very itchy bumps and lines in the genitals and other areas of the body* (the webs between the fingers, wrists, belt line, buttocks, ankles, and armpits, among others). The bumps appear about two to four weeks after the initial infection, but they can appear sooner in someone who has previously been infected. The itching tends to be *worse at night and after a shower.*

Syphilis. The skin symptoms of syphilis vary depending on which stage of the infection is present. In primary syphilis, a *single painless ulcer* called a *chancre* can occur on the genitals (or other areas of the body) where infection took place. It can occur internally—for example, in the vagina or on the cervix in women, or in the anus in men and women—and may not be noticed because there is no pain. There may be more than one lesion, and swelling of the lymph nodes of the groin is also common. In secondary syphilis, there can be many genital skin changes, ranging from *lesions that resemble genital warts (hard, painless bumps)* to *skin rashes that look like flat red patches or are raised and scaly like those of psoriasis,* among others. Sometimes the rashes itch. A rash that occurs on the *palms and soles* is characteristic of secondary syphilis. All of these skin changes will usually vanish on their own, even if the person does not receive treatment for syphilis, but the underlying infection is still present.

Warts. Genital warts are *usually symptom-free bumps* that can occur in the genital and anal area. They are *harder than the surrounding skin* and *can either have a cauliflower-like appearance or be flat.* They *itch slightly* in about 20 percent of people who have them and can bleed if scratched or picked at. They may resolve spontaneously, stay the same size, or grow slowly over time.

Yeast. Both men and women can contract yeast infections in the genital area. One type of yeast, *Tinea cruris,* causes a *red, scaly, itchy rash in the genital area and groin,* known as *jock itch.* Men and women can also become infected in the genitals with the fungus *Candida albicans.* Women who are infected may have a clumpy white discharge from the vagina. In men, the rash is often red and flaky. Men who have not been circumcised are more likely to get a fungal rash on the penis, particularly under the foreskin.

SWELLING OF THE LYMPH NODES

Lymph nodes are found in the groin at the juncture of the leg and the trunk, as well as in other areas of the body, such as the neck and the armpits. They are part of the lymphatic system, through which circulate cells of the immune system that are important in fighting off infection and cancer. Basically any infection in the genital area can result in swelling of the lymph nodes in the groin. Once lymph nodes swell, they may not return to their normal size. Swollen lymph nodes are usually rubbery in texture and do not hurt. This list is by no means all inclusive, but it summarizes the most important causes of genital lymph node swelling. An examination by a health care provider is necessary to make a definitive diagnosis.

Cancer in the genital area. Because the lymph nodes in the groin receive drainage from all the pelvic structures, cancer in any of the genital organs may cause the lymph nodes in that area to swell. Lymph nodes enlarged as the result of a malignancy are usually hard and not moveable. Lymph node swelling in young adults is rarely caused by cancer; more often it is the result of an infection, but an examination is best to be certain. Lymph node swelling that results from infection usually subsides considerably when the infection is treated. A lymph node biopsy—in which a small piece of tissue is removed and then examined under the microscope—can be performed to rule out cancer if there is a question.

Conditions that can cause lymph node swelling throughout the body. Systemic (whole-body) infections such as mononucleosis, HIV, and secondary syphilis, as well as malignancies such as lymphoma (a cancer of the lymph nodes), can cause swelling in lymph nodes throughout the body (neck, armpits, and other areas in addition to the groin). Other symptoms are usually also present. Mononucleosis usually causes lymph node swelling in the neck and armpits.

Infection in the genital area. Any genital infection can cause lymph node swelling in the genital area. This includes bacterial infections such as gonorrhea, chlamydia, lymphogranuloma venereum, chancroid, syphilis, and donovanosis, as well as the syndromes PID and MPC in women and NGU in men. The viral infection herpes and the protozoan infection trichomoniasis can also cause lymph node swelling. Even a bladder infection can result in groin node swelling.

MOUTH AND THROAT SORES AND LESIONS

Several sexually transmitted infections can cause lesions or sores in the mouth or throat.

Aphthous ulcers. At one time or another, everyone gets aphthous ulcers—those painful little ulcers that commonly occur on the inside of the lips or on the gums, last a few days to a few weeks, and then disappear on their own. Many people confuse these with herpes lesions, but they are different. Although the cause of aphthous ulcers is not known, they are not transmitted sexually.

Cancer. Oral cancer can occur anywhere in the mouth, but the most common location is under the tongue. It is much more common among smokers or people who chew tobacco. The most common symptom is a *painless, nonhealing sore or ulcer in the mouth.*

Gonorrhea and chlamydia. Although they cannot be transmitted by kissing, gonorrhea and chlamydia can develop in the throat in someone who performs oral sex on a partner who has an infection in the genital area. Infections such as these in the throat are more common in a woman or man performing oral sex on a man (where there is penis-throat contact) than in a man or woman performing oral sex on a woman. *These infections usually do not cause symptoms in the throat.* Occasionally, though, there can be a *sore throat and redness and white or yellow patches on the back of the throat.* These symptoms are similar to those of a "strep throat," caused by a bacterial group called *group A streptococci,* which is not sexually transmitted. However, the treatment is different for streptococcus and the STDs, so testing must be performed to reach a definitive diagnosis if a person with a sore throat has a history of performing unprotected oral sex.

Herpes. There are two types of herpes, type 1 and type 2. Type 1 usually causes oral infection, and type 2 usually causes genital infection, although type 1 can occur in the genital area and type 2 can occur around the mouth. The symptoms caused by oral herpes are *redness, bumps, or blisters on the outside of the lips,* although occasionally the symptoms can occur on the *roof of the mouth, the gums, and the throat.* Sores on the inside of the lips are usually caused by aphthous ulcers, not herpes. Most people contract type 1 herpes in childhood, although only about a third ever experience symptoms. If a person does not have type 1 herpes in the mouth, he or she may acquire type 2 herpes in the mouth in adulthood by performing oral sex on a partner who has genital type 2 herpes. However, type 2 herpes infection in the mouth usually does not cause symptoms.

Syphilis. The sore of a primary syphilis infection, called a *chan-*

cre, is usually a painless ulcer that occurs where infection took place. Therefore, a person who performs oral sex on a partner who has syphilis may acquire syphilis infection in the mouth, which would manifest itself as a *painless ulcer on the tongue or gums or in the throat.* A person may not notice this sore, because it is painless.

Systemic conditions that cause mouth ulcers. Many systemic (whole-body) conditions can cause mouth ulcers, including inflammatory bowel diseases such as Crohn's disease and ulcerative colitis, infections such as those caused by coxsackievirus, and autoimmune conditions such as Behçet's syndrome. All of these systemic conditions generally produce other symptoms as well.

Yeast. Although a yeast infection in the mouth is a more common infection among people who have a compromised immune system (such as those with AIDS), occasionally people with normal immune systems may get fungal infections in the mouth, particularly after taking antibiotics. *Anyone with a fungal infection in the mouth should be tested for HIV,* unless there is another clear reason why the infection could have occurred. *Soreness, redness, and white patches* will usually be seen. A scraping from the mouth usually shows yeast under the microscope.

IF YOU HAVE any of the symptoms described in this chapter, if you have any concerns about having had unprotected sex, or if you just want to have peace of mind, you should see a health care provider for a complete STD examination. The next chapter describes what's involved in such an examination.

WHAT TO EXPECT DURING AN STD EXAMINATION

Seeking advice about a problem related to sexuality can be difficult. Because of this, many people with sexual health concerns never seek help. Others go to their health care providers, but once they get there they are too embarrassed to mention what is really worrying them. Some people who do try to get proper care find that their health care provider is also embarrassed or doesn't have expertise in issues related to sexual health, so they don't get the attention, understanding, or treatment that they need. Finally, there are those who never have themselves tested for a possible sexually transmitted infection because they are afraid of what the results might be.

There are many good reasons to overcome embarrassment and fear and seek medical advice if you suspect that you may have a sexually transmitted disease. Someone who is infected but doesn't know it, for example, can still infect his or her sexual partners, and pregnant women who are infected with certain STDs may pass the infections to their babies during the pregnancy or at delivery. Certain infections of the reproductive tract can cause infertility in both men and women if they are not detected and treated in time. Some STDs can cause cancer or death. Many infections are curable, however, so early detection and treatment are essential for your long-term health.

If you are convinced of the importance of early detection of sexually transmitted infection, and if you are committed to being vigilant about your sexual health, what should you do? You may decide that you want to be tested regularly, say every six months to a year, especially if you are sexually active and not in a steady, monogamous relationship. People who are in steady, monogamous relationships may want to be tested before they become sexually intimate, or they may learn about the importance of STD screening after they've become intimate and decide then. You may want to make STD screening part of your annual physical examination. If you have many partners, or anonymous partners, or use substances that may cloud your judgment when having sex, you may want to consider being screened more often, possibly every three to six months. These are all good ideas, and so is getting tested after any unprotected sexual contact with a partner whose status for infection is unknown or if you have symptoms.

Because regular STD check-ups are an important part of maintaining sexual health, it is crucial for you to find a health care setting where you feel comfortable discussing issues of sexual health.

> Regular STD check-ups are an important part of maintaining sexual health, for both men and women.

All adolescents and adults must have a health care provider with whom they can talk. The person you choose to provide you with medical advice in the area of sexuality may or may not be your regular health care provider. Sometimes people do not feel comfortable bringing up these issues with a long-time health care provider or someone who also provides health care to other family members. Another consideration in choosing a medical person to advise you in the area of sexual health is that certain family practitioners, internists, and pediatricians who don't specialize in STDs may not have access to the most up-to-date information about them.

After a sexual encounter about a week earlier with a woman he had met in the local tavern, Darryl became worried when he began having burning with urination and a discharge from his penis. Both Darryl and his partner had been drinking, and they didn't use a condom for either oral or genital sex. The next day, Darryl realized that he had put himself at risk, and he was not surprised when a few days later he began to have these symptoms. He had had gonorrhea in the past and was sure he had it again. He went to see his internist, who told Darryl that he didn't do much screening for sexually transmitted infections but would run a urinalysis. A few days later, the nurse called to let Darryl know he did not have a urinary tract infection. She didn't mention anything about sexually transmitted infections.

Darryl was still having symptoms, so he decided to go to a clinic that specialized in the diagnosis and treatment of STDs. Another urine sample was taken, and Darryl was told that this test would specifically look for gonorrhea and chlamydia. The next day he found out that the test showed gonorrhea.

Darryl was given a shot and some pills to take over the next week. He was also counseled about safer sex practices, and it was recommended that he seek help for his alcohol use, since it had increased over the last few years and often contributed to poor decisions about sexual partners. He also had tests performed for other STDs and scheduled a follow-up visit in a few months for additional tests.

Unless you talk honestly about your sexual health, your health care provider may not be aware that you need or want to be screened for STDs. Some health care providers don't routinely screen their patients for STDs unless they think the patient is at high risk. Don't assume that your health care provider has performed an STD screening just by looking at the genital area or by doing a Pap smear. The physical examination is just one of the steps in the screen. Specific tests must be done to screen for most STDs. Ask your health care provider what tests have been done.

A full STD screen includes evaluation for the following (the diseases are listed in alphabetical order, not in order from most to least common or vice versa):

1. Bacterial vaginosis, for women (not an STD)
2. Chancroid, donovanosis, and lymphogranuloma venereum. (These are not routinely screened for in most areas of the country because they are very rare. You may be screened if you are at risk, or if you show symptoms of these STDs on examination. See the descriptions of specific STDs in Part II to determine if you are at risk.)
3. Chlamydia
4. Genital warts, and a Pap smear, a screen for cervical cancer, for women if one has not been performed in the past year

5. Gonorrhea
6. Hepatitis B and possibly A or C
7. Herpes
8. HIV
9. Intestinal infections for recipients of anal sex or those who practice oral-anal sex
10. Lice and scabies
11. Molluscum contagiosum
12. Mucopurulent cervicitis (for women)
13. Nongonococcal urethritis (for men)
14. Pelvic inflammatory disease (for women)
15. Syphilis
16. Trichomonas
17. Yeast (not an STD)

Clinics that specialize in treating sexually transmitted infection and promoting sexual health may be a good alternative to the family physician. You can find listings for them in the phone book for your community under "sexually transmitted diseases," or you may want to contact one of the national hot lines in the reference section of this book, which can assist you in finding a local provider. There are family planning clinics, state and county health department STD clinics, infectious disease clinics, women's health clinics, and private STD clinics from which to choose. Many clinics offer these services at reduced fees or on a sliding-fee scale.

It's extremely important to feel comfortable with your health care provider and to trust that person to provide sound advice and good medical care. Only under these circumstances can you be honest about what's worrying you and about your symptoms. And only if you are honest can a health care provider help you. Health care providers aren't mind readers—they make decisions about your care based not only on what they find during the examination, but also on what you tell them. Keep in mind, too, that your health care provider is bound by the rules of practice to protect your privacy. This also goes for adolescents: All adolescents in the United States have the right to diagnosis and treatment of sexually transmitted infections without the consent or knowledge of their parents or guardian.

Testing can be done confidentially or, in some instances, anonymously. *Confidential testing* means that your medical records are not released to anyone without your written permission. Most medical records are confidential; however, the people who work where you were tested, and possibly your insurance company, will have access to your records. *Anonymous testing* means that you do not use your whole name when you are tested. You may use only your first name, or you may use a name other than your real name. You may be assigned a number that corresponds to the number on your tests, and you must give this number to receive your results. In this case, there is complete anonymity, and only you know that you are being tested and what the results of the testing are.

However, in every state in the United States, when a person is diagnosed with gonorrhea, syphilis, AIDS, or chlamydia, this fact must be reported to the state or local health department. This information is important in helping to develop programs in that area to help stop the spread of these infections. The health department will also assist those who have been diagnosed with these infections in contacting partners to be tested and treated. This partner notification is done anonymously: The health department contacts partners and tells them, "Someone you have been intimate with has been diagnosed with an STD, and you should be tested and treated, too." The name of the person diagnosed with the infection is not revealed, and this information is not released to any other individuals or organizations, such as insurance companies. This is a very important way to help make sure that people get treated. The laws governing the reporting of STDs, including HIV, vary from state to state. Talk with your health care provider about the requirements for your state.

A final thought: Health care providers should not try to impose their own beliefs about sexuality or religion on patients. To be effective, the health care environment must be supportive and nonjudgmental. If it is not, you would be well advised to find another health care provider.

> It is important to find a health care provider who provides supportive, nonjudgmental sexual health care and counseling. If your provider does not, find another health care provider.

MEDICAL HISTORY

Usually the first thing that happens when you visit a health care provider is that he or she takes a medical history by asking a lot of questions about your health, your behavior (for instance, "Do you smoke?"), and your family's health. When you are seeking advice about sexual health, some of the questions you will be asked may seem embarrassing. It may seem that a health care provider is prying, but that is usually not the case. These questions help the health care provider assess your risk for a sexually transmitted infection. Remember that what you discuss is confidential. Here are a few of the questions you may be asked:

1. When was your last sexual contact with a partner? With your steady partner? With a casual partner?
2. What kind of sexual contact have you had? Oral? Anal? Genital? (Knowing where on the body you have had sexual contact will help the health care provider know where to look for evidence of infection.)
3. How many sexual partners have you had in the last two months? In the last twelve months? In your lifetime?
4. For heterosexual persons: Do you use any type of birth control, such as a condom, diaphragm or cervical cap, or birth control pills? For all sexually active persons: What method do you use to prevent STD transmission, such as condoms, spermicides, or dental dams? Did you use this method during your last sexual contact?
5. Are your partners male, female, or both? (Certain health care providers may use terms that label people in terms of their sexual orientation, such as *gay* or *homosexual* for those who have sex with same-sex partners, *straight* or *heterosexual* for those who have sex with opposite-sex partners, or *bisexual* for those who have sex with both male and female partners. This approach may make some people less willing to answer this question. Certain health care providers make assumptions; in other words, they may assume that if you are male, you only have sex with females. You must make clear what type of sexual *practice* you have engaged in, so that your health care provider will have accurate information.)

6. Are you concerned that your partner may be having sex with other partners?
7. Are you having any symptoms in the genital area? (See Chapter 2 for a description of worrisome symptoms.)
8. Have you had a history of a sexually transmitted infection in the past, and if so, when? Have you ever been tested for STDs?
9. Do you use injection drugs? Do you have a sexual partner who uses injection drugs?
10. Have you ever had a blood transfusion?
11. Do your partners (or partner) have a history of sexually transmitted infections? Are they having symptoms now?

You will also usually be asked about your understanding of sexually transmitted infections—what causes them, how they are transmitted, and so on—and be given a chance to have all your questions answered. This is a great time to get accurate information about STDs; with that information, you can make changes in your life that will put you at lower risk for acquiring an STD.

If your health care provider does not bring up these questions, you may want to bring up the topic yourself. Here are examples of ways in which you might start off the discussion:

> The questions you will be asked may seem embarrassing. However, answer as honestly as possible, since honest answers are essential to receiving adequate care.

— "I have just started a new relationship, and my partner and I have decided that we want to be tested for sexually transmitted diseases."
— "I have concerns about sexually transmitted infections. There are a few questions I want to ask you."
— "Is there anything unusual that you noticed during the examination today? I have concerns about sexually transmitted infections."

In addition to the questions listed, you will be asked about your medical history regarding nonsexually transmitted infections or other illnesses. You will be asked what medications you take and if you are allergic to any medications. You will be asked if you have taken any antibiotics within the last month or so, since this may influence which tests are done and when. (If you took an antibiotic within the previous few weeks, you may test negative for certain bacterial STDs even if you do have the infection.)

If you are a woman, you will be asked when your last period was, if you have ever been pregnant, and if so, how the pregnancy turned out. Did you have the baby, miscarry (a spontaneous abortion), or have an abortion (an induced abortion)? You will also be asked when you last had a Pap smear and if you've ever had an abnormality on a Pap smear (the section on genital warts in Part II explains why this question is important).

Before you leave the office or the clinic, try to express all your concerns. It may take a while during the visit before you feel comfortable, however, and it's possible that you'll overlook something. Find out how to contact your health care provider after you leave. That way, you can call if any more concerns or questions occur to you later.

If your health care provider does not seem to have the answers you are looking for, or if you feel uncomfortable for any reason, you may want to consider a visit to another clinic or health care provider to get the help you need.

THE PHYSICAL EXAMINATION

Knowing what to expect during an examination helps make people feel less afraid or embarrassed. Many health care providers explain everything they are about to do during the examination for just this reason: so that there are no surprises. If your health care provider doesn't do this, ask him or her to take a few minutes to explain what is involved in each step of the examination.

MEN

For men, the examination usually consists of the items listed below, which are not necessarily performed in the order shown here. The man may be asked to remove his clothing and put on a gown so that the health care provider can perform a thorough evaluation.

1. The skin is examined. This is necessary because certain STDs cause rashes on the body as well as in the genital area.
2. If you are having symptoms in the mouth and throat or have per-

formed oral sex on a partner, the health care provider will inspect those areas with a bright light and may swab the throat to obtain samples to test for infections such as gonorrhea and chlamydia.

3. The skin of the genital area is examined for rashes, sores, or bumps, some of which may be very small or may not be causing any symptoms you can feel, so you may not even know they are there. If a health care provider finds something, he or she may want to swab the area to facilitate specific tests to help in diagnosis. Sometimes a biopsy of a lesion is necessary to make the diagnosis. To take a biopsy, a small piece of tissue is removed and then examined in the laboratory. Some skin bumps—such as those caused by the virus that causes genital warts (human papillomavirus) or molluscum contagiosum—may be treated at this time.

    The lymph nodes of the genital area are also examined. These glands are part of the immune system and sit at the top of the legs, in the groin area; they may be swollen and tender when infection is present.

4. The testicles are examined for any bumps, tender areas, swelling, or redness. This is done by gently feeling the contents of the scrotal sac between the fingers. Certain infections and other conditions, such as testicular cancer, can be detected in this way. This is usually not a painful part of the examination.

5. If a man is uncircumcised, the foreskin is retracted to look for any bumps or sores or rashes. The urine opening (urethra) is gently opened to see if there are any skin changes there and any discharge from the penis. Sometimes the urethra is "milked" to look for any discharge. This involves gently pushing on the underside of the penis to see if discharge can be expressed. Either the health care provider or the patient can do this.

6. There are several ways to check for infection of the urethra. If there is discharge, a small amount is put on a swab, and tests can then be performed to check for various specific causes of urethral infection, such as gonorrhea and chlamydia. If there is no discharge, then a small swab is inserted about 2 cm into the urethra and quickly removed; the swab is wiped on a slide, which is examined under a microscope for pus (white blood cells) cells. The

swab can cause pain, but the procedure is done quickly and the pain is usually brief. Another way of examining the urethra is to collect urine from the very first part of the stream and look for pus cells in this sample. A newer and more sensitive test also allows testing for gonorrhea and chlamydia from a first urine sample. (Whether or not a swab or urine sample is taken, it is very important that a man not urinate for four or more hours—and preferably overnight—before this part of the examination, since urination may wash out evidence of infection.) After this, a midstream urine sample may be tested to look for evidence of a bladder infection, a rare occurrence in men.

7. The anal area and buttocks are examined for any rashes, bumps, or sores. Swabs may be taken from this area (to test for gonorrhea and chlamydia) if a man has been the recipient of anal sex or has STD symptoms in the anal area. If the man has diarrhea, a stool sample may be obtained to test for evidence of intestinal infections. Whatever a man's sexual orientation, an anal examination is an important part of the screening. For example, genital warts and herpes lesions can occur in this area even if a man has never received anal sex. A procedure called an *anoscopy* may be performed if there are symptoms in the anal area or if the man has diarrhea. In an anoscopy, a small plastic speculum is inserted into the anal area and the health care provider looks for changes in the lining of the rectum or for skin lesions such as warts. If there are no symptoms in this area, this is not a routine part of the examination.

8. A prostate examination may be performed. (This is not routinely done during an STD screen unless symptoms indicate a need for it.) The health care provider asks the man to bend over the table and then inserts a gloved, lubricated finger into the anal area. Not only can abnormalities of the wall of the rectum be felt, but the prostate gland can also be felt to determine whether it is swollen, tender, or irregular in shape. This part of the examination may cause brief discomfort. The man may be asked to provide a sample of urine after this part of the examination to test for evidence of prostate infection. This is best done after the earlier urine samples have been collected to evaluate for urethral infection and for bladder infection.

9. Men who perform oral sex on a male partner will also have a test of the throat for gonorrhea and chlamydia.

WOMEN

For women, the physical examination usually consists of the items listed below, which are not necessarily performed in the order shown here.

A woman may be asked to remove her clothing and put on a gown so that the health care provider can perform a thorough evaluation. She may also be asked to provide a urine sample before the examination, which will make the examination more comfortable for her and also make it easier for the health care provider to feel her internal organs. Urine from the very first part of the stream may be used to test for infections such as gonorrhea and chlamydia. If there is concern about a urinary tract infection, then a midstream sample may be collected after the woman has cleansed the area around the urethra, following her health care provider's instructions. The urine sample is examined microscopically and chemically for any abnormalities— blood, white blood cells, or bacteria—that could be signs of infection. A pregnancy test can also be performed on the urine.

1. The skin is examined. This is necessary because certain STDs cause rashes on the body as well as in the genital area.
2. If you are having symptoms in the mouth and throat, or have performed oral sex on a partner, the health care provider will inspect those areas with a bright light and may swab the throat to obtain samples to test for infections such as gonorrhea and chlamydia.
3. The skin of the genital area is examined for rashes, sores, or bumps, some of which may be very small or may not be causing any symptoms, so you may not even know they are there. If a health care provider finds something, he or she may want to swab the area for specific tests to help in diagnosis. Sometimes a biopsy of a lesion is necessary to make the diagnosis. To take a biopsy, a small piece of tissue is removed and then examined in the laboratory. Some skin bumps—such as those caused by the virus that causes genital warts (human papillomavirus) or molluscum contagiosum—may be treated at this time.

The labia majora are spread to see if there are any rashes,

bumps, or sores on the labia minora or at the opening of the vagina.

The lymph nodes of the genital area are examined. These glands are part of the immune system and sit at the top of the legs, in the groin area; they may be swollen and tender when infection is present.

4. A speculum, an instrument made of plastic or metal, is slowly inserted into the vagina and then gradually opened so that the health care provider can see the vaginal walls and the cervix, which sits at the end of the vagina. The health care provider will examine the vagina for sores or bumps, redness, swelling, and discharge and will examine the cervix for sores, bleeding, or discharge. Swabs are usually taken from the vaginal walls to test for yeast, trichomonas, and bacterial vaginosis, and a swab is inserted into the opening of the cervix (the os) to test for specific infections such as gonorrhea and chlamydia. If the woman has not had a Pap smear done within the past year, one can be done at this time. Cells from the inside and outer parts of the cervix are removed gently with a brush and spatula and are sent for laboratory examination.

5. The anal area and buttocks are examined for any rashes, bumps, or sores. If there are symptoms in the anal area, or if the woman has diarrhea or evidence of infection on examination, then the area may be wiped with a swab to collect a sample for testing. If a woman has received anal intercourse, then swabs may be taken to test for gonorrhea and chlamydia, whether or not she has symptoms. If a woman has diarrhea, a stool sample may be obtained to test for evidence of intestinal infections.

An anal examination is an important part of the check-up. Even if a woman has never received anal intercourse, certain STDs, such as warts and herpes, can reveal signs of infection in the anal area. If a woman has a gonorrhea infection in the cervix, for example, the anal area can become infected from secretions, even if she has not received anal sex.

If the woman has diarrhea or anal symptoms, a procedure called an *anoscopy* may be performed. This involves inserting a small plastic speculum into the anal area and the health care provider looks for changes in the lining of the rectum or for skin lesions such as warts. This is not a routine part of the examination if a woman is without symptoms in this area.

A rectal examination may be performed. In this procedure, the health care provider inserts a gloved, lubricated finger into the anal area to feel for masses or bumps.

6. A bimanual examination is performed. In this procedure, the health care provider inserts one or two gloved, lubricated fingers into the vagina to feel the cervix, and then gently presses on the pelvic area with the other hand to feel the shape and contour of the uterus and ovaries. In this way, any swelling or tenderness of these organs can be detected. This part of the examination is important in detecting pelvic inflammatory disease.

Bridget and Alicia had met during an evening art class six months ago and were very happy together. One day Alicia told Bridget that she would be home late from work because she was going to her gynecologist for her Pap smear. She explained that she went every year, ever since she had had an abnormality on her Pap smear about five years ago, which fortunately had turned out not to be serious. Bridget was surprised. She had never had a Pap smear, because her doctor and her friends had told her that women whose sexual partners were other women did not need to get them, since they were not at risk for cervical cancer. But Alicia said that her gynecologist had told her that all sexually active women needed to be tested regularly, since the human papillomavirus, which can cause cervical cancer, can be transmitted through genital rubbing and not only through intercourse. Bridget decided to set up an appointment for herself the following week, and she asked Alicia to go with her, since she was nervous about having her first gynecological exam.

BLOOD TESTS, DIAGNOSIS, AND TREATMENT

After the examination, blood tests for infections such as HIV, syphilis, hepatitis, or herpes may be performed. A health care provider will explain all the tests, what a positive or negative result means, and how much they cost, and will decide with you which tests need to be done.

Some blood tests may be performed at the time of your examination, and may need to be repeated later to make sure they are accurate. For instance, it can take up to three to six months after infection to show a positive blood test for HIV. Your health care provider will explain when you need to return for additional tests.

Make sure you know how you are going to find out the results of your tests. Are you supposed to call or is your health care provider supposed to call you? Do you need to return to the office or clinic to learn the results of your tests? If you don't get a telephone call, don't assume that everything was normal. Sometimes offices and clinics are understaffed, and making even important phone calls can be overlooked. Be sure to find out your results.

> Wanda and Mike were relieved when they went to pick up their HIV results and found out they both had tested negative. They had decided that if they were going to be sexually involved, they first wanted to be tested for HIV and know that "everything was O.K." Although the nurse who tested them explained that HIV tests were only one part of an STD screen, they weren't interested in testing for other infections, because "only HIV can kill you."
>
> They became sexually intimate without using condoms. Six months into their relationship, Mike developed small, painful blisters on his penis that, on culture, tested positive for herpes simplex 2. Wanda had a herpes blood test, which showed that she, too, was positive for herpes simplex 2, although she had never shown any symptoms. She had most likely transmitted the infection to Mike, since Mike's blood test for herpes was negative. (See the section on herpes in Part II; it may take weeks to months to develop antibodies after a new infection.) If they had been tested earlier in their relationship, and had found out that Wanda was positive for herpes and Mike was not, Mike and Wanda could have decided whether they wanted to take precautions to help decrease the chance that Mike would become infected.

After the physical examination has been completed and blood has been taken for testing, your health care provider will explain what he or she has seen on the examination and what diagnoses have been made, and then will discuss treatment, if any is needed. (You may need to wait until the results of tests are available before you receive a diagnosis and can begin treatment.) You may be offered printed information about subjects that were discussed or about the findings of the examination.

The health care provider may give you samples of medication to treat your infection or a prescription to take to a pharmacy. Make sure your provider explains how to take the medication, any potential side effects, and whether it interacts with any of the medications you are already taking. It is very important to take the complete course of medication that is prescribed. Find out what to do if symptoms recur, or if the medicine doesn't seem to be clearing up the symptoms. If follow-up visits were recommended, make sure you set them up before you leave the clinic, and mark them on your calendar so you'll remember.

If you are diagnosed with an infection, your health care provider may recommend that your partner be screened or treated for that infection. If this presents problems—because of any number of issues that can arise in intimate relationships—you can ask your provider for suggestions about the best way to handle the situation. Sometimes role playing, with the health care provider acting as your partner, can help you find an effective way to communicate this news. You may want your provider to call your partner for you, or you may want to come to the office or clinic with your partner so that everything can be explained. As discussed earlier, in some instances the local or state health department will help you notify your partner or partners. It may or may not be possible to determine who had the infection first, and in any case that's not the most important thing: the most important thing is for both partners to receive treatment. It is a sign of respect and concern for your partner to let him or her know what is going on with you. Lack of symptoms doesn't always mean lack of infection: even without symptoms, he or she could have the infection too. Chapter 4, on sexual communication, discusses this topic more fully.

This is the time to ask any questions, no matter how silly they may seem. The provider is there not only to diagnose and treat your infections, but also to educate you about STDs and help prevent you from putting yourself or anyone else at risk in the future. Abstinence and safer sex practices will usually be discussed (these are covered in Chapter 5). Health care providers expect to receive phone calls from patients, so if you have questions about what was discussed during the examination, do not hesitate to contact your health care provider.

Regular sexual health care check-ups are as important a part of maintaining your health and well-being as a blood pressure check or a cholesterol screen. If you are currently sexually active, or are thinking about becoming active, find a health care provider in your community with whom you feel comfortable discussing these issues. Your health is worth it.

SEXUAL
COMMUNICATION
COMMUNICATE NOW, NO REGRETS LATER

alking about sex can be very difficult, so many people—regardless of their gender, age, or sexual orientation—avoid the subject altogether. For example, an American Social Health Association survey of women attending college showed that although 81 percent, on entering into a sexual relationship with a man, asked their partner how many partners he had had in the past, only slightly more than half asked if he had ever had a sexually transmitted infection or had ever had unprotected sex. Fewer than a third asked whether their partner had ever had a same-sex partner or had ever used intra-

> Despite the bombardment of sexual imagery and innuendo to which we are subjected by the media and the frequency with which sex is discussed in the abstract, people still have a hard time discussing safer sex with partners.

venous drugs. And these are the findings on how women behaved when they knew their partner *fairly well* before entering into the sexual relationship. When women were entering into a new sexual relationship with a *casual* partner, even fewer of them asked these important questions. Finally, although about 85 percent of the women in this study were sexually active, fewer than half of them used any method to protect against sexually transmitted infections, and about a quarter had never had a pelvic examination.

Talking with a partner about these issues *before* you become sexually active has been proven to help prevent infection with STDs, no matter what your age or sexual orientation. Study after study confirms that communicating with a partner increases the chance that

> Talking with your partner before you become sexually active helps protect against STDs and unwanted pregnancy.

steps will be taken to guard against STDs and unwanted pregnancy. However, poor communication with a partner increases the likelihood that you will contract a sexually transmitted infection.

As noted earlier, screening for sexually transmitted infections is the only way to know for sure whether or not a person has been infected. The goal of this chapter is to help prepare you to become a better communicator about sexual health. The chapter begins with a discussion about why it is so difficult to communicate and then suggests ways to make communication easier. For many people, talking about sex is easier if you practice communication skills beforehand. If you have thought about what your partner may tell you, and what you would say in response, you will be better prepared for any situation that may arise. You can also learn from your past mistakes. If in the past things did not turn out exactly as you would have wanted, think about what you might do differently now and in the future and identify the communication patterns you want to change. You do not have to keep on making the same mistakes. You owe it to yourself to be safe.

> If you have been in situations with a sexual partner in which things did not turn out as you wanted, think about ways in which you could avoid similar situations in the future.

WHY IS IT SO HARD TO TALK ABOUT SEXUAL HEALTH AND STDs?

Why is it that we often have difficulty communicating honestly and openly with a partner in general, much less on subjects such as sexual health and STDs? A few of the many reasons are described in this section. As you read through it, see how many of these issues have crossed your mind. Do you see yourself in any of the following scenarios? Knowing *why* you have difficulty talking about safer sex with your partner will help you make changes. Especially in the era of HIV infection—a life-threatening sexually transmitted infection for which there is as yet no cure—people must be able to talk comfortably about safer sex.

THE SEX TALK TABOO

Most people have not been raised to discuss sexual topics openly. In fact, while they are growing up, most people are not even allowed to discuss genital anatomy using the appropriate terms, and if these terms are mentioned it is often with an embarrassed giggle—sometimes even by adults. Nearly everyone we know has been raised in this culture, and they find talking about sexual topics as difficult as we do. As a society, it is time for us to grow up and start talking about sex and STDs in a more mature way. We must also start talking to our children earlier and more openly, so that they can make informed decisions when they reach sexual maturity. Then, once they enter into intimate relationships, it will not be so difficult to discuss these issues.

LACK OF INFORMATION

Because of misinformation or lack of information, people may not even know that they need to discuss safer sex with their partners. To understand that they do need to communicate, and to communicate effectively, couples must have accurate information about sexual health.

Many people get their information about sex from the media: from television, books, and magazines. This information may or may not be correct. In the advertising world, sex is a commodity—it sells products. And sex always looks great and risk free when it is being used to sell something. But that's not the real world. Young people often get much of their information about sex from their peers or from family members, who may be misinformed. Sometimes even health care providers may have difficulty talking about sexual health issues or may not have the most current information. Thus many people may not be aware that they are practicing unsafe sex. The HIV epidemic that began in the early 1980s promoted more open discussion about sexual issues, but the depth of discussion in our society about STDs and condom use is still woefully inadequate.

Current public service announcements about sex on U.S. television rely on generalities, such as "Be careful out there." Although these may increase public awareness of STDs, vague warnings are often of limited use, especially for young people. What is needed is accessible, accurate information about how to prevent infection. Education about STDs must be started early and include information about abstinence, as well as ways to protect oneself from becoming infected with an STD if one is sexually active. More and more young people are becoming sexually active at younger ages. Whether or not this is a good thing, it is a fact: teenagers account for about three million of the twelve million people infected with STDs in the United States each year, and two-thirds of those infected each year are younger than twenty-five.

> Sitting on the sofa with Peter, her new boyfriend, Holly was incredibly embarrassed when a public service announcement came on the TV: "Some things about sex are not sexy—like sexually transmitted diseases," the movie-star spokesperson said. Holly had been planning to tell Peter about her past history of genital warts and to discuss this issue before having sex with him. Her health care provider had explained warts and the virus that causes them, and had told her how common the disease was. Yet after hearing the TV announcement, Holly was convinced that the general public still didn't get it. The ad made her feel unattractive and alone with her condition. She decided she couldn't talk to Peter about her sexual health—at least not yet.

Abstinence (not having sex) until you are older and better informed is the best solution. Waiting to have sex allows a young person to develop as an individual and to focus on school and other interests. Young people

Talking to young people about sex, STDs, and condom use does not make young people more sexually active.

who are already sexually active, however, need information on how to protect themselves from infection and pregnancy. Studies have shown that children who take sex education classes are actually less likely to engage in sexual activity, and if they do, they are more likely to use condoms. Education about STDs and safer sex is the first step in helping prevent infection.

THE "PLANNED SEX IS NOT GOOD SEX" THEORY

In the movies, as the waves rush over the embracing couple, they kiss passionately, limbs entwined. How romantic to be swept away by unplanned passion! Many people think that the best kind of sex is experienced when one is swept away in the moment and that talking with a partner before sex about condom use and STDs will somehow rob the event of its magic. Others may deliberately choose to be unprepared, because they won't feel guilty if they believe that they have no control over whether or not they have intercourse: "I didn't plan it, so I'm not a bad person." But in real life, people can contract sexually transmitted infections, or become pregnant, by not thinking before they have sex.

Planned sex can be every bit as good as unplanned sex—even better. For one thing, knowing for certain about sexually transmitted infections lets your relationship move ahead without any nagging doubts. For another, being honest with a partner, and sharing your thoughts and concerns, often leads to a closer relationship and is the first step toward real intimacy.

> Planned sex doesn't mean bad sex. By decreasing your anxieties about STDs and pregnancy, planned sex may actually be more fulfilling.

TRUST

Some people think that if you trust a partner, you don't need to talk about these things, and they worry that communicating with a partner about sexual health issues may cause that partner to leave. The problem with this approach is that, in an effort to show your partner that you trust him or her by having unprotected sex, you could acquire an infection that could impair your ability to have children in the future (gonorrhea or chlamydia) or shorten your life (HIV). You could end up with a lasting and painful reminder of the relationship. Diving into a relationship such as this with unrealistic optimism, hoping that you are somehow immune, is naive. On the other hand, talking about sex and sexual health shows that you care enough about your partner and yourself to do what is necessary to protect both of you.

CULTURAL OR RELIGIOUS TABOOS

There are particular cultural taboos against using condoms and talking about sexual health. In certain cultures, whether people are living in their country of origin or elsewhere, women are not permitted to request that a condom be used. And some men refuse to use condoms, because they believe that doing so diminishes their manliness. In other societies sexual intercourse is perceived as the exchange of energy, which a condom blocks. Furthermore, in certain religions, using birth control methods such as condoms is not acceptable, so preventing the transmission of STDs with a condom is not possible. Some people may also believe that if they choose partners of their own ethnic or cultural background they will not contract an STD, because STDs are infections that only "others" get. It can be difficult to bridge these cultural gaps, but through education about sex and STDs there are those who may decide to alter their behavior and also find partners who are willing to practice safer sex.

NOT BEING PREPARED

Many people have their own guidelines about when they will become sexually active. Some want to be sexually active only when they are in a committed, mutually monogamous relationship, or when they are married. Others may decide they want their partners to be tested for STDs before they become sexually active together. All of these guidelines are reasonable, and yet it is still a good idea to think about what kind of birth control and STD prevention method you will want to use if you do become sexually active, just in case this happens before you thought it would.

Even if you don't expect to have sex with a new partner for a long time, it makes sense to be prepared and to talk with your partner about safer sex before you become sexually active. Whether you are a man or a

> Carrying condoms with you in case you become sexually active with a new partner does not make you promiscuous. It makes you prepared.

woman, it's a good idea to have condoms available, in case you want to have sex. (A woman should not always assume that her male partner will bring a condom.) Condoms, if used consistently and correctly, are one of the best ways to avoid becoming infected with STDs. Learning how to use a condom is also important, because it is well known that most condom failures result from incorrect use, not defects, and that the risk of a condom breaking or coming off is higher if one has little experience using it. Men can practice putting condoms on before becoming sexually active, and women can practice putting them on a male partner, possibly by using a banana or a cucumber. Other barrier methods are available for couples. (See Chapter 5 to learn more about how to use a condom and other barrier methods.)

Another way to be prepared is for both of you to be tested for all sexually transmitted infections before you become sexually active. Make sure it has been long enough for each of you since your last sexual contact with other partners, or other potential sources of infection, for the test results to be accurate. And make sure that you have only each other as partners. If you can feel fairly sure

> Just talking about safe sex is not enough to prevent infection.

that both of you are uninfected, and if you remain mutually monogamous, then from the standpoint of STDs you are in good shape. If you find out that one of you has a treatable STD, then treatment can be started and transmission of the infection avoided. If you find out that one of you has a chronic STD, knowing this beforehand is better than finding out later in the relationship. If you have both been tested, but you cannot be sure that your partner does not have other sexual partners, then continuing to use barrier methods makes very good sense. Heterosexual couples who opt not to use condoms for preventing STD transmission may still want to consider the use of condoms (or another option) for birth control.

"THE RISK IS WORTH IT"

Some people hurtle full speed into sexual relationships without stopping to think about the consequences. They may convince themselves that the relationship or the sex is so terrific that it's worth any risk— even worth dying for. Even if that seems true in the heat of the moment, in reality no relationship is worth sacrificing your health. No relationship is worth becoming infected with HIV or acquiring an infection that prevents you from having children.

> Sometimes logic goes out the window when people are passionately involved in a new relationship. Use your head. Be safe.

DENIAL

Certain people, especially teenagers, may believe that although the risk of acquiring a sexually transmitted infection exists, they are somehow immune from getting one: "It couldn't happen to me." When the reality of the risk of overwhelming, it may be easier to think that one is "magically" protected than to deal with the responsibility of protecting oneself. And there are those who have the misperception that only promiscuous people get STDs. These myths can give people a false sense of security, and therefore they don't perceive themselves to be at risk for getting a sexually transmitted infection.

It's time to dispel these myths. *Each year twelve million people in the United States acquire a sexually transmitted infection.* Many more than that are dealing daily with chronic STDs such as herpes and genital warts. A variety of people in a variety of circumstances contract STDs. It only stands to reason that the more partners you have, the more likely you are to become infected with an STD. But even if you have only one partner, and that partner has had sex in the past and did not use protection, then you could be at risk of infection. And some STDs, such as genital warts and herpes, may be transmitted even when you use a condom.

> People from all walks of life, not only promiscuous people, get STDs.

We have by now been through almost twenty-five years of the AIDS epidemic, and the incidence of STDs is still increasing at an alarming rate. People fondly recall the "carefree" 1960s and 1970s, when sex was "risk free"—meaning that there was no perceived risk of HIV infection. It's true that HIV has changed our ideas about sex and safer sex, but *sex was never risk free.* There have always been sexually transmitted infections. There have always been emo-

> Denial is dangerous when it comes to STDs.

tional risks as well. For heterosexual couples there has always been the risk of an unwanted pregnancy. But you have the ability to protect yourself—beginning by recognizing that there is a risk.

"I'M NOT WORTH IT"

Lack of self-esteem can be a big problem in sexual communication. For example, a person with low self-esteem may be more vulnerable to being bullied by a sexual partner into doing things that he or she doesn't want to do. If a partner says, "You would have sex with me if you loved me" or "If you don't have sex with me, it means you're frigid," a person with low self-esteem may do what the partner wants instead of being able to recognize these lines for what they are: unfair pressure to have sex. A person who lacks self-esteem may feel that he or she doesn't even deserve to express his or her needs, much less insist on having those needs honored. There are those people who feel so bad about themselves that they may think they deserve to become infected if it happens, so they don't protect themselves at all.

By practicing what to say in various situations, you can prepare yourself to respond in a way that produces the best outcome for you. If you are in a relationship with someone who contributes to your feelings of low self-esteem and who is unwilling to change, think about finding a new partner. You may also want to think about seeking counseling, to sort out why you feel that you don't deserve to have your needs met. There are also self-help books that may enable you to begin developing a better sense of yourself and to become more confident and assertive in your relationships. By learning to care for yourself and about yourself, you can learn to make smart decisions, and thus keep yourself healthy.

> Low self-esteem often contributes to poor decision making about sex and the inability to communicate about your needs.

ALCOHOL AND DRUGS

Use of alcohol and drugs makes it harder to make good decisions and often leads to risky behavior—such as driving too fast or spending the night with a relative stranger. The combination of not thinking clearly and being in a situation in which sex is involved can make a person very vulnerable. It's hard, in such a situation, to ask questions or prac-

tice safer sex, or even to remember that a person can become infected with an STD from a single
unprotected sexual contact. If
you have a problem with drugs
or alcohol, seek help and counseling.

**Alcohol and drugs can
impair your decision-making
ability and make you
vulnerable to becoming
infected with an STD.**

> Arthur had known he was HIV positive for four years. He heard
> through the grapevine that his last partner, Bill, whom he'd been with
> for three difficult years, was also HIV positive. Arthur's health had
> been good; he saw his physician regularly and tried to live a healthy
> life, but sometimes the stress of his situation got the better of him,
> and he drank to cope. He was lonely and didn't feel comfortable
> telling people about his infection. One evening he went to a bar and
> drank until he was drunk. That night, he met a man named Chuck,
> who had also been drinking heavily. Chuck made him laugh, which
> he hadn't done for a long time. There was a mutual attraction. They
> continued to drink together until the bar closed, then went back to
> Chuck's apartment and had sex. When Arthur woke up the next
> morning, he dressed quickly and left for home while Chuck was still
> asleep. Arthur couldn't remember whether he had used a condom,
> but he didn't think he had. He felt horrible. How could he have done
> this? He had put Chuck at risk for acquiring HIV.

TALKING ABOUT SEX

Talking about sexual health with a partner shows that you care about
yourself and your partner and that you want to share information to
safeguard both your own and your partner's health. Your personalities
as well as the nature and length of your relationship will have a lot to
do with when and how you choose to talk about the subject. The best
time to have the talk is well before becoming sexually involved. It is
more difficult to talk about safer sex in the heat of the moment, when
you're about to engage in sex. Although this may seem obvious, many
people find themselves making this mistake over and over again.

WHEN YOU'RE READY TO TALK

When you and your partner have gotten to know each other and feel
comfortable talking about becoming intimate, choose a time when
you are together in private and won't be interrupted. It's a good idea

to have your options clearly in your mind as well as some general guidelines about what you do—and don't—want to do. Make up your mind that you're not going to allow yourself to feel pressured into doing anything you don't want to do. Although it may not always work out that way, it's almost always best to let relationships take time. If a partner is worth getting to know better, he or she will stay around without sex. Indeed, you may decide after getting to know a partner that you don't want to become intimate.

> **Waiting to have sex until you know the person well, and feel comfortable enough to talk about sex and safer sex, is a very good idea.**

If you do decide that you want to enter into a sexual relationship with a person, here are a few ways to get the conversation started:

> "I'm starting to feel close to you, and before things go any further, I want to talk about safer sex. Is this a good time for you?"

> "I want to talk with you about a topic that's a bit uncomfortable for me to discuss, but I think it's important. I want to talk about safer sex and using condoms. Is that O.K. with you?"

If your partner is uncomfortable or is not ready to talk about sex, let him or her know that you understand, that these are difficult topics to discuss, and that whenever he or she is ready to talk about them, you are ready to talk, too. But let your partner know that you don't want to have sex until you have had this discussion.

When you and your partner do have the discussion, keep in mind that what you want is a dialogue, in which both of you can express your feelings on these topics. Blanket or judgmental statements—such as "Everyone who has sex without a condom is stupid"—rarely lead to an open discussion. Try to be honest about your own thoughts and goals. Don't say things to impress your partner. Use "I" statements (such as "I would like to use a condom"); they allow you to express your feelings openly and clearly. Then you can ask your partner about his or her feelings, using open-ended questions such as "What are your thoughts?" If you are having this conversation, the odds are that both you and your partner have been thinking about these issues and want to find out specific information about each other. Answering the questions listed here will provide the information you will want to have before beginning a new sexual relationship. It is important to be honest. Intentionally misleading your partner will only weaken the foundation of your relationship.

Rather than reading the questions off like a laundry list, or interrogating your partner in a way that makes him or her uncomfortable, you may simply want to cover these topics in the course of your conversation. However you and your partner go about discussing these subjects, it is helpful to get answers to the following questions:

1. How many sexual partners have you had in the past?
2. Have you had any partners of the same sex?
3. Have you ever had unprotected sex with a partner?
4. Have you ever used injection drugs? Did you ever share needles?
5. Have you ever received a transfusion of blood or blood products? (The U.S. blood supply began to be screened for HIV in 1985; the risk of acquiring HIV infection from blood transfused since 1985 is very low.)
6. Have you ever been tested for sexually transmitted infections?

WHEN YOUR PARTNER WON'T COOPERATE

What if your partner never wants to discuss sex but still wants to have sex? Possibly he or she has difficulty with open, honest discussion. This may make the relationship difficult in other respects as well. Possibly your partner doesn't understand the importance of the discussion and is poorly informed about STDs. This may mean that he or she has engaged in risky behavior in the past and may now put you at risk as well. Maybe your partner is afraid to talk about the issue for other reasons. Without talking about it, it's hard to know. Having sex with someone who won't discuss sexual health probably doesn't fit into anyone's plans for keeping safe. Remember: the decision about whether or not to become intimate with this person is yours. If you decide not to go any further, say no in a clear and unmistakable way to let your partner know where you stand.

Certain partners may try to make you feel embarrassed or awkward for bringing the topic up, or even try to make you feel that you are unusual for raising the issue. Such a person may not be the one for you. Consider the following ten statements from a person who is pressuring someone to have sex without talking about safer sex first, or is pressuring someone to have unprotected sex. Each of the statements is followed by a response that might be helpful, if not in convincing your partner, then at least in helping you keep your priorities straight.

1. "People who are in love don't need to use condoms."
   "Being in love doesn't protect anyone from getting an STD."

2. "A condom will spoil the mood and make it less pleasurable for me and for you."
   "Getting infected with an STD would be an even bigger mood spoiler. It's important to me that we use condoms."

3. "Talking about this means you must have slept around."
   "No, it doesn't. It means that I care enough about myself and about you to talk about a difficult topic."

4. "You don't want to have sex with me because you're uptight."
   "Name-calling won't make me want to have sex with you."

5. "If I withdraw before ejaculation you can't get an STD."
   "That's not true. Pre-ejaculate can still transmit infection. If we have sex, we need to use a condom for the entire time, not just during ejaculation."

6. "Sex is best without a condom. It's more spontaneous."
   "The best sex is when you don't need to worry about getting an infection or getting pregnant. We need to use a condom."

7. "I won't have sex with you if we need to use condoms."
   "Then we won't have sex. My sexual health is more important to me then having sex with you tonight."

8. "I've never used condoms before, and I never got an STD."
   "People can have STDs without having any symptoms, and you wouldn't know you were infected unless you got tested. Since neither of us has been tested recently, for both of our sakes, it would be best to use a condom to be safe."

9. "Not using a condom is a way to show me that you love me."
   "No, it means I care about both of us if we *do* use a condom."

10. "Only homosexuals [or heterosexuals, or promiscuous people, or people living in the city, or whatever other myth is out there] get STDs, so we don't need to use a condom."

"The truth is that anybody can get an STD, no matter what their sexual orientation or where they live. We need to be responsible and use condoms."

You must decide what you need to do to keep yourself sexually healthy, and then stick to your plan. Your sexual health, and possibly your future, depends on it. It doesn't matter what anyone else says, or what anyone else is doing. Even if your peers are practicing unsafe sex and putting themselves at risk, that doesn't mean you have to make the same mistakes. It might even mean that you have to be more careful than ever.

> Everyone is different, and everybody has a different perspective about life—including sex. What works best for you may not work for someone else. You must decide how to keep yourself safe, and stick to your plan.

WHEN YOU'RE READY TO HAVE SEX, HAVE YOURSELF TESTED

Let's say that you and your partner have discussed sex and your sexual health, and you are ready to begin an intimate relationship. What's next? Unfortunately, talking doesn't guarantee safety. For one thing, if your partner has had sex with another person in the past, just because your partner doesn't have any symptoms of a sexually transmitted infection doesn't necessarily mean that he or she is not infected (see Chapter 2 and Part II). Another consideration is that, even if you and your partner agree always to use a condom, you are not 100 percent safe: condoms sometimes fail because they are improperly used, and sometimes they break. Certain sexually transmitted infections, such as herpes and genital warts, can be transmitted even when condoms are used, although condoms certainly decrease the risk.

The bottom line is that if you have had sex in the past, *the only way to know for sure whether or not you are infected with an STD is to be tested.* If both you and your partner are properly tested at the time intervals at which any infection is likely to show up, and you are both negative for all infections, and you are both mutually faithful and don't engage in other risky behavior, then you may want to consider not using condoms for STD prevention. (See Chapter 5 for an explanation of the time intervals required to ensure accurate testing and discussion of "risky behavior.") Under any other circumstances, you may want to assume that your partner may be infected with a sexually transmitted infection and therefore keep yourself safer by using condoms. If you or your partner have not been tested, or if you or your partner have other partners, or engage in risky behavior, then it is best to use condoms.

One important note: Because of the media attention devoted to HIV, many couples consider getting screened for HIV before becoming sexually involved, which is a great idea. Of all the sexually transmitted infections, this is the one of which most people are aware, and the one that most people are afraid of because it is life-threatening and incurable. Although *testing for HIV is very important* for any sexually active adult, testing for HIV alone is *not* a complete screen for all of the sexually transmitted infections. (See Chapter 3 for a description of what is involved in a complete STD screening.) You may actually be at higher risk for acquiring other STDs (such as chlamydia or herpes) than HIV, so it is important to get a complete screening.

AVOIDING OTHER PITFALLS, MAKING OTHER CHOICES

Sometimes two people have been together for a certain period of time—months or years—and have been monogamous. They trust each other and want to stop using a barrier method of preventing the spread of STDs. But either or *both* of them might have acquired a sexually transmitted infection from a previous partner, even if they don't have any symptoms. Getting a complete STD screening before starting a sexual relationship is the only way to avoid unknowingly passing any such infection along.

After using condoms for six months, Mandy and Alan decided that they didn't want to use them any more. Mandy started taking the pill as her birth control method. She and Alan thought it was safe to stop using condoms because they had been together so long that they thought they would have symptoms by now if either of them was infected with an STD from a previous partner. About two weeks later, Alan began experiencing a burning sensation when he urinated. He was diagnosed with nongonococcal urethritis. Mandy was surprised when her gynecologist recommended testing for STDs and treatment as well, even though she hadn't had any symptoms. Although each denied it, both she and Alan were concerned that the other had been unfaithful. Testing showed that Mandy had chlamydia, which hadn't caused any symptoms. Most likely, she had been infected by a previous partner, and all the time she and Alan had been using condoms she was symptom-free and unaware of the infection. Alan had been protected until they stopped using condoms.

Casual sex presents plenty of risks, but if you are planning to have casual sex with a partner with whom you do not intend to build a relationship, then be prepared. Think about how you are going to protect yourself, such as

> **Because most STDs can be symptom free, don't assume that your partner is not infected just because he or she doesn't have symptoms.**

having a condom available. Sensual massage, mutual masturbation, and other alternatives to intercourse or genital-oral contact are not nearly as risky as other practices, so you might strongly consider these alternatives whenever you find yourself without a condom or with a partner whom you don't know very well.

Suppose that you do have an episode of unsafe sex. Everyone makes mistakes or makes decisions that in hindsight may not seem wise. If you have put yourself in a situation in which you could have been infected with an

> **If you find that you have put yourself in a situation in which you could have been infected with an STD, have yourself tested promptly.**

STD, have yourself tested. Talk with a health care provider who specializes in the diagnosis and treatment of STDs to decide which tests you need, and don't put it off. Also, think about ways in which you can avoid being in the same situation again. Your sexual health is worth it.

WHAT IF YOU GET AN INFECTION?

Robert decided that he wanted to "be responsible" and get tested for infections before having sex with his new partner, Lauren. He didn't want to risk infecting her with an STD. He had just read in a magazine article that most sexually transmitted infections can be symptom free, and because he had been sexually involved in the past without using condoms, he decided to be tested for all infections. He went to a local family planning clinic, where he was diagnosed with chlamydia by a urethral swab test. He had never had any symptoms of infection in the urethral area, such as discharge or burning with urination, but he found out that about half the men with this infection don't have any symptoms.

Robert was given an antibiotic to treat the infection and was told it was important he contact his last sexual partner to inform her of the diagnosis. He had broken up with his partner of two years, Linda, about two months ago. Although it was difficult for him, he realized that this infection could cause infertility if not treated, and he called Linda to inform her. She was initially surprised but was very grateful to hear from him. She realized that although it must have been difficult for him to call, it meant he cared enough about her and her future to do so.

What if, despite being very careful, you are diagnosed with an STD anyway? How could this happen? One possibility is that your partner has had another partner while he or she has been with you. Or, as was the case with Mandy and Alan, you or your partner may have had an infection without knowing it. When someone who is in a long-term relationship is diagnosed with an STD, it can lead to problems in the relationship. This is one reason why a health care provider must go over all the possibilities when you are diagnosed with an infection. Many

> Because certain STDs can be present for years before they become symptomatic, one partner developing an STD in a relationship does not automatically mean that one of the partners has been sexually involved with someone else.

people ask, "Does this mean my partner has been with someone else?" Not always. It is occasionally difficult to tell who was infected first. The person who has been diagnosed with the infection is not always the person who brought the infection into the relationship. In either case, the most important thing is for both parties to be treated.

If you are diagnosed with an infection, you need to talk honestly with your partner. Your health care provider can tell you whether or not your partner (or partners) must be tested and treated. Particular sexually transmitted infections—such as gonorrhea, chlamydia, and syphilis—are reportable in most states to the state health department, where a program is in place to notify and treat partners. Even if a partner does not have any symptoms of an STD, he or she could be infected and needs to be tested and possibly treated.

Do not avoid telling a partner because you are uncomfortable or embarrassed. Many sexually transmitted infections, even if they are symptom free, can progress to serious complications if left untreated.

When you talk with your partner, make sure you are alone in a quiet place with little chance of being interrupted. Explain as calmly as you can what your health care provider told you. Explain what your diagnosis was, how you are being treated, and what your provider recommended for your partner. You may want to talk with your partner about whether or not he or she has been with someone else. You may need to tell your partner that you have been intimate with someone else. If there has been another partner, the discussion may be very emotional and almost certainly will be difficult. Try not to make things worse by adding blame and guilt, tempting as this may be. If the idea of facing your partner with this information is overwhelming, you can ask your health care provider to talk to you and your partner together, to explain what is going on.

> **Even though neither you nor your partner may have had other partners while in your relationship, you may still have to deal with an STD.**

Your partner may deny having an infection because he or she has no symptoms. You may need to point out that the lack of symptoms doesn't necessarily mean a lack of infection. If it is not clear to you and your health care provider who had the infection first, explain this to your partner. This conversation may bring up difficult issues in the relationship. But first things first. First, make sure your partner is tested and treated, that you both abstain from sex during the treatment process, and that you both schedule follow-up examinations, if necessary, to verify that the treatment has worked. An important point about treatment: *Never share your medication with your partner.* Each partner must be evaluated as an individual and take the medication that will best treat his or her infection.

> **Talking with your partner about an STD diagnosis can be difficult. The important thing is that both of you get proper medical treatment.**

If you are not currently with a partner, your last partner (or partners) may need to be treated, even if you are not in contact with them any longer. Talk with your health care provider about how far back you should go to inform previous partners about your diagnosis. It may be a few months for some infections or possibly years for other infections. For certain infections, your provider or the state health department may be able to notify partners for you in an anonymous manner.

> It is important to let previous sexual partners know if you have been treated for an STD. If you prefer, your health care provider may do this for you.

Being diagnosed with an STD does not mean that you are a bad or immoral person. STDs are caused by germs with which people can become infected while having sex. Some are curable; some are not. If you are diagnosed with an STD, you may want to evaluate your sexual practices and think about how to make yourself safer in the future. Being diagnosed with an STD causes many people to become more open in their discussion of STDs with new partners, and this frankness can lead to safer sexual relationships and, often, better relationships. It does not mean you can never have sex again, even if you are diagnosed with a chronic STD. You may need to take more precautions, but for most people it does not mean the end of their sex life.

SPECIAL CONSIDERATION FOR PEOPLE WITH CHRONIC STDs

People with chronic sexually transmitted infections, such as herpes and genital warts, face additional challenges in talking with partners. Not only do they need to think about all the issues discussed in this chapter, they also need to decide how and when to talk with new partners about these conditions. If you are in this situation, an open discussion about STDs is important for the benefit of your partner as well as for you. You must still think about safer sex to limit your chances of acquiring another sexually transmitted infection. People with genital herpes, for example, may be more vulnerable to acquiring other STDs, because breaks in the skin make acquisition of certain other STDs easier.

> Five months ago, John was diagnosed with genital herpes after being together with Susan for about two years. Susan never told John that she had herpes, because she thought she could always tell when she had an outbreak and could therefore protect him from becoming infected by being careful. Although she knew it was possible to

pass on herpes even without an outbreak, she was afraid that partners would not want to be with her if they knew she was infected.

When John was diagnosed he was devastated, and it made it
worse that Susan had not been honest with him early in their relationship. Susan explained why she hadn't told him about her herpes,
but he found it difficult to trust her after that. Things were not going
well in their relationship for other reasons as well, and they broke up
about three months later. John decided to become as informed about
herpes as possible, and he made up his mind to tell future partners
about his herpes before becoming intimate with them.

The challenge of discussing a chronic infection with a new partner can seem overwhelming. Some people decide that they don't want
to discuss the topic—ever—but there are two good reasons for bringing the topic up before becoming intimate. First, most potential partners respond favorably and are glad you cared enough about them to
be honest. Few people decide not to pursue a relationship because of
this one issue. Second, if partners are not told and later find out, or are
told after becoming intimate, they may feel betrayed. Trust can be
lost. Telling before you become intimate also allows you to deal with
the issue as a couple, rather than putting all the responsibility for preventing transmission on the person who has the infection. Honest discussion often allows people to
develop a more intimate relationship. You may encounter a partner who does not respond favorably, and this can be painful.
Consider in advance how you
will take care of yourself if you
get a negative response.

> Talking with a new partner about
> a chronic STD can seem
> overwhelming, but it is always
> better to talk about this subject
> before you have sex.

Before you discuss issues of sexual health and become intimate
with a new partner—whether or not part of the discussion involves
sharing information about a chronic STD—it is a good idea to establish the groundwork for a relationship. As you get to know the person
better, you may find that you don't want to pursue the relationship
any further, and you don't want to have sex with that person. In that
case, you may have discussed these issues unnecessarily. If you get to
know a person before becoming sexually intimate, it will be easier to
tell the person about your STD. Don't put off discussing this until the

heat of the moment, however, because your partner will need time to process the information. Telling him or her as you are about to become intimate can be very awkward.

John met Sandra a few months after he broke up with Susan, and he told her before they became intimate that he had herpes. Sandra didn't know much about herpes, so John spent a lot of time discussing herpes and his own history of becoming infected. He gave her reading material about herpes and let her have some time to digest it. However, he still viewed the virus as his responsibility, and his alone, in the relationship. "The last thing I want to do is give this to Sandra. I don't want her to have to go through what I went through."

But Sandra would not have to go through what John went through, because John had informed her before they became sexually active that he had herpes, and she had made the decision to proceed with the relationship. She knew that the responsibility was a shared one, and she reassured John that she wanted them to deal with this issue together. Making decisions together, as a team, helped Sandra and John lay a solid foundation on which to build other aspects of their relationship.

When you do decide to tell someone about your STD, be well informed about the infection and have literature available for your partner so that any questions can be answered. How you present the information about your infection will have much to do with how your partner views it. If you tell your partner, "This is the worst thing that has ever happened to me," he or she may view it that way, too. It may take your partner a few days to process all the information. Give your partner time. He or she may not see the infection as a big deal or may even tell you that he or she also has the infection. About one-fourth of sexually active adults have genital herpes, for example, so there is a good possibility that your partner may also be infected, even if he or she doesn't know it. You may want to go together for counseling with a health care provider who is well informed about STDs. Or your partner may want to visit a health care provider alone to have some of his or her

> As with all discussions about sexual intimacy, discussion about a chronic STD usually goes better if you have gotten to know your partner well enough first and have established the foundation for your relationship.

questions answered. It's up to you and your partner. Thousands of issues make up a relationship, and an infection such as herpes is just one of them. By following the suggestions presented here, you increase the likelihood that your relationship will continue to grow and move forward.

C H A P T E R 5

WHAT IS
"SAFER SEX"?

Most people are aware that having unprotected sex with a partner carries a risk for infection with HIV and other sexually transmitted infections. Nevertheless, more than twelve million people in the United States are infected with an STD each year. Why is this? Are they misinformed about STDs and how they are spread? Do they think they are not in a risk group? Do they deny the risk in the heat of the moment? Do they not understand what "safer sex" is and what it isn't? All of these reasons and more explain why there is an epidemic of STDs in this country even in an age of increased media attention to the problem.

> Despite more discussion about STDs and safer sex after the discovery of HIV, the number of people infected with all STDs continues to grow.

Roughly 50 percent of people diagnosed with a sexually transmitted infection are between the ages of fifteen and twenty-four. Since adolescence is a time when experimentation with sexuality begins, teenagers don't have much chance of avoiding infection with an STD unless someone talks with them clearly and accurately about sexually transmitted infections and about exactly how to have safer sex. As earlier discussions in this book have made clear, the health and other consequences of STDs range from minor nuisances to major threats, even death. To protect yourself from infection is the first step. *Acting* on that understanding *by only having sex that is as safe as possible* is an investment in your future health, your ability to have children, your relationships, perhaps your livelihood, and even your life. In this chapter I explain what safer sex practices are and which practices are absolutely unsafe.

> Although anyone, of any age, can become infected with an STD, teenagers are particularly vulnerable because of lack of information.

First a word of caution about what follows. Some of it may be overwhelming. As I have said before in this book, having sex always involves some risk, if not for a sexually transmitted infection, then an emotional risk or unintended pregnancy. But it would be absurd to suggest that people should avoid sex altogether forever, for it is a natural part of life for most people. Rather, my intent is to teach those who are sexually active how to recognize the symptoms if they have an STD (Chapter 2), how to obtain appropriate testing and treatment to maintain sexual health (Chapter 3), how to communicate about sex in a way that will help protect them from getting an STD (Chapter 4), and, in this chapter, how to practice safer sex—which really means things people can do to lower their risk of acquiring an STD.

> The purpose of this chapter is to give you the tools to keep yourself safer if you decide to have sex.

Driving cautiously can reduce your risk of being in an automobile accident, and using seatbelts can decrease the chance that you will be injured if you are in an accident. Sex can be approached in the same way. By taking certain precautions, you can significantly reduce your chance of becoming infected with an STD. You need to know how to keep yourself safer and then decide what level of risk you are willing to take. What may be an acceptable level of risk for one person may not be acceptable to another. If you need absolute cer-

> Decide what level of risk in sexual relationships you are willing to take, and then take precautions accordingly.

tainty on this issue, you may decide to abstain from sex, or at least abstain until you meet a partner who has also never had sex or who, if he or she has had sex, agrees to undergo complete testing for infections and is found to be uninfected and is mutually monogamous. Or you may decide to use some form of protection, such as condoms, to help protect yourself from acquiring an STD.

I hope you will think carefully about the discussion that follows and choose strategies that can keep you safer. The guidelines offered in this chapter are *general* ones—rules to follow when entering into a sexual relationship when you don't know whether your new partner has any STDs. The general guideline that is easiest to remember is that *sexual practices in which semen, vaginal secretions, or blood come into contact with mucous membranes (such as those in the genital area, rectum, and mouth) or another vulnerable area (such as cuts or breaks in the skin) could potentially result in the transmission of an STD if one of the sexual partners is infected.*

Having said that, it's important to repeat that every STD is different and can be transmitted in different ways. Part II of this book discusses each STD *specifically* and explains how transmission of that STD takes place. This is important for couples who know that one of them has an STD, or who suspect that an STD may have been transmitted from one of them to the other. Part II will help explain how they can protect themselves or how transmission may have taken place.

Finally, unprotected sex is not unsafe for two people who are mutually faithful, have tested negative for all of the STDs, and are beyond any waiting periods that are necessary for a positive test for infection to show up, as long as neither of them has other risk factors for infection (such as a recent exposure to infected material by a health care worker, or intravenous drug use and needle/works sharing).

Before turning to the more general guidelines, I list the practices that we know *put you at risk* for acquiring an STD if you are having sex with a partner whose status for infections you don't know:

- —Receiving vaginal sex without a condom
- —Giving vaginal sex without a condom
- —Giving oral sex without a condom or barrier
- —Receiving oral sex without a condom or barrier
- —Receiving anal intercourse without a condom

—Giving anal intercourse without a condom
—Oral-anal contact (rimming) without a barrier
—Contact with your partner's blood

The following practices are *possibly unsafe* and should be avoided with a partner whose status for infections you don't know:

—Hand contact with your partner's genital or anal area without a glove
—Sharing sex toys without cleaning them or using a new condom on the toy

In the following list of *safer* practices, the first five are unsafe if the condom or barrier breaks. Even with the condom intact, some STDs, such as herpes, may be transmitted. In the first three examples, condoms or barriers must be used for the entire contact, since pre-ejaculate (the small amount of fluid released prior to ejaculation) can transmit infection. Wet kissing is possibly safe if neither person has bleeding gums or other open sores in the mouth.

—Anal intercourse (giving or receiving) with a condom
—Vaginal intercourse (giving or receiving) with a condom
—Oral sex with a condom or barrier
—Oral-anal contact with a barrier
—Sharing sex toys with a barrier
—Wet (French) kissing

Finally, practices that we know are *safe* are the following:

—Masturbation in each other's presence (touching *your own* genitals, *not* your partner's)
—Sensual massage
—Dry kissing
—Hugging
—Fantasizing together
—Rubbing clothed bodies together (without genital-genital contact)
—Bathing together (without contact with a potentially infected area of a partner)

The first section of this chapter discusses a dozen things you can do to help protect yourself from contracting a sexually transmitted infection. Later in the chapter I provide details about how to be safer by using barrier methods of protection such as condoms, how to be safer during oral sex and anal sex, information specifically for same-sex couples, and a discussion of special considerations during pregnancy. By following these recommendations, you will significantly decrease your chances—or your child's chances—of becoming infected with an STD. The chapter ends with some information about notifying partners about a sexually transmitted infection.

TWELVE GUIDELINES FOR SAFER SEX

ABSTINENCE

The only absolutely positive, 100 percent sure way to avoid acquiring a sexually transmitted infection is never to have sex. Most people at some point in their lives do decide to have sex, but certain people decide for various reasons, often religious ones, never to become sexually active. For some people, practicing abstinence is what they want to do during a specific time in their lives, whereas at other times they choose to be sexually active. They may decide that they don't want to have sex unless they are in a committed relationship, or until they and their partner have been tested for STDs, or until they are married (their spouse may still need to be tested). These are all very individual decisions.

The media bombard us with sexual images and messages, which may cause people to think, "Everybody but me is having sex all the time with lots of different partners." Obviously that's not true. It's important not to be pressured—by potential partners, by your peers, by the media—into doing anything that you don't want to do.

> You must decide when it's right for you to have sex and not allow yourself to be pressured by a partner or peers or the media.

There is a specific circumstance in which abstinence is recommended, and that is when one or both partners are being treated for a sexually transmitted infection. Make sure that both partners have been treated and cured, with all symptoms resolved, before resuming sexual contact. If they are not, then there is a good chance of becoming reinfected. In the case of the chronic STDs, such as herpes and genital warts, for which there are no cures, things are not so easy, but the diagnosis of these infections does not mean that one can never again have sex! (See the entries on these diseases in Part II for more information.)

MONOGAMY OR LIMITING THE NUMBER OF YOUR SEXUAL PARTNERS

Monogamy means having sex with only one partner who only has sex with you. This strategy dramatically reduces your likelihood of acquiring an infection. Having partners outside your primary relationship puts both you and your steady partner at risk for acquiring a sexually transmitted infection. The fewer partners people have, the less likely they are to become infected with an STD.

> **Monogamy can significantly reduce your risk of acquiring an STD.**

Having sex with one partner can still pose a risk if that partner has had unprotected sex with other partners in the past or has engaged in or continues to engage in other high-risk activity, such as sharing equipment for injection drug use. The only sure way to know if a partner is infected with STDs is for that partner to be tested. Otherwise it is a good idea to abstain from sex, or to use barrier methods such as condoms, to keep yourself safer.

Some people, particularly some teenagers, believe that having sex with only one person at a time, even if it's only for a few weeks at a time, will prevent them from becoming infected with an STD, and that it is therefore safe not to use condoms. This practice, called "serial monogamy," does not offer any protection against getting an STD, since any partner could be infected with an STD from a previous relationship and not know it. If there is any risk of having acquired STDs in the past, even if both partners are symptom free, employ safer sex practices or abstain from sex until both partners have been tested. If a partner refuses to be tested and you decide to have sex with that partner, continue to practice safer sex.

> **Monogamy itself is not a guarantee against becoming infected with an STD if your partner has been at risk for STDs in the past or engages in other risky behavior during your relationship. He or she may be infected and not know it.**

AVOIDING SEX WITH
AN INFECTED PARTNER

That everyone should avoid having sex with an infected partner sounds obvious, but it is not always. People who are infected with STDs may or may not know it. It's highly unlikely that someone who has never had sex (oral, genital, or anal) will be infected with a sexually transmitted infection (except, rarely, by being infected through a blood transfusion or health care accident, or by his or her mother at birth; see the section "Special Issues Concerning Pregnancy and STDs" later in this chapter). But anyone who has had sexual relations may possibly have a sexually transmitted infection, even if he or she is completely symptom free.

If your partner has used condoms or other barrier methods during every sexual contact with other partners, it is less likely that he or she has acquired an infection, but this also is not guaranteed. Certain infections, such as herpes or genital warts, may spread even with condom use. Being tested for all of the sexually transmitted infections before becoming sexually active is the only way to know for sure. If you are not certain that your partner is not having sexual contact with other partners, then it is wise to continue to practice safer sex to protect yourself.

Testing for sexually transmitted infections will allow both you and your partner to know if either one of you is infected with STDs and to deal with it before you become intimate.

If your partner has any symptoms, or if you notice anything about your partner's body that worries you, such as rashes or sores or discharge, it's best to delay having sex until the symptoms have been evaluated by a health care provider. Inspecting your partner's genitals before you become intimate can help you detect potential problems, including things that your partner hasn't noticed or realized could be a problem. This examination doesn't have to be done in a scientific way. During foreplay, if adequate lighting is available, you can usually briefly examine your partner without being obvious about it.

Sometimes couples visit a health care provider before starting a sexual relationship so that both can be tested for sexually transmitted infections. (See Chapter 3, "What to Expect during an STD Examination.") This is a good idea. If a treatable infection such as chlamydia is diagnosed, then medication can be administered before the couple becomes sexually active. If a chronic infection such as herpes is diagnosed, then counseling can be given on ways to decrease the risk of transmission and to deal with the resulting emotional is- sues. Chronic infections such as herpes and human papilloma- virus (HPV, the virus that causes genital warts) are very common.

> **Knowing about sexually transmitted infections before you become intimate can prevent a painful discovery later. Even for the chronic STDs, knowing—and then dealing with the problem—is usually better than not knowing.**

Many people enter into a relationship with a partner who has a known, chronic infection, such as herpes or HPV, because these two infections are very common in the United States (see the sections on herpes and genital warts in Part II). Most of the time, this piece of in- formation is not a "make or break" issue for the relationship, so long as the issue is discussed openly and honestly. It is only one of a mul- titude of factors that go into a relationship. Becoming informed about these infections allows couples to make choices and decide together on ways to help decrease the chance of passing on the infection. Mil- lions of couples deal with chronic sexually transmitted infections every day and continue to have healthy, fulfilling sex lives.

Discovering a sexually transmitted infection once the sexual relationship has already begun—and perhaps especially when the dis- covery is made as a result of one partner being infected by the other— can be much more upsetting than knowing at the beginning and decid- ing right from the start what you want to do as a couple. Not knowing from the beginning can mean a painful discovery later in your rela- tionship. Concerns about infidelity may surface, and there may be a break in the trust that has developed. (See the sections on specific chronic STDs in Part II of this book for more information, as well as Chapter 4 for suggestions about how to discuss sexual health with your new partner.)

REGULAR VISITS TO A HEALTH CARE PROVIDER

Many people don't think about getting regular check-ups for sexual health. They know about the importance of getting a blood pressure or cholesterol check or (for women) a mammogram and Pap test regularly, but issues of sexual health are often overlooked or ignored. Getting regular check-ups can detect problems early, however, possibly even before a person knows that he or she is infected with an STD. It is also very important for women to understand that Pap smears, which are a screen for cervical cancer and are extremely important, are *not* a complete screen for sexually transmitted infections.

Men and women alike tend to seek advice about or testing for STDs only when they have symptoms, but (as is discussed throughout this book) many infections can be present without symptoms. For men and women alike, being informed about STDs and being aware of what's involved in a full screen for infections makes them better informed recipients of health care. You can request these tests from your regular health care provider or you can go to a provider or clinic specializing in STD testing. Either way, make sure that you're getting an appropriate screen for infections. (See Chapter 3, "What to Expect during an STD Examination," for a complete explanation of what's involved and how you can receive proper testing, treatment, and advice.)

> **Both men and women must have regular sexual health check-ups, even if they are symptom free. This is just as important as a regular blood pressure or cholesterol check.**

When she began a new relationship, Andrea went to an anonymous testing center to get an HIV test. Both Andrea and her new partner felt that this was an important step before becoming intimate. The physician's assistant who did the test explained that there were other tests that both Andrea and her partner might want to consider, such as tests for herpes and chlamydia. Andrea didn't think there was any need for this. "I've had a Pap smear every year, and my doctor would have told me if anything else was wrong," she said. When asked whether tests for STDs had been performed on those visits, Andrea said that she didn't know. Andrea was therefore encouraged to talk with her regular health care provider. It turned out that she had not been tested for other sexually transmitted infections, and she decided to have some additional tests performed before becoming sexually intimate with her new partner.

LEARNING ABOUT
SEXUALLY TRANSMITTED INFECTIONS

Most people have incomplete or inaccurate information about sexually transmitted infections, how they are transmitted, and what they can do to prevent themselves from becoming infected. As I have emphasized so often in this book, *having complete and accurate knowledge is essential for your health and well-being. This knowledge is power*—power to keep yourself and your partner healthy. And sex that is free of the anxiety of contracting an STD is better sex.

Some people have claimed that if we teach people, especially young people, about sex and how to prevent STDs, then they will become more sexually active. Nothing is further from the truth. Studies have shown that the level of sexual activity among young people who are provided with sexual education either stays the same or decreases, and that *all people who are taught about sexual health have fewer sexual partners*. In addition, *the degree of condom use and reliance on other safer sex practices increases* among people who are already sexually active. It's time to make this information more widely available, and to provide it in a way that is free from moralizing about whether or not sex is right and which types of sex are "good" or "bad." Whether or not to have sex, and which sexual practices to engage in, are an individual's decision. But if you decide to have sex, then you need the tools to stay healthy. In this book I provide this information—these tools—in the same way I usually provide it to my patients. This information will help you protect yourself, and it will help you communicate better with your health care professional about testing and other issues.

> **When people learn the facts about STDs and how to prevent them, people generally act in ways that keep them safer.**

Arnie was still feeling blue after his separation from his lover following a relationship that had lasted for several years. After the breakup, Arnie decided that he didn't want to date for a while and that he would concentrate on other aspects of his life—his job and friends and family. A few months later Arnie's friend Alex invited him to a party. Not expecting to meet anyone new, Arnie was pleasantly surprised to meet Kyle, who was new in town.

After a few dates, things started to get serious, and after one romantic evening Arnie sensed that they were moving toward a sexual relationship. He told Kyle that he thought it would be a good idea if they used condoms when they had sex. Kyle was offended. "Why do you want to use condoms? It spoils the pleasure. Do you think that means I have an STD?" Arnie had always been very careful in the past, and he had never had a partner complain about condom use. He knew that even people who look and feel healthy can still be infected with an STD, and he worried that if Kyle was willing to have unprotected sex with him, it probably meant that he'd had unsafe sexual encounters in the past.

Kyle and Arnie decided to end the evening without becoming intimate. When they met for lunch the next day, Arnie explained what he knew about sexually transmitted infections and condom use, and how it meant that he cared enough about himself, and Kyle, to want to be safe. Kyle's earlier comments, Arnie realized, indicated that Kyle had incomplete knowledge about STDs, but Kyle was willing to listen to the information Arnie provided. They decided to go to a local STD clinic and be tested for infections before becoming intimate.

GOOD COMMUNICATION

It should be obvious that to know definitely whether or not a partner is infected, some discussion must take place about STDs and the use of barrier methods, and about your partner's sexual history. Such a discussion can be very difficult for most of us. However, overcoming the awkwardness has its rewards. By communicating effectively with your new partner, you can make informed decisions about your risk of acquiring an infection and decide together what you do and do not want to do. Most people, possibly including your partner, also feel awkward about this topic, and they may actually appreciate your openness. It is a sign of respect and caring to bring this issue up, especially in the era of HIV. It can be difficult, but it may save your life. (Chapter 4 explains when and how to discuss these issues with your partner in a way that's most likely to lead to the best outcome.)

> Being able to talk with your partner about sexually transmitted infections decreases the likelihood that you will become infected.

AVOIDING HIGH-RISK BEHAVIORS
AND HIGH-RISK PARTNERS

Several behaviors put people at highest risk for STDs, including having unprotected sex, having unprotected sex with a prostitute, and sharing needles during injection drug use. A woman whose male partner has sex with other men may be at higher risk for becoming infected with an STD if her male partner has had unprotected sex with male partners either while they are together or in the past. In addition to avoiding these behaviors yourself, you must choose your partners wisely, because not only are partners who engage in high-risk activity at risk for acquiring an infection themselves, they may infect *any* sexual partner they are with. A partner who has sex with other partners while you are together puts you at risk for sexually transmitted infections.

People who exchange sex for money or drugs, such as prostitutes, are at very high risk for acquiring and transmitting STDs. Those who have sex with prostitutes have a high risk of acquiring infections. Any type of sexual contact—oral, anal, or genital—with a prostitute is high risk. If protection is used, then this risk is decreased, but condoms may break or leak, so there is still risk. Some people are under the erroneous assumption that receiving oral sex without a condom from a prostitute is safe. But if a person performs unprotected oral sex on many people, his or her throat can become a harbor for infection just like the genital or anal area.

> Martin had been with the company for about a year when he was invited to attend a yearly conference out of town. His wife, Becky, was four months pregnant with their first child, and although he felt a little anxious leaving her, he thought he had to go in order to keep moving up in the company. It was also exciting to travel to a new city.
>
> On the first night of the conference, his co-workers invited him to a local brothel, which they said was a "company tradition." Martin had never been to a prostitute, but, not wanting to seem different, he went along. While there, to decrease his anxiety, he got drunk, as did the other men. His co-workers kept encouraging him to do things he thought weren't safe, but they promised him that receiving oral sex from a prostitute was safe—it was genital sex that was risky. With the alcohol clouding his judgment, he received oral sex from a prostitute. The next morning he felt terrible, not only from the hangover but also from the feeling that he had betrayed Becky.
>
> Three days later, on the plane trip home, Martin started noticing

a burning, itching sensation inside his penis. After he got home, he also noticed a yellow discharge. He decided not to have sex with Becky until he had been checked out. He went to an STD clinic and was diagnosed with gonorrhea. He was given antibiotics, and he learned that if a partner has performed unprotected oral sex on other partners, the throat can become infected with sexually transmitted bacteria such as gonorrhea and chlamydia. Other STDs, including HIV, can also be transmitted through oral sex. He knew that he wouldn't learn whether he had acquired other infections from that contact, such as HIV, until several months down the road.

Now Martin had another problem: Should he abstain from sex or use condoms to protect Becky and their child until he knew he was not infected with other STDs, such as HIV (which would mean explaining why they needed to do this)? Or should he hope that the gonorrhea was the only infection he had acquired and not do anything differently? Although it was difficult, he decided to talk to Becky, because he didn't want to risk infecting her or their child.

Another cause of poor decision making is alcohol or drug use. Like Martin, some people only feel comfortable in social situations if they are using alcohol or drugs. Others may go to a social event not expecting to have a sexual encounter, but then cloud their judgment by drinking or using drugs and end up doing things they wouldn't have done if they were sober. These contacts can be very risky for STD transmission. If a person engages in casual, unprotected sex with you, there is a good chance that he or she has engaged in casual, unprotected sex with others. Some people engage in such behavior over and over again, realizing they are putting themselves at risk but not feeling they can do anything about it. If you are in this situation, it is important to realize that you must get help for your drug or alcohol problem, and that only through overcoming your problem will you be able to have control over all your sexual encounters.

> Use of either alcohol or drugs can impair your decision-making ability and make you very vulnerable to acquiring a sexually transmitted infection.

If you use injection drugs, get help for your addiction in a drug treatment program and absolutely *never* share your equipment with others. In some areas of the country, needle exchange programs are available. If you must share, disinfecting your equipment first with bleach *may* help decrease the risk of acquiring infection, but this is not a guarantee.

Finally, some people have a sexual addiction. They put themselves in dangerous situations over and over again—for example, choosing high-risk partners or engaging in risky anonymous sexual encounters with partners—despite recognizing the hazards involved. People who are putting themselves and possibly their partners at risk by such behavior may benefit from counseling to break this cycle and regain control over their lives.

Before moving on, it's important to emphasize that people *can* leave behind high-risk lifestyles for safer ones. If a partner has a high-risk background but is not currently engaging in high-risk activity, and has had a full screen for STDs and been found free of infection, and if you and that partner are mutually monogamous, then you may feel more at ease with this partner.

VACCINES TO PROTECT AGAINST SOME COMMON STDs

There is a vaccine available that offers lifelong protection against acquiring hepatitis B, a common, sexually transmitted type of hepatitis. All newborns and children are now being vaccinated as part of their routine immunization series to offer them protection later in life, and all sexually active adults should consider being vaccinated. The vaccine is given as a three-shot series over a six-month period and is well worth the effort and cost. Some facilities, such as county health departments, may offer the vaccine at a reduced cost.

In addition, for those who engage in oral-anal contact as part of their sexual practice, a vaccination against hepatitis A should be considered. Hepatitis A is usually thought of more as a food-borne infection (usually transmitted through fecal contamination of food), with occasional outbreaks at restaurants. However, it can also be transmitted sexually through oral-anal contact with a partner who is infected. People receive two vaccinations: an initial one and then a second one six to twelve months later as a booster. This series should also offer lifelong protection. (For more information about hepatitis A and hepatitis B, see Part II.)

Recently a new vaccine has become available to prevent infection with four of the most common types of HPV, the virus that causes genital warts and cervical cancer. Talk with your health care provider about whether or not this vaccine would be of benefit to you (see the section on genital warts in Part II).

DON'T SHARE SEX TOYS

Some people find that their sexual pleasure is enhanced by the use of sex toys such as dildos and vibrators. If they are used back and forth by a couple during sexual contact, the sex toys can transmit infection. If you and your partner are going to share a sex toy, consider putting a barrier, such as a new condom, on it each time each individual uses it. Or else avoid sharing altogether, with each of you using your own sex toys.

EXPLORING "OUTERCOURSE" INSTEAD OF INTERCOURSE

Not all sexual pleasure has to derive from penetrative intercourse, although as a culture we are often programmed to think this. *Outercourse* is a term used to describe sexual contact that does not include penetrative anal, oral, or genital intercourse and the exchange of body fluids. Many people have found creative ways to derive pleasure through outercourse in the era of HIV. Masturbation in each other's presence, sharing fantasies, hugging and dry kissing, the use of sex toys that are not shared, and sensual massage are all options for safer sex.

Masturbation is a safe option for sexual pleasure, whether or not a person is in a sexual relationship. Masturbation can be done either alone or with a partner, either masturbating individually in each other's presence or masturbating each other, a practice called "mutual masturbation." Masturbation is a normal release of sexual tension and pleasurable for both men and women. Many people masturbate, but there is still a taboo about discussing it, and a number of people still grow up thinking that it is "dirty" or immoral. In fact, masturbation allows a person to explore his or her own genital area and learn what is sexually pleasing, and it provides a safe and healthy alternative to sex with a partner if a person is not currently in a relationship. All the myths about physical harm coming to people if they masturbate are simply that: myths. They have no basis in fact.

Touching your partner's genitals or anal area during masturbation could possibly result in STD transmission, particularly if your skin has breaks or tears. You may want to use some method of protection, such as latex gloves for the whole hand or a finger cot for just the finger. Latex gloves can be purchased in most pharmacies, and finger cots can be purchased from stores or mail-order businesses that sell sex toys. Lubricants can be used with these devices to enhance sexual pleasure. Oil-based lubricants may cause latex products to break more easily, so be sure to use a non-oil-based lubricant with latex gloves (and with latex condoms as well).

Sensual massage is another option. Many people derive pleasure from being sensually touched in areas other than the genital area. This can be done before intercourse, as a form of foreplay, or instead of intercourse. Sensual massage allows people to explore other types of sexual pleasure that can enhance their sex lives. It is also a safe sexual practice if no body fluids are exchanged.

There are many other outercourse options, limited only by your imagination. These contacts are generally safe, and they can also be a lot of fun.

> Sexual pleasure does not have to come from intercourse alone. Many people use their imaginations to discover other ways in which to experience sexual pleasure.

NO DOUCHING BEFORE OR AFTER SEX

Douching has been promoted in the media by the makers of douches as a necessary part of feminine hygiene, but the truth is that vaginal douching has been linked to pelvic and vaginal infections. Rectal douching is also practiced by some men and women after anal intercourse, but this practice can lead to infection in the rectal area. The vagina and the rectum do not need our help to "cleanse" themselves. Their natural secretions are already able to do this adequately.

Douching in the vagina can disrupt the normal secretions and bacterial environment and promote yeast infections and bacterial vaginosis. A more serious consideration is that it can lead to pelvic inflammatory disease, which in turn can lead to scarring, chronic pelvic pain, and infertility. Furthermore, the mucosal tissues that line the vagina and rectum are very delicate, and douching

> Douching before and after sex does not protect against infection and in fact may promote infection after exposure to STDs.

may tear the linings, allowing potentially harmful viruses and bacteria from a recent or subsequent sexual contact a better chance to take hold and cause infection. Douching before and after sex has also not been found to prevent infection after someone has been exposed to an STD. Therefore, for many reasons, douching before or after sex is not a good idea.

USE OF BARRIER METHODS

Finally, if you are sexually active, using barrier methods such as condoms during sexual contact is the best way to reduce your risk of acquiring or transmitting an STD. The details of barrier methods are the topic of the next section.

BARRIER METHODS

Barrier methods include condoms (both the male and female kinds), diaphragms and cervical caps, and dental dams or other barriers for oral sex. With practice and the use of a little creativity, many people find that they can incorporate these protective devices into their sex lives without much loss of pleasure. The following sections of this chapter explain how to use them effectively for safer sex. Remember that nonbarrier forms of contraception—such as intrauterine devices (IUDs); the contraceptive hormones, including birth control pills (taken orally), Depo-Provera (injected), or Norplant (implanted under the skin); and surgical procedures, including hysterectomy and surgical sterilization ("tubes tied")—do not offer any protection against sexually transmitted infections.

MALE CONDOMS

Condoms have been around in one form or another since the pyramids were built in Egypt. Originally they were made from animal skins or animal bladders. Rubber condoms became available in the late 1800s (thus the common name "rubbers"), and latex condoms became available in the 1930s. Today most condoms are made of latex, though newer condoms made of plastic (polyurethane) are also available for men and women. Condoms can be purchased in most pharmacies and grocery stores. Latex and plastic condoms offer protection against many of the sexually transmitted infections; condoms made of lambskin are still available, but although they do offer some protection against pregnancy, they do not protect against sexually transmitted infections. There are many different brands of condoms. Check the label to learn exactly what your condoms are made of.

Latex and plastic condoms offer protection against most of the STDs. Animal skin condoms do not.

To help prevent the transmission of most STDs, including the spread of HIV, condoms must be used correctly and consistently. Male latex and plastic condoms help protect against the transmission of HIV as well as other STDs, such as chlamydia, gonorrhea, trichomoniasis, and, probably, pelvic inflammatory disease (PID); latex condoms have been tested more extensively, and nonlatex condoms have a higher breakage and slippage rate than latex condoms. Even though condoms may help protect against the transmission of viral STDs, such as the viruses that cause genital warts and herpes, they do not offer complete protection (see the sections on genital warts and herpes in Part II). They are most effective at preventing infections that are transmitted by fluids from mucosal surfaces. If condoms are used only some of the time, or are used incorrectly and break, then they offer no protection. Condoms should be used for any penetrative intercourse (oral, anal, or genital) with a partner who has not been tested for sexually transmitted infections.

Some people have the mistaken belief that if their partner doesn't ejaculate, they can't become infected with an STD. This is not true. Pre-ejaculate can also transmit infections. If a person starts having penetrative sex

Starting to have sex without a condom, and then using a condom for the rest of the sex, is essentially unsafe sex.

without a condom, and then uses a condom for the rest of the intercourse, that person has had unsafe sex.

People come up with many different reasons to justify not using condoms. Some of the most common are the following:

> —They're uncomfortable.
> —They're unattractive.
> —They decrease my pleasure in sex because they decrease sensation.
> —I'm afraid they won't work.

—I'm embarrassed to buy them.
—I'm embarrassed to put them on in front of my partner.
—I'm afraid they'll spoil the mood.
—I'm on the pill, so my partner doesn't have to use condoms for
   protection against sexually transmitted infections.

My answer to all these arguments is that there are two important reasons for using condoms:

—They can protect you from an unwanted pregnancy.
—They can protect you from acquiring a sexually transmitted
   infection, which could make you infertile (e.g., pelvic
   inflammatory disease) or cause your death (e.g., HIV).

Practicing with condoms usually helps a man use them more effectively and feel less awkward about it. Studies show that most condom failures are a result of inexperience in using them, or using them incorrectly, not flaws in the condoms themselves.

Most men can find a brand of condom that works well for them. If not, then female condoms (discussed below) may be an option for heterosexual couples. There is no difference in effectiveness between the different name brands of latex condoms. Some men find that they like the newer plastic condoms better than the latex ones, because they believe that sensation is improved with the plastic ones. Some individuals have an allergy to latex, which prevents them from using latex condoms, and the plastic ones offer an alternative. The best suggestion is to try different types and see which one works best for you and your partner.

All condoms are regulated by the U.S. Food and Drug Administration, and each individual condom is tested to make sure it is not defective. You do not need to "test" the condom yourself before using it, and in fact this may cause the condom to break during use. Do not leave condoms exposed to the air or sunlight for lengthy periods of time, because they can become brittle and break more easily.

Condoms with spermicide (nonoxynol-9) are not any more effective in preventing pregnancy or STD transmission than condoms without it. In fact, spermicides such as nonoxynol-9 may

> All condoms are tested
> to make sure that they
> do not have defects.
> Failure of the condom usually
> results from misuse.

actually *increase* the risk for sexually transmitted infections. Non-oxynol-9 has recently been found not to protect against cervical gonor-rhea, chlamydia, or HIV infection in women, so it is no longer recom-mended as a method of STD or HIV prevention. In fact, nonoxynol-9 may act as an irritant to the skin and mucosal membranes, some-times causing breaks in the skin, which may *increase* the risk of transmission of infections such as HIV in women receiving vaginal intercourse from men and possibly in men receiving anal intercourse from a male partner. According to the Centers for Disease Control, condoms lubricated with spermicides cost more, have a shorter shelf-life, and may irritate the skin and cause urinary tract infections, so condoms *without* spermicide are the best option for all sexual ac-tivity.

When condoms are used correctly, and used every time you have sex, the failure rate from a condom breaking is usually less than 2 per-cent. In other words, condoms break about twice out of every one hun-dred times they are used. However, in the real world, condoms fail more often, sometimes ten out of every one hundred times used. Not surprisingly, this is usually because they are not used correctly or con-sistently. Here are the "top twelve rules" of male condom use. These rules apply to both latex and plastic condoms except where differences are specifically noted.

1. *A new condom should be used for every sexual contact with a person whose status for STDs is not known. This includes oral, anal, and genital contact.* If you or your partner uses a condom only "some of the time," then you are not protecting yourself against STDs. It can take only one unprotected sexual encounter to transmit an STD.

2. *Condoms should be put on before any genital contact.* It is not enough to use the condom only during ejaculation and not during the earlier sexual contact. Pre-ejaculate can also cause pregnancy and transmit STDs if a male partner is infected.

3. *Latex condoms should not be used with any oil-based lubricants,* such as mineral oil, vegetable shortening, massage oil, or petro-leum jelly, because these will increase the chances of their break-ing. Only water-based lubricants, such as those that are glycerin

based, are recommended for use with latex condoms, since these do not increase the risk of breakage. Watch out for lubricants that say they are "water soluble." This is not the same as water based, and water-soluble lubricants may actually contain oils and are therefore not to be used with latex condoms. *Plastic or polyurethane condoms can be used with either oil- or water-based lubricants.*

4. *Latex condoms should not be stored in a warm or hot place,* such as a wallet or the glove compartment; heat will increase the risk of breakage. *Plastic condoms are not destroyed by heat exposure.*

5. *Check the expiration date on the package before use.* If the expiration date has passed, making the condom more vulnerable to breaking, use a newer condom instead.

6. *Condoms should be completely unrolled onto the erect penis,* otherwise they may fall off during the sex act. This is a common cause of condom failure. Men who are not circumcised should pull back the foreskin before putting on the condom. Leave a small space at the tip of the condom as a reservoir for semen. Some condoms have a built-in reservoir.

7. Make sure there is *no air trapped inside the condom,* since air inside the condom is another common cause of condom breakage and failure.

8. Make sure there is enough lubrication; *dryness may increase the risk of the condom breaking.* If you are using a latex condom, then make sure you do not use an oil-based lubricant, which, as mentioned earlier, can cause the condom to break. Liberally apply the lubricant to the outside of the condom and onto your partner's genital or anal area before insertion; this will help ease penetration and therefore help decrease the chances of breakage. Spermicides such a nonoxynol-9, as noted earlier, may increase the likelihood of STD transmission and are not recommended.

9. Be careful opening the condom package so that you do not accidentally break the condom. *Do not use your fingernails or teeth or nail clippers to open the condom package.*

10. If the condom breaks during intercourse, *withdraw the penis and continue with a new condom if desired.* Consider being tested for STDs if your partner has not been tested.

11. *Use a new condom with every act of intercourse.* This may seem like common sense, but it's worth emphasizing. A used condom has semen on the outside of the condom that could cause infection or pregnancy. Throw used condoms away.

12. *Hold the condom firmly at the base of the penis during withdrawal to prevent it from falling off, and withdraw the penis with the condom while the penis is still erect.* If you wait to withdraw the penis until after the erection is gone, there is a higher risk that the condom will fall off.

FEMALE CONDOMS, DIAPHRAGMS, AND CERVICAL CAPS

Introduced in 1994, *female condoms* are inserted into the vagina to offer a protective sheath and are an option for women to decrease their risk of unwanted pregnancy or infection if their male partner can't, or won't, use a condom. No study has yet been conducted to compare the effectiveness of female condoms and male condoms.

The female condom available in the United States is made of plastic or polyurethane and is lubricated with a silicone-based lubricant. It consists of a pouch with a ring at each end. One ring is inserted into the vagina and fits around the cervix as does a diaphragm. The outer ring covers part of the labia, providing protection of the covered areas from some sexually transmitted infections that require skin-to-skin contact for transmission. These types of condoms may offer more protection than male condoms against infections that are transmitted through skin-to-skin contact, such as herpes and genital warts, although this has not yet been proven. The female condom can be inserted up to two hours before sexual contact and is removed after sexual intercourse. It is also used just once.

Because it is made of plastic, the female condom is not damaged by heat as is the male latex condom, and it can be used with either oil- or water-based lubricants. It prevents penetration by common sexually transmitted bacteria and viruses, but there are few studies to show that female condoms protect against STDs, including HIV, in real life. Each female condom costs a bit more than a male

> **The female condom offers an alternative for women who want protection against unwanted pregnancy and STDs.**

condom. The failure rates resulting in pregnancy are similar to those for the diaphragm and cervical cap—about 15–18 percent. This failure rate may be due partly to incorrect use, as with male condoms, and this percentage may well decrease as a woman gains experience in using the female condom.

Diaphragms and cervical caps are devices women insert into the vagina and fit around the cervix to protect against pregnancy. They are usually used in conjunction with spermicidal cream or gel. The amount of spermicide is small; although spermicides are not recommended at this time as a method to prevent infection with STDs, the small amount used with diaphragms and caps is unlikely to cause a problem. They have typical failure rates for pregnancy of about 15–20 percent. They may help protect against some of the sexually transmitted infections, such as gonorrhea, chlamydia, and trichomonas, because they offer some barrier to the semen reaching the cervix. However, they do not offer protection as thorough as that provided by a barrier method (male or female condom). In addition they do not provide any protection against the other sexually transmitted infections, such as HIV. If a woman uses a cervical cap or diaphragm while her male partner uses a condom, this is a good combination. However, how spermicides and cervical caps and diaphragms affect the transmission of infections from women to men is unclear; spermicides and diaphragms both seem to *increase* the risk of bacterial urinary tract infections in women; and there is evidence that spermicides may *increase* the risk for sexually transmitted infections if you have sex with an infected partner.

Diaphragms and cervical caps come in different sizes, and therefore a woman must be fitted for one by her health care provider. They are often made of latex and therefore should not be used with oil-based lubricants.

> Diaphragms and cervical caps may offer some protection against bacterial STDs such as gonorrhea and chlamydia, but barrier methods are superior for this purpose.

A promising new area of research is the development and study of "microbicides," which are gels that a woman can use to prevent acquiring a sexually transmitted infection during vaginal or anal sex when a male partner refuses to use a condom. However, no microbicides are available at this time.

BARRIER METHODS FOR PROTECTION
DURING ORAL SEX

Oral sex involves placing your mouth to a partner's genital area. Many couples take great pleasure in oral sex. Performing oral sex on a female partner is called *cunnilingus*, and performing oral sex on a male partner is called *fellatio*. STDs can be transmitted through oral contact, however, so you must know how to help protect yourself from becoming infected in this way.

Many people still think that STDs, particularly HIV, cannot be transmitted through oral sex. This may be assumed by some because, early in the HIV epidemic, unprotected anal and vaginal intercourse were seen as high-risk behaviors, and unprotected oral sex was seen as low risk or no risk, since saliva does not carry a sufficient quantity of HIV for it to spread infection. The risk of HIV transmission is probably lower with oral sex than with anal or vaginal sex, but it is not zero.

There are documented cases of HIV transmission from both receiving and giving oral sex, though there are few studies of how often people become infected after a certain type of sexual contact. Obviously it is not ethical to perform studies in which people are exposed to HIV from a particular sex act to find out how many of them become infected, so reliable statistics are not available. The Centers for Disease Control includes oral sex on its list of risky behaviors for acquiring HIV. But HIV is not the only sexually transmitted infection to consider; others—such as gonorrhea, chlamydia, and syphilis—can be transmitted via oral sex with an infected partner as well.

The risks from unprotected oral sex may be acceptable for some people but not for others. Use of a condom or dental dam is recommended, to afford some protection against STD transmission via oral sex if your partner has not been screened for infections or has a chronic STD.

Oral-anal contact, known as *analingus* or *rimming*, is a sexual practice common among men who have sex with other men, but heterosexual couples can also find pleasure in this type of sexual contact. This practice in-

> For oral-anal and oral-genital contact, barriers are recommended to help prevent STD transmission if your partner's status for infections is unknown.

volves placing your mouth to a partner's anal area. Again, precautions must be taken to prevent the transmission of infection, not only with the organisms that cause STDs (such as gonorrhea, chlamydia, and HIV) that can be transmitted through genital contact, but also with hepatitis A and all the infectious intestinal organisms, such as salmonella and giardia, that can be transmitted through contaminated feces in the anal area. Once again, if you are unsure of your partner's status for these infections, it's a good idea to use a barrier method during oral-anal contact. The barriers used are the same as those used for oral-genital contact, and they are described later in this section.

If a person has breaks in the skin of the mouth (such as chapped lips or a cold sore) or bleeding gums, this may increase the likelihood that he or she will become infected with an STD while performing oral sex on a partner, since breaks in the skin can make transmission easier. Using a barrier method can provide protection. Do not floss your teeth before or after an oral sexual contact, since the resulting disruption of the gum tissue may increase the chance of becoming infected with an STD through oral sex.

Many sexually transmitted infections can be transmitted through oral sex, including HIV.

Several methods have been used to protect against STD transmission during oral sex with a partner whose status for STDs is not known or who is known to have a chronic STD. For women or men who perform oral sex on male partners, condoms are the best option for protection. You may want to try using unlubricated condoms, since spermicide has an unpleasant taste for many people and, as discussed above, spermicide may increase STD transmission. Both latex and plastic condoms can be used for this purpose. Flavored condoms are also available, and these may be an option for those who do not like the taste of latex or plastic. As discussed earlier in this chapter, animal skin condoms do not provide an effective barrier against STDs.

A dab of lubricant inside the condom can help improve sensation. Be sure not to use too much lubricant, since the condom may fall off. (As mentioned earlier, latex condoms can only be used with water-based lubricants; plastic condoms can be used with either oil- or water-based lubricants.) The condom should be used for the entire sexual contact. Herpes (particularly type 1 herpes, the most common form of

oral herpes) can be transmitted through kissing the genitals and therefore can be spread even without penetration. Oral-genital contact even
with a condom carries a risk of transmitting herpes, but it is probably
less likely with a condom. (See the section on herpes in Part II.)

For men or women performing *oral-genital sex on a female partner or oral-anal sex on any partner,* latex barriers will offer the most
protection against transmission of sexually transmitted infections.
One type of latex barrier used for this purpose is the dental dam, which
is a small (6-inch) square of latex commonly used in dentists' offices
to prevent splattering of oral secretions into the dentist's face during
procedures. Many people also use them for protection during oral sex
by placing the dam over the female partner's genitals or the female or
male partner's anal area before beginning oral sex. They come in different flavors, which can make using them more fun. You may want
to wash off the dam before use, since sometimes there is a dusting of
powder on it, to which some people may have an allergic reaction. In
addition, it's a good idea to put a dab of water-based lubricant on the
side that comes into contact with the partner's genital or anal area,
since this enhances the pleasure. Dental dams tend to be thicker than
condoms or gloves and therefore may offer less sensory pleasure. Dental dams are available from stores that sell dental supplies or stores or
mail-order businesses that sell sex toys.

Another option for oral–female genital or oral-anal sex is cutting
open a condom or a latex glove and using it in the same way. Again,
because spermicide tastes bad to many people, and because spermicides may increase the risk of STD transmission, unlubricated condoms are a better choice for this method than lubricated ones. Condoms can be purchased in most pharmacies and grocery stores, and
latex gloves are also available in most pharmacies.

There are plastic options as well. Plastic may offer better sensory
stimulation, since it is thinner than latex, yet it probably provides the
same degree of protection. It is a good option for those who have a sensitivity to latex. The newer plastic condoms can be split down the
middle and placed over a partner's genitals or anal area to permit the
performance of safer oral sex. Another alternative is household plastic wrap. Although there aren't any scientific studies to show that
plastic wrap offers good protection, it is probably better than no pro-

tection, and it offers the option of using as big a piece as you need. You may want to use more than one layer of plastic wrap for extra protection. Plastic barriers can be used with water- or oil-based lubricants, and putting a small amount on the side that touches your partner can enhance his or her pleasure.

When using any of the barrier methods described for oral-genital or oral-anal contact, it is important to use the barrier only once, and, if it comes off, to reapply it with the same side touching your partner. If you switch back and forth between one side and the other, it is essentially like not using any protection at all. If you can no longer figure out which side is which, simply use a new barrier.

> Latex and plastic barriers can help prevent against the transmission of sexually transmitted infections through oral sex.

BARRIER METHODS FOR PROTECTION DURING ANAL SEX

Receptive anal intercourse is practiced by both men and women, though many opposite-sex couples are reluctant to admit that they practice anal sex because they fear its stigma as a "gay" sex practice and its reputation as a route for transmitting HIV. Nevertheless many couples, whatever their sexual orientation, find pleasure in anal intercourse. But with the onset of the HIV epidemic, the practice of casual anal sex has become less common, especially among men who have sex with men, because of the risk of HIV transmission from an infected partner. On the other hand, some heterosexual couples, particularly teenagers, operate under *the mistaken belief that anal sex is "safe sex"* because there is no risk of getting pregnant!

Receiving anal sex from and giving it to an infected partner is the highest-risk sexual practice for becoming infected with HIV and other STDs, with receiving anal sex a higher risk than giving it. This may be because there is a

> Unprotected anal intercourse with a partner whose status for STDs is unknown is the highest-risk sexual practice.

higher risk for small tears to occur in the anal mucosa while receiving anal sex, and these tears can facilitate the transmission of infection. Having unprotected anal sex with a partner whose status for infections is unknown puts you at risk for acquiring a sexually transmitted infection.

If a couple has a monogamous relationship and both partners have been tested for HIV and other infections and are not infected, then anal sex is safe and can be practiced if it is mutually enjoyable to both partners. (This last condition, of course, applies to all types of sexual practice.) Once again, if you are not certain that your partner is or will be faithful, then it is a good idea to stay safe and use condoms.

Condoms without spermicide should be used during anal intercourse with anyone whose status for infection is not known. Spermicides (such as nonoxynol-9) should not be used for anal intercourse because, as mentioned above, they increase the risk of STD transmission. The only way to know a person's status is for her or him to be tested for STDs (all of them, not just HIV); being symptom free is not enough. If the person has not been tested, or has been tested and is known to have an infection, then condoms with adequate lubrication offer the best protection against becoming infected during anal sex. As noted previously, condoms are not 100 percent reliable, but they are the best protection available for anyone engaging in anal sex with unknown or untested partners.

SAME-SEX COUPLES

Those with same-sex partners face specific STD risks. Some misperceptions must also be discussed, and I try to address them here as clearly as possible. Although nearly 10 percent of sexually active adults engage in sexual activity with partners of the same sex, considerable misunderstanding and stigma about same-sex relationships persists among the general public, in the media, and among health professionals as well. Some people in same-sex relationships find it difficult to discuss their sexuality openly with a health care provider or are discouraged in their efforts because the health care provider is so clearly uncomfortable. Under these circumstances a person is less likely to receive the high-quality health care that he or she deserves.

Until fairly recently, there had been little research into the sexual health risks faced by same-sex couples. In the United States, awareness of HIV and the prevalence of this infection among men who have sex with other men has led to more sexual health–related research in the last twenty-five years, but there has still been remarkably little re-search addressing lesbian women and their risk for acquiring STDs. The sections that follow cover some of these specific risks.

WOMEN WHO HAVE SEX WITH OTHER WOMEN

Studies indicate that about 4 percent of women in the United States label themselves as "lesbian." This statistic probably significantly un-derestimates the number of women who have sex with other women; one study showed that up to 18 percent of women experienced at-traction to other women or were in sexual relationships with other women. When labels are assigned to a minority group, and especially when those labels have certain negative connotations, people may be hesitant to claim membership in the group.

Many women who have sex with female partners believe they are not at risk for sexually transmitted infections, and health care pro-viders may also believe that these women are not at risk. This is partly because there have not been many studies of the rates of STDs among lesbians,

Fear of homophobia may prevent many lesbian women from seeking adequate health care.

but it may also be because of bias against those in same-sex relation-ships, or lack of knowledge. Even if lesbian women do turn to tradi-tional health care providers for care, they may experience the homo-phobia of a health care provider or receive incorrect advice, such as "gay women don't need Pap smears." Many lesbian women find a more open approach at clinics that specialize in the health care of women.

Here's the truth about the risk for sexually transmitted infections in woman-to-woman sex as we know it today: Some infections—such as herpes, syphilis, and genital warts—can be transmitted by genital rubbing and do not require heterosexual penetrative intercourse for transmission. Therefore, if two women engage in genital rubbing, one of the women may acquire an STD from the other, even if neither of the women has ever had sexual contact with a man. Furthermore, some infections, such as oral herpes (herpes virus type 1, or HSV-1), can also be transmitted through oral-genital contact. A person with oral HSV-1 may pass this infection to the genital area of a partner, even if there is no obvious cold sore (see the section on herpes in Part II).

Sex toys, or vaginal or anal contact with the hands, can also pass infections, such as trichomoniasis, bacterial vaginosis (BV), and even HIV infection (as discussed earlier).

Another factor to consider is that many lesbian women report having had a sexual relationship with a man at some time in the past, and about 25 percent of lesbian women report "occasionally" having sex with men. These women may be at risk for infections such as gonorrhea, chlamydia, trichomoniasis, hepatitis, and HIV, and so may their sexual partners.

Women who have sex with other women are also at risk of becoming infected with STDs in the ways that any person could become infected, such as receiving a transfusion of a blood product that was not adequately screened for infection, sharing injection drug works, and receiving tattooing or body piercing with unclean equipment. Lesbian women can also become infected with STDs through artificial insemination with semen from a man who has not been adequately screened for infections.

The reality is that there is inadequate information on the frequency of STDs in lesbian women—how often transmission takes place and how likely transmission is with each type of sexual practice. Studies of these questions are currently under way, but in the meantime this type of information must be extrapolated from data from heterosexuals and from the few studies of gay women that have been done. We do know that lesbian women have a high rate of bacterial vaginosis infection between sexual partners and that BV may be a sexually transmitted infection among them, which is not the case among heterosexual women. In one study, 18–29 percent of lesbian women who had not had sex with men within the last year were found to have BV, and about 73 percent of the sexual partners of these women had BV as well.

In addition, the human papillomavirus, the virus that causes genital warts (probably the most common STD in the United States), is also very common among women who have sex with other women. Studies have shown that more than 70 percent of sexually active adults have antibodies to the virus that causes genital warts. One study among lesbian

> Women who have sex with other women can become infected with STDs and need to have yearly Pap smears as a screening test for cervical cancer.

women revealed a similar prevalence of the virus, with about 62 percent of women having antibodies on a blood screen for HPV. As with heterosexuals, the types of the virus that are linked with cervical cancer are those that are the most common. This finding underscores the need for *yearly Pap smears for all women, including those who have sex with other women.* Unfortunately, lesbian women are often told that they don't need Pap smears, in the mistaken belief that only women who have sex with men can get cervical cancer.

In addition to routine screening for STDs, safer sex practices are recommended for women who have sex with women, just as they are for any sexually active person. This means using latex barrier methods for any genital-genital, oral-genital, hand-genital, or oral-anal contact with a partner whose status for sexually transmitted infections is not known. As discussed earlier in this chapter, options include dental dams and condoms that have been cut open, or latex gloves can be used for hand-genital contact. If any sex toys are used, it is a good idea to cover them with a new condom before they are used by each partner, or each partner can use her own sex toy and not share. As mentioned earlier in the chapter, spermicides are no longer recommended to decrease STD infection.

If partners have been fully screened for sexually transmitted infections and are beyond the waiting periods for infection to show up as positive on the tests, and if they are mutually monogamous, then it is safe to have unprotected contact.

MEN WHO HAVE SEX WITH OTHER MEN

Depending on the study consulted, between 2 and 10 percent of the general population of men in the United States have sex with other men. They may be homosexual (have sex only with other men) or bisexual (have sex with both men and women). Some men may see themselves as heterosexual (having sex only with women) but occasionally have sex with male partners as well. Like lesbian women, men who have sex with other men have often had to evolve as sexual beings in an environment that has told them that what they are doing is wrong or immoral. That social pressure—along with the HIV epidemic, which in the United States and Europe initially hit the male homosexual population the hardest—has made life difficult for many gay men in the last two decades.

Many men who have sex with other men have often felt marginalized because of prejudice and excluded from traditional health care settings because of homophobia or the unvoiced assumption on the part of their health care providers that they are heterosexual. Health care providers do, unfortunately, sometimes bring their own prejudices into the work setting. Many health care providers do not receive education about STDs, let alone sensitivity training in dealing with sexual minority groups. This is not an excuse, but rather an unfortunate reality—one that is changing slowly.

For issues of sexual health, men who have sex with other men may choose to seek health care providers other than their regular providers, with whom they may feel uncomfortable being open about their sexuality. Clinics that provide health care primarily to men in same-sex relationships have come into existence since the 1980s for just this reason. Some men may feel more comfortable seeking sexual health care in county or city STD clinics, or in other settings where anonymity can be guaranteed and the attitude is nonjudgmental. It is important for any person, irrespective of sexual orientation, to seek and receive care from a nonjudgmental health care provider with whom he or she feels comfortable discussing these issues (see Chapter 3).

Men who have sex with other men are individuals, with individual characteristics and lifestyles. After the existence of HIV had become widely acknowledged, some gay men changed their sexual behaviors and began to practice safer sex, and the rates of bacterial STD infections and new HIV infections have decreased over the last twenty years. However, more recently there has been a rise in syphilis, gonorrhea, and chlamydia infections among men already infected with HIV, possibly because of the extended survival and improved quality of life of men receiving therapy for HIV, or because of "safe sex burnout."

Men who have sex with other men confront specific health care problems. Receptive anal sex may increase the risk of acquiring sexually transmitted infections, because of the tears in the rectal mucosa that may occur; these tears make it easier for bacteria or viruses to enter a person's body. Furthermore, through oral-anal contact, some men may be more vulnerable to such infections as hepatitis A (see the sections on hepatitis A and on proctocolitis, proctitis, and enteritis in Part II). It is recommended that men who engage in oral-anal contact with a partner be vaccinated against hepatitis A. (All sexually active adults should consider being vaccinated against hepatitis B as well.) In addition, a man who performs anal intercourse on a male partner may acquire a nongonococcal urethral infection from the bacteria found in stool and not from the more common sexually transmitted bacteria, such as chlamydia. All of these possibilities must be taken into account when sorting out the potential causes of symptoms in a man who has sex with other men. Therefore, it is a good idea for the man to have a health care provider with whom he feels comfortable discussing his sexual practices, so that the correct diagnoses can be made and the discussion about how to remain safe can be appropriate within the context of his sexual orientation.

Men who have sex with other men and are not in a stable, mutually monogamous sexual relationship, in which both men have been tested, should consider having the following tests at least each year: HIV, syphilis, gonorrhea, and chlamydia (see separate sections on each infection in Part II).

SPECIAL ISSUES CONCERNING PREGNANCY AND STDs

Sexually transmitted infections and pregnancy share a connection on several levels. Certain STDs can make it difficult or even impossible for a woman to get pregnant. Others may make a woman more likely to lose a pregnancy, and still others may cause infection of the baby either in the womb or at delivery, resulting in lifelong problems for the child. It is often a very painful connection, made more so because many of these complications could be avoided through education and routine screening during pregnancy.

Many pregnant women are not adequately screened, because of the assumption on the part of their health care providers that "nice women" don't get STDs—which, as I emphasize throughout this book, is not the case. Anyone can contract an STD if she or he is not aware of the risks. Furthermore, many women do not or cannot get adequate health care during their pregnancies, and simple, potentially lifesaving screening is therefore not performed. Health care providers must become better educated about STDs, be able to advise patients wisely about the risks they face, and be on the lookout during pregnancy for any potential problems.

What follows is a summary of some of the links between STDs and pregnancy. For a more detailed discussion about each STD and its effects on pregnancy, see the corresponding entry for that STD in Part II.

BEFORE PREGNANCY

To protect a woman's fertility for the future, safer sex practices are mandatory. One episode of chlamydia-induced pelvic inflammatory disease decreases a woman's likelihood of becoming pregnant in the future by 20 percent, and each episode of PID makes a repeat episode more likely because of the scarring that occurs.

Unfortunately, many women experimenting with their first sexual experiences in young adulthood are not adequately informed about STDs and how to keep safe. It is young people, and young women in particular, who suffer the brunt of the consequences of the STD epidemic. Young women are more vulnerable than older women to becoming infected with bacterial STDs such as gonorrhea and chlamydia, because the anatomy of the cervix makes it more susceptible to infection in adolescence and the twenties than in later adulthood. Even though women may not be thinking about pregnancy at this early point in their lives (in fact, they may be trying their best not to get pregnant), what about five or ten or twenty years later? The actions taken by a young woman now could affect her chances of getting pregnant later, when she wants to.

Many women are becoming sexually active at earlier ages but are delaying marriage and childbirth until later—a life choice that leaves them with more time for sexual activity and more opportunity to acquire a sexually transmitted infection. Abstinence is the best way to prevent becoming infected with an STD. But if you decide to become sexually active, education can equip you with the tools to protect your fertility for later in life, and getting regular STD screens will help to detect most infections early, while they are still treatable and reversible.

> Some STDs, such as gonorrhea and chlamydia, can impair a woman's ability to become pregnant in the future. Being safe now will help her keep her options open later in life.

DURING PREGNANCY

If a woman becomes pregnant while she is infected with certain STDs, or acquires them during the pregnancy, there is an increased risk that she will not be able to carry the pregnancy to term. For example, gonorrhea and chlamydia can cause preterm delivery, miscarriage, premature rupture of the membranes, and infection in the uterus after the delivery. Syphilis (discussed in more detail later in this section) can also cause miscarriage and preterm labor. Bacterial vaginosis, a common and usually benign infection of the vaginal area (which is usually not considered a sexually transmitted infection), can cause similar problems in pregnancy, as can trichomoniasis, which is a sexually transmitted vaginal infection.

The herpes virus, which causes a very common genital infection that is often symptom free and thus remains undiagnosed, can adversely affect pregnancy. Infection during the first trimester increases a woman's risk of miscarriage. A woman who becomes infected with herpes while she is pregnant is at risk of transmitting the virus to the child (either in the womb or at delivery), especially if she becomes infected during the last trimester of the pregnancy. Women who become infected with herpes *before* their pregnancy transmit the virus to their child much less frequently. (See the section on herpes in Part II for a detailed discussion of this topic.)

Women who are pregnant should be screened for evidence of infection and use a barrier method or abstain from sex during the pregnancy if their partner's status for infections is not known. Routine screening of both the woman and her partner in the early stages of pregnancy will help to avert many problems. If a woman continues to be at risk during the pregnancy, then screening for STDs should be repeated during the pregnancy and safer sex practices should be used (as discussed earlier).

Women who are in stable relationships and are considering becoming pregnant should ask their partners to be tested for sexually transmitted infections if they have not been in the past. This should be considered even if the man does not have symp-

> Routine screening for sexually transmitted infections before and during the pregnancy, for both the woman and her partner, is the only way to know for sure about these infections. In this way a lot of heartache can be avoided.

toms. You are in this together, and the only way to know about your risk for infections is for both of you to be tested and be educated about STDs. There is enough to worry about during the pregnancy without having to worry about sexually transmitted infections.

What does a complete screening for pregnant women consist of? The Centers for Disease Control recommends the following tests: HIV, syphilis, hepatitis B and C, chlamydia, and gonorrhea, as well as screening for BV (which is not an STD but can cause complications during pregnancy; see the section on bacterial vaginosis in Part II) and a Pap smear (if none has been done in the year before the pregnancy). Herpes screening should also be considered, with culture testing of any lesions present during delivery (see the section on herpes in Part II). If you are pregnant, have a frank discussion with your health care provider about whether you have been screened for these infections. Your own and your baby's health may depend on it. Also, if your tests show you are uninfected, but during your pregnancy you have sexual contact with someone new or someone who has not been tested, talk with your health care provider. Chances are you will need to be screened again to be safe.

EFFECTS ON THE CHILD

Some of the consequences of maternal STD infection for the fetus and child can be devastating. (See the individual sections on these infections in Part II for more information.) With the increase each year in the numbers of people becoming infected with STDs, and with increasing numbers of women becoming infected, more and more babies are being born infected with STDs. This is an especially distressing situation because so often such infection is completely preventable with education and proper screening.

The risk with bacterial infections such as gonorrhea and chlamydia occurs as the baby passes through the infected birth canal. Infection of the eyes or anal-genital areas often occurs in the newborn. The infection of the eyes can cause blindness if not treated promptly. Chlamydia can also cause infection of the lungs in the newborn. In addition, babies born to mothers with gonorrhea and chlamydia are more likely to be born prematurely and thus face all of the health consequences associated with prematurity.

Another bacterium, the one that causes syphilis, can have devastating consequences. With the resurgence of syphilis, especially among heterosexual women (often those who engage in illicit drug use or have partners who do), there has been an increase in the number of cases of neonatal syphilis (syphilis of the newborn). This can result in many developmental problems, including mental retardation; physical deformities of the nose, legs, and other organs; liver enlargement; and skin rashes.

The protozoan trichomonas can cause infection of the genital area in newborn girls, as well as problems related to premature delivery.

Bloodborne infections, such as HIV and hepatitis, can also cause infection of the fetus in the womb. With HIV, no developmental problems are associated with the infection itself, but there is about a 25 percent risk of a child acquiring HIV if born to a mother who is HIV positive and is not being treated with HIV medications. Mothers who are HIV positive can reduce the risk of transmission of the infection to their child by taking HIV medications during the pregnancy. (See the section on HIV infection and AIDS in Part II for more information.) Combination therapy (with more than one HIV medication) is offered in many settings. Children who are born to mothers with hepatitis B may be protected from acquiring the infection if they are immunized against the infection at birth. If a child acquires hepatitis B at birth, there is a high risk that the child will become a lifelong carrier of the infection.

Children who are infected with herpes in the womb, at delivery, or after birth may experience problems that range in severity from a mild skin infection to mental retardation and death. Again, knowing your own and your partner's status for herpes prior to and during the pregnancy, and taking appropriate precautions, can decrease these risks. Most problems occur when a woman does not know she has herpes during the pregnancy and therefore takes no precautions, or when she becomes infected while she is pregnant, which poses a greater risk for

> Not only can STDs prevent a woman from getting pregnant and from having a normal full-term pregnancy, they also can have lifelong consequences for the child. Screening and education can help prevent this.

transmission. This is why women's partners must also be tested. There is also a risk of infection after the delivery from well-meaning but uneducated friends and relatives, who may pass the virus to the baby by kissing the baby, especially if they have an active cold sore.

The human papillomavirus, which causes genital warts, may cause vocal cord infection in a newborn during the child's passage through the infected birth canal. Considering how common genital infection with this virus is, this type of neonatal infection is a rare occurrence.

PARTNER NOTIFICATION

To effectively treat a sexually transmitted infection, both partners must be treated for the infection, not only to prevent reinfection but to prevent infection of any new sexual partners. If only one partner is treated for the infection and the couple continues to have unsafe sex, the treated partner will be reinfected. New partners of the sexual partner are also at risk if he or she is not treated.

People being treated for infections may wish to tell their partners directly, but they may be reluctant to do so, for many reasons. If you find out you are infected and are reluctant to inform present or former partners, your health care provider, or the state health department in the state where you live, can assist in anonymous partner notification. This means that a partner is notified, without being given your name: for example, "A partner of yours has been diagnosed and is being treated for 'X' infection; you also need to be treated." The person will be located based on name, address, description, or any other information you can provide.

In every state, a health care provider is required to report treatments for the following sexually transmitted infections: syphilis, gonorrhea, chlamydia, chancroid, and AIDS. HIV infection is reportable in most states, and states vary in their reporting rules for other STDs. However, these reports are not made public; they are kept confidential (meaning your name is not reported to insurance companies, partners, etc.).

Talk with your health care provider about any concerns that you have, but *please don't avoid getting tested.* In most situations, treatment can be provided, and confidentiality maintained, for both you and your partner(s). Furthermore, with a few exceptions, *all adolescents in the United States can consent to the confidential diagnosis and treatment of infections without parental consent or knowledge, including testing for HIV.*

P A R T

ENCYCLOPEDIA
OF STDs

BACTERIAL VAGINOSIS

incidence: very common
cause: bacteria such as *Gardnerella* and *Mycoplasma*
symptoms: vaginal discharge, fishy odor
treatment: antibiotics

WHAT IS IT?

The vagina normally contains a combination of several kinds of bacteria, including the most common vaginal bacterium, *Lactobacillus*. *Bacterial vaginosis* (BV) is a bacterial syndrome that occurs when other bacteria that also occur normally in the vagina—such as *Gardnerella vaginalis*, and *Mycoplasma hominis*, among others—begin to reproduce rapidly and replace the normal bacteria. BV, then, is a syndrome caused by an overgrowth of bacteria in the vagina that disturbs the normal balance of bacteria there. It is sometimes referred to as causing an *imbalanced ecosystem*. Occurring exclusively in women, it is the most common vaginal disorder.

> **BV is a syndrome caused by an imbalance of bacteria in the vagina.**

In the past, BV was called *Gardnerella* (referring to only one of the bacteria that can cause this infection) or *nonspecific vaginosis* (a term that has gone out of use since the causes of BV have been determined).

HOW COMMON IS IT?

Although many women have never heard of it, BV is the most common disorder of the vagina. Many women will develop BV at some point in their lives, and about half of the women who visit their health care provider because of a vaginal discharge have it. For unknown reasons women of color seem to have a slightly higher risk of BV.

A woman does not get BV from sexual contact with an infected male partner, but women who are sexually active, particularly women with multiple partners or new partners, are more likely to have the infection. Women who have sex with other women may transmit the bacteria that cause BV back and forth, especially if they share sex toys.

Rarely, women who have never been sexually active and women in stable relationships can develop BV, as can women who have not had sex for a long period.

> BV has been associated with sexual activity, the presence of other genital infections, douching, and the use of an IUD.

BV also seems to occur more often in women who have other genital infections (such as chlamydia), women who douche (douching disrupts the normal bacterial population and allows the "bad bacteria" to overgrow), and women who use an intrauterine device (IUD) as a birth control method.

WHAT ARE THE SYMPTOMS?

As many as half of the women with BV have no noticeable symptoms, and the diagnosis is often made when a woman has a routine gynecological examination or an examination for other reasons. If BV does produce symptoms, they are often subtle and include a thin white to gray discharge from the vagina and a "fishy" odor. The odor is stronger after sexual intercourse and during a period. BV does not cause inflammation of the vagina or labia but may cause mild itching. These symptoms may cause more psychological than physical stress, especially if the infection recurs frequently.

> Most women with BV have only mild symptoms. A "fishy" odor from the vagina, often after intercourse, is a sign of BV.

Despite its mild symptoms, BV can cause serious complications when a woman who has the infection undergoes an invasive procedure such as an abortion, a biopsy of the endometrium (the lining of the uterus), placement of an IUD, or hysterosalpingography (a procedure in which dye is inserted into the uterus and Fallopian tubes to help visualize abnormalities). Although BV usually does not cause infection above the vagina, under these circumstances it can cause infection higher up, in the cervix or uterus, which can result in pelvic inflammatory disease (PID). (See the section on pelvic inflammatory disease.) Any woman who has BV, whether or not it is symptomatic, should be treated for the infection before having an abortion.

BV has also been associated with several complications of pregnancy, including preterm delivery, delivery of a low-birth-weight infant, premature rupture of membranes, premature labor, and infection of the uterus and amniotic fluid. Between 12 and 22 percent of pregnant women have BV, so many women and infants are potentially at risk. Many specialists recommend treating the infection in pregnant women, particularly those who are in the high-risk category and have delivered a premature infant in the past.

HOW IS BV TRANSMITTED?

Bacterial vaginosis is not really transmitted from one person to another, except possibly in women who have sex with other women. Although it occurs more commonly in women who are sexually active than in women who have never been sexually active, there is no evidence that the causative bacteria are transmitted from men to women. Rather, BV is an imbalance that occurs in the vagina in which the bacteria that are normally there are overgrown by other bacteria, such as *Gardnerella*, which are also normally found in the vagina but usually in lower numbers. This imbalance can occur in women who are not currently sexually active. Why some women develop this imbalance is not clear, but, as mentioned earlier, there are several circumstances—such as genital infections, douching, IUD use, and sexual activity—that make it more likely that a woman will develop BV.

TESTING FOR BV

An examination is important to determine what is causing a discharge from the vagina, because there are many possible disorders. Some (such as gonorrhea and chlamydia) originate in the cervix, and others (such as BV, yeast, and trichomoniasis) are vaginal disorders. Women may have BV along with other infections (such as chlamydia and trichomonas), and the only way to sort out the situation is through an examination. There are essentially four diagnostic clues for BV: (1) evidence of discharge during a pelvic examination, (2) a vaginal pH level that is abnormally high, (3) a fishy odor that can be detected on examination of the vaginal fluid, and (4) abnormal appearance of the cells that line the vaginal wall. Growing cultures for vaginal bacteria is not a helpful diagnostic procedure in this case, since the bacteria associated with BV are often found in cultures from women who do not have BV. A Pap smear may or may not detect BV.

A health care provider who has experience in vaginal infections

will have little difficulty diagnosing BV. Diagnosis usually doesn't
require any elaborate or expensive tests. Furthermore, the
health care provider can usually

**An examination is required to
detect BV. Testing is usually rapid
and inexpensive.**

diagnose the infection during the office visit, so there will be no delay in starting treatment. An evaluation for STDs is often a good idea
if BV is diagnosed, especially if the woman is sexually active with a
new partner, because BV can sometimes be a marker for other infections, such as chlamydia.

If a health care provider doesn't have access to a microscope to diagnose BV, he or she can use some of the newer tests that involve sending a vaginal specimen (taken
with a swab) to the laboratory for
testing. BV is diagnosed in these
tests by looking for the most
common bacteria that cause BV
or for the changes in the vaginal
fluid that BV causes.

**Any woman with symptoms of
discharge or odor should be
screened for BV. Because BV can
cause complications in pregnancy,
all pregnant women should be
screened for BV.**

TREATMENT

The goal of treatment of BV is to rebalance the bacteria in the vagina,
so that the predominant bacteria are once again the "good" bacteria,
Lactobacillus, and the numbers of the "bad" bacteria are decreased.
(Even a woman without BV may have some of the "bad" bacteria in
her vagina, but unless they predominate they will not cause BV.) There
are several ways to treat BV, using either topical creams or oral medication.

The treatment of BV relieves symptoms, so that if a woman has
BV but is symptom free, she may choose not to treat the condition.
There are two exceptions. As mentioned previously, if an invasive
genital procedure, such as the insertion of an IUD or a uterine biopsy
is to be performed, which may cause the bacteria to travel up into the
pelvic region, then the symptom-free woman with BV should be
treated. In addition, in pregnancy, treatment should be considered because of the risks that the infection poses to both the mother and the
child if left untreated, especially if a woman has delivered a premature infant in the past.

BV can be treated topically by applying cream or gel or orally by taking pills. Topical treatments include metronidazole gel and clindamycin cream; they are applied in the vagina for five days and seven days, respectively. A cream that was used in the past, triple-sulfa cream, is still prescribed by some health care providers, but it is not effective. If a woman is pregnant, clindamycin cream is usually not used because it isn't as effective and may cause problems in the pregnancy.

Oral metronidazole can be taken by mouth for seven days. Although in the past oral metronidazole was not thought to be safe for women during the first trimester of pregnancy because of its potential for harming the infant, the likelihood of any harm coming to the fetus from this drug has recently come into question and it is a recommended treatment for pregnant women. However, as mentioned above, clindamycin cream may cause problems in pregnancy and isn't recommended.

Which medication is chosen depends on the woman and her situation. She and her health care provider should discuss the treatment options, including a thorough discussion of the risks and benefits of each choice.

All medications have potential side effects. Topical creams generally have fewer side effects than oral medications. Metronidazole pills, for example, should not be taken with alcohol, since the combination can cause severe nausea and vomiting. If a woman will be consuming alcohol during her treatment, then topical treatment with either metronidazole gel or clindamycin cream is the preferred course. Metronidazole pills can also cause stomach upset and a metallic taste in the mouth. Clindamycin cream may weaken condoms and diaphragms made of latex.

Even with treatment of BV and the relief of symptoms, recurrences can occur, and treatment with an alternative medication is usually recommended if this happens. Women who have had BV once tend to have recurrences, and relapses of the disorder after treatment can be frustrating. Why these recurrences happen is not clear, although research is now under way to help answer this question.

> **BV can be treated with antibiotic pills or vaginal creams, but recurrences are common.**

Some studies have tried to replace the *Lactobacillus* in the vagina and eliminate the "bad" bacteria through a diet containing yogurt or nutritional supplements (such as acidophilus-containing milk, yogurt, or pills). So far this strategy has been unsuccessful, because the *Lactobacillus* in yogurt is different from the *Lactobacillus* in the vagina. Currently, there is no effective way to replace this type of *Lactobacillus* in the vagina by simply putting it there, although studies continue.

Another "treatment" often prescribed to women, or initiated on their own, is douching. *Douching should absolutely be avoided by all women.* Not only does douching put women at higher risk for pelvic infections, it only masks symptoms and thus prevents many women from seeking health care for potentially serious problems.

Male partners of women with BV do not need to be treated. There is no evidence that treatment of male partners changes the course of the infection in women, nor does it prevent recurrences of BV. If a woman with a male sexual partner is diagnosed with BV, however, it is reasonable to test both the woman and the man for other sexually transmitted infections, such as chlamydia, since a chlamydia infection can trigger BV in women, as mentioned previously. Pregnant women who are treated should see their health care provider after completing the treatment to make sure the therapy was effective.

A case can be made for treating female partners of women who have BV, especially if there is evidence of the infection in the partner. Among women who have sex with other women, BV may be considered a sexually transmitted infection, since female partners of women with BV have a high rate of infection themselves. This may occur through vaginal fluid transmission from the sharing of sex toys.

For any woman being treated for BV, it is a good idea to abstain from sex during the treatment.

CHANCROID

incidence: very rare in the United States
cause: bacteria (*Haemophilus ducreyi*)
symptoms: genital ulcers, lymph node swelling
treatment: antibiotics

WHAT IS IT?

Chancroid is a sexually transmitted infection of the genital area caused by the bacteria *Haemophilus ducreyi*. The primary symptom of chancroid is painful genital ulcers. Having any sexually transmitted disease that causes genital ulcers makes a person more susceptible to acquiring HIV infection, because breaks in the skin make it easier for HIV to be transmitted.

HOW COMMON IS IT?

In the United States, chancroid is not a common STD. It is more common in the tropical and subtropical developing world, such as Africa, where it is the most common cause of genital ulcer disease (in the United States the most common cause of genital ulcer disease is herpes). The late 1980s saw an increase in the incidence of chancroid in the United States, with about 5000 people diagnosed a year. Since then there has been a slight decline in the number infected each year.

Given the low incidence of chancroid in the United States, who is at risk for contracting the infection? It's important to know, first of all, that people who continue to have sex when they have chancroid sores—most often sex workers and those who visit them, especially in urban areas in the East and South—easily spread the disease. *Having sex with someone who has sores increases your chances of contracting this infection.* In addition, individuals who use crack cocaine or abuse other mind-altering substances, including alcohol, are less likely to use good judgment and more likely to have unprotected sex with high-risk partners. Men are more commonly infected than women; not being circumcised increases the risk of acquiring this infection. Finally, anyone living in the United States who travels to other areas of the world where infection is common and engages in unprotected genital or anal sex with high-risk persons is at risk.

The incidence of chancroid in this country may be higher than statistics indicate. The diagnosis may be missed because the symptoms are very similar to those caused by herpes and syphilis (which are more common STDs in the United States), and because the bacterium that causes chancroid is hard to culture.

WHAT ARE THE SYMPTOMS?

The ulcers in the genital area caused by chancroid are usually painful and look very similar to the ulcers of genital herpes and the first stage of syphilis, although the ulcer from syphilis (the chancre) is usually painless. One difference between chancroid and herpes is that herpes sometimes causes whole-body symptoms, such as fever and headache, and chancroid does not. Chancroid ulcers vary in size from small to very large. They usually start as a red bump, which then erodes, drains pus, and becomes an ulcer. Sometimes—and more often in women than in men—the lesions do not hurt.

About one-third of people with chancroid also develop swelling in the lymph nodes in the groin area. Lymph nodes that are draining pus are characteristic of chancroid and unusual for syphilis or herpes simplex. These symptoms usually take about a week to show up after infection.

Men and women may experience bleeding and pain from the rectum if that is where the ulcers are. In addition to the ulcers and lymph node swelling, women may notice a vaginal discharge and pain with intercourse, and men may have a discharge from the penis and burning with urination. If the lesions are not treated, they may last for one to three months and then resolve, yet they may recur at a later time. The ulcers may appear in the mouth, if that is where infection occurred.

> **The most common symptoms of chancroid are genital ulcers and lymph node swelling in the groin.**

HOW IS CHANCROID TRANSMITTED?

Chancroid is transmitted through genital, oral, or anal sexual contact with an infected person. Chancroid is usually transmitted by a person who has a sore or sores, but the disease can be transmitted by someone who has no sores. Condom use decreases the risk of transmission but may not eliminate it if a person has sores outside the area that a condom protects.

> **Chancroid is transmitted only through sexual contact. Using condoms decreases the risk of transmission.**

There is no evidence that the disease can be transmitted from one person to another by nonsexual contact, but an infected person can rarely spread the infection to other areas of his or her body by touching infected genital skin and then touching the other areas.

TESTING FOR CHANCROID

The specific tests for chancroid involve taking material directly from ulcers and culturing it using a special medium for the bacteria. Blood tests designed to detect the body's immune response (antibodies) to the infection may also help with the diagnosis. The cultures are not always positive when a person has the disease (tests demonstrate the infection less than 80 percent of the time), so a negative culture is not definitive. For this reason, if the infection is strongly suspected, treatment may be started even if the culture is negative.

Newer technology using the polymerase chain reaction test, which looks for the genetic material of the bacterium is available in some laboratories.

A person who is being tested for chancroid should simultaneously be tested for the more common causes of genital ulcers, herpes and syphilis, as well as other STDs. The less common causes of genital ulcers in the United States, lymphogranuloma venereum and donovanosis (see the sections on these topics) may also be tested for, depending upon the person's history.

> Testing involves either culturing the bacterium that causes chancroid from the lesion or performing a blood test for antibodies to the infection.

TREATMENT

Chancroid is treatable with antibiotics, but recently there has been increasing bacterial resistance to some of the older antibiotics, such as the sulfas. Treatments that are generally effective include azithromycin, ceftriaxone, erythromycin, and ciprofloxacin. People who have had sex with an infected person within ten days of the time that person developed symptoms must be treated as contacts for the infection and receive medications for treatment, even if they do not show symptoms.

> Antibiotics are used to treat persons infected with chancroid and their partners.

The symptoms usually disappear within a week or two, although scarring can remain after treatment. Treatment failures are common in people with HIV or other individuals with poorly functioning immune systems, and those with HIV may require additional courses of therapy. If the lymph nodes are pus-filled, draining them may help with healing. All people diagnosed with chancroid should be tested for HIV. Also, because 10 percent of people infected with chancroid also have syphilis or herpes, they should be tested for these infections as well.

CHLAMYDIA INFECTION

incidence: very common
cause: bacterium (*Chlamydia trachomatis*)
symptoms: burning with urination, discharge (but often none)
treatment: antibiotics

WHAT IS IT?

Recognized since 1970, chlamydia infections are among the most common genital infections. They are caused by the bacterium *Chlamydia trachomatis*. In addition to genital infections, chlamydia can also cause eye infection in newborns.

Some types of *Chlamydia trachomatis* can cause lymphogranuloma venereum (LGV), another sexually transmitted infection (see the entry for this disease). Other species of *Chlamydia* cause different infections. *Chlamydia pneumoniae*, for example, causes respiratory infection, and *Chlamydia psittaci*, which is transmitted from birds to humans, also causes a respiratory illness. Here the discussion is limited to sexually transmitted *Chlamydia trachomatis* infections.

HOW COMMON IS IT?

Chlamydia is the most common sexually transmitted bacterial disease in the industrialized world, with the highest rates among men and women aged twenty-five years or younger. Estimates are that between four and six million people are infected each year with chlamydia in the United States, but this may be an underestimate. Many people are symptom free and are never diagnosed or reported. Studies have shown that 3–5 percent of men and women in general medical clinics and about

> Chlamydia is the most common sexually transmitted bacterial infection in the developed world and is particularly common among young people.

15–20 percent of men and women attending STD clinics are infected. Studies of symptom-free people in various areas of the country have found that between 5 and 50 percent of those tested are infected with chlamydia. About half of those infected are teenagers, and about one-third are between twenty and twenty-four years old.

Even though chlamydia is a common infection of adolescents and young adults in the United States, any sexually active person can become infected. Younger women are more likely to become infected with chlamydia if exposed, because the anatomy of the cervix makes them more vulnerable.

Because many people have chlamydia without experiencing any symptoms, it is an infection that is frequently passed between sexual partners unknowingly. People of any sexual orientation can become infected with chlamydia, although it seems to be more common among those who have opposite-sex partners. Women who have sex with other women may be the least likely to become infected, although there may be a small possibility of infection if they share sex toys. Routinely screening those at high risk for chlamydia is the only way to halt the spread of this epidemic.

WHAT ARE THE SYMPTOMS?

Most chlamydia infections don't cause any symptoms! Half of men and three-quarters of women with chlamydia infections in the genital area are *completely symptom free.* Therefore, many people at risk for infection with chlamydia may mistakenly believe they don't need to be tested. A person with chlamydia infection may remain symptom free for his or her entire life or may start to show symptoms weeks, months, or even years after infection.

> Most people who have chlamydia are completely symptom free. Many people who have infection never even get tested.

Women

A woman with chlamydia infection can have infection of the uterus and Fallopian tubes (pelvic inflammatory disease, or PID), of the cervix (mucopurulent cervicitis, or MPC), and/or of the urethra (urethritis). Rarely, in PID, infection can occur around the liver (called

Fitz-Hugh Curtis syndrome). If she is going to develop symptoms, they usually appear one to three weeks after infection. The symptoms include the following:

—discharge from the genital area
—burning with urination
—pelvic pain
—bleeding between periods or after sexual intercourse

(See the sections on pelvic inflammatory disease and mucopurulent cervicitis for a more thorough discussion of these syndromes.) About half the time, chlamydia infection that seems to be limited to the cervix is actually causing silent (symptom-free) infection in the uterus. For all women, the urethra is a potential site of infection with chlamydia; the only symptom may be burning with urination. This may be the only symptom in infected women who have had a hysterectomy.

Men

A man with chlamydia in the genital area can have infection in the urethra (urethritis), the epididymis (epididymitis), the prostate (prostatitis), or a combination of these. If he is going to develop symptoms, they usually appear one to three weeks after infection, but they may take longer. The symptoms include the following:

—discharge from the penis, which can range from clear to yellow
—burning with urination
—an "itchy" or "irritated" feeling in the urethra
—redness at the tip of the penis

Pain and swelling in the testicles can occur if the chlamydia infection travels to the scrotum and causes epididymitis. Chlamydia infection of the prostate may cause pain between the scrotum and anal area, and difficult or frequent urination (see the section on epididymitis). Chlamydia infections (other than LGV, which is rare in the United States) do not cause ulcers in the genital area.

Men and Women

Chlamydia infection of the eye usually produces redness, itching, and pain in the lining of the eyelids, called *conjunctivitis*.

A man or woman who becomes infected with chlamydia in the anal area after receiving anal intercourse from someone who is infected may develop a mucous rectal discharge, rectal bleeding, diarrhea, and pain with bowel movement. Or there may be no symptoms.

Finally, the throat can also be a site of infection with chlamydia, usually in someone who performs oral sex on a man who is infected. Men who perform oral sex on women are usually not at high risk, since there is no direct contact with the cervix, which is the usual site of infection in women. Kissing is not a risk factor for chlamydia. Although throat irritation can occur with chlamydia throat infection, usually there are no symptoms when someone has a chlamydia infection of the throat.

> Chlamydia infection can occur in the throat, the eyes, and the genital and rectal areas of the body.

Both men and women have a risk of sterility with chlamydia infection, so prevention, diagnosis, and treatment are extremely important.

Reiter's Syndrome

Reiter's syndrome is an uncommon complication of chlamydia infection or infection with other organisms, such as salmonella and shigella. It occurs in about 1 percent of people infected with chlamydia and is more common among men than women. Most people who develop this syndrome have a genetic predisposition to it.

Reiter's syndrome is characterized by urethritis (urethral discharge and pain with urination), arthritis (joint inflammation), conjunctivitis, skin rashes, and other symptoms. It may occur even after the underlying infection has been treated with antibiotics. The syndrome is diagnosed when a person with urethritis or cervicitis also has arthritis for longer than a month. Why Reiter's syndrome occurs following these infections is not clear. One theory is that it occurs when the body is creating proteins, or antibodies, to fight off the chlamydia or other infections; these antibodies mistakenly consider normal tissues in the body as foreign and mount an immune response to them, causing the symptoms listed above.

Reiter's syndrome is treated with anti-inflammatory medication, such as ibuprofen; relapses are possible even after the initial symp-

toms resolve. Sometimes
stronger medications are needed
to treat the disease. It is a disorder that is best managed by a
rheumatologist (a doctor who
specializes in joint diseases). Of
course, the underlying infection
that triggered the Reiter's syndrome must be treated as well.

> **Reiter's syndrome—a condition of recurrent episodes of urethritis, arthritis, conjunctivitis, skin rashes, and other symptoms— can follow chlamydia infection even after treatment.**

HOW IS CHLAMYDIA TRANSMITTED?

Chlamydia is transmitted through sexual contact with a person who is infected, whether or not that person has symptoms. It can be transmitted through oral, genital, or anal sex, and possibly by sex toys. Some people think that if a male partner does not ejaculate, then infection with chlamydia (and other STDs) cannot take place. This is not true! Condoms help prevent transmission of chlamydia and should be used consistently and correctly, and with every contact for oral, genital, or anal sex when a partner's status for infection is unknown.

An infant born to a mother who has chlamydia can become infected when passing through an infected birth canal. Such an infant may develop infection in several different areas. About 50 percent of newborns of mothers with chlamydia in the cervix acquire a chlamydia eye infection when passing through the birth canal. About 10 percent have infection in the lungs, often developing symptoms several months after birth. Occasionally children who are born to infected mothers develop infection in the vagina and rectum, but child abuse must always also be considered when infection of these areas occurs. Chlamydia can also cause miscarriage, premature rupture of membranes, preterm delivery, and delivery of a low-birth-weight infant.

TESTING FOR CHLAMYDIA

First, a word about the woeful *lack* of routine testing for chlamydia. Unless a person is being seen in a clinic that specializes in STDs, chlamydia testing is usually offered only if the health care provider notices an obvious symptom, such as discharge or irritation of the cervix, during a routine gynecological exam. Since women and men can have chlamydia without having symptoms, waiting for a health care provider to notice a symptom is not a good idea. Unless you are specifically told that you are being screened for chlamydia, it usually means that you are not. It is also not true that a woman's annual Pap smear provides a screen for such STDs as chlamydia. (For more about the Pap smear, an important screen to detect cancer of the cervix, see the section on genital warts.)

Who Should Be Tested?

The following people should consider being tested for chlamydia:

1. Anyone who has had unprotected sex in the past with a partner whose status for infections was not known.
2. Any person twenty-five years of age or younger who is sexually active. If the person has had a negative test in the past and does not have a new sexual partner or any new risk or symptom, then it may be reasonable to skip screening unless or until these factors change.
3. Any person who is diagnosed with another STD.
4. Anyone diagnosed with MPC, PID, nongonococcal urethritis, epididymitis, or proctocolitis.
5. Anyone who has had a new sexual partner within the past sixty days.
6. Anyone who has had more than two sexual partners in the past six months.
7. Any woman who is pregnant or planning on becoming pregnant.
8. Any woman who is planning to have an intrauterine device inserted.
9. Anyone who has been infected with chlamydia or any other STD in the past twelve months. (Reinfection from continuing risky sex practices or from resuming sex with untreated partners is, unfortunately, very common.)
10. Anyone who is not consistently using barrier methods of infection control with new partners.

> Talk with your health care provider about whether or not you should be tested for chlamydia. Routine testing and diagnosis of this treatable infection can help preserve your health and fertility for the future.

The Tests

In the past ten years, testing for chlamydia has become easier and better. The best tests (called "nucleic acid amplification tests," or NAATs) look for the genetic material (the nucleic acids) of the bacterium and, for both men and women, can be done on a urine sample or swabs from infected areas. These tests detect infection in more than ninety of a hundred people who are infected. Culture and other tests that look for the body's immune response to the bacteria, or for proteins on the surface of the bacteria, are less sensitive, although these tests may be used if NAATs are not available. For throat or anal chlamydia, culture is still the preferred test.

When someone is found to have chlamydia, decisions about what kind of medication is to be used, how long it is to be used, and what kind of follow-up is necessary depend on the extent of the infection. In order to determine the extent of the infection, *a physical examination is needed in addition to the screening test.* For women may test positive for chlamydia and have no evidence of infection on examination, whereas others have cervicitis or PID. In men who test positive for chlamydia, an examination may show no evidence of infection, or there may be signs of urethritis, epididymitis, or prostatitis.

TREATMENT

Chlamydia is completely treatable with antibiotics, but the consequences of the disease, such as scarring, may not be treatable. The antibiotics most commonly used for uncomplicated genital chlamydia infections in men and women are doxycycline (which is taken for a week) and azithromycin (taken as a single dose by mouth). Alternatives to these, for people who can't take the preferred antibiotics, are erythromycin, ofloxacin, and levofloxacin. Because reinfection rates are high (meaning many women are reinfected from the same or another partner) and the consequences are potentially severe, it's a good idea for men and women to be retested in the next three to twelve months.

Azithromycin may be the best choice for some people in the long run, since individuals sometimes do not take the full week-long course of the medication, and as a result do not receive adequate treatment and can still have infection and complications later. A medication that treats the infection with just a single dose can avoid this problem. *However, it is important to abstain from sex for a full week after taking the single-dose treatment of azithromycin,* because it stays in the system for quite a while (actually up to a week) and is actively treating the infection during that time. Resuming sexual activity sooner than this can reinfect partners.

It is especially important for someone being treated for sexually transmitted infections to take the medication as prescribed and take all of it. If a woman with infection is found to have PID from chlamydia, or a man is found to have infection of the epididymis or prostate from chlamydia, then a longer course of antibiotics must be used (see the sections for these STDs).

Any partners within the past two months (or more than two months, if that was the most recent sexual contact) should also be treated as contacts to infection, even if they do not have symptoms or evidence of infection on examination.

Talk with your health care provider about whether you need to follow up after treatment for chlamydia to make sure the infection is gone. In most cases, it is not necessary. However, pregnant women should always have a follow-up test to make sure the treatment for chlamydia has been effective. Erythromycin is the medication best suited for the treatment of chlamydia during pregnancy; the others may be harmful to an unborn child.

> Follow-up testing to ensure that chlamydia has been successfully treated may be necessary, especially during pregnancy.

Tests for chlamydia usually prove negative about three weeks after treatment. You may want to consider getting tested again to make sure the treatment has worked, particularly if you are pregnant. In addition, if you are at continued risk for infection, or reinfection, you should continue to be screened regularly by your health care provider.

DONOVANOSIS

incidence: very rare
cause: bacteria (*Klebsiella granulomatosis*)

symptoms: ulcers
treatment: antibiotics

WHAT IS IT?

Donovanosis, also called *granuloma inguinale,* is caused by the bacterium *Klebsiella granulomatosis.*

HOW COMMON IS IT?

In the United States, fewer than fifty people are infected with donovanosis each year; the infection is also uncommon in Europe and other parts of the developed world. Infection is more common in Papua, New Guinea; Southern Africa; India; and central Australia. In some areas of the world, it is the most common cause of genital ulcers (in the United States the most common cause of genital ulcers is herpes).

Studies have shown that donovanosis may significantly increase the risk of a person becoming infected with HIV if exposed. Controlling the spread of donovanosis and other genital ulcer diseases may help to prevent the spread of HIV.

WHAT ARE THE SYMPTOMS?

Symptoms of donovanosis usually appear between eight and eighty days after infection. The most common symptoms are persistent ulcers, which continue to grow, at the site where infection occurred (genitals, anal area, or mouth); the ulcers are dark red and can cover a large area. They usually start as red nodules or bumps under the skin, which then ulcerate. The ulcers can grow together and form even larger ulcers, and the tissue can become thickened and heaped up around the ulcers,

The symptom of donovanosis is chronic ulcers in the area where infection took place (genitals, anal area, or mouth).

which often bleed easily. Unlike in other genital infections, lymph nodes are usually not swollen in the area of the infection.

The ulcerous lesions are usually mildly tender if tender at all; they may persist and progress over many years and can become infected with skin bacteria. Permanent scarring in areas such as the urethra is common, and the drainage of lymphatic fluid may be obstructed, leading to swelling of the genital tissues, a condition called *genital ele-*

phantiasis. Without treatment of the infection, the ulcers can become so extensive that they destroy parts of the genitals.

It is possible for the bacteria to spread through the blood to the liver and bones and cause infection there. Women can also have infection on the cervix, which may cause bleeding between periods or after intercourse.

HOW IS DONOVANOSIS TRANSMITTED?

Transmission occurs only through oral, genital, or anal sexual contact with an infected partner. It usually but not always takes several exposures for transmission to take place. Correct use of condoms helps prevent transmission of this infection.

TESTING FOR DONOVANOSIS

There is no reliable blood or culture test; testing for donovanosis requires a biopsy of an infected area of skin, in which a piece is removed for analysis. Special tests must generally be performed in the laboratory to detect evidence of the bacterium that causes this infection, though the infection is sometimes detected in women through Pap smears.

> Testing involves taking a biopsy of the lesions and testing the tissue for the bacterium.

Because someone with donovanosis is also more likely to be infected with other sexually transmitted diseases, a complete STD screening is recommended for anyone with this diagnosis. Other infections that are often confused with donovanosis are chancroid, syphilis, and lymphogranuloma venereum (see the sections on these individual diseases). It can also be mistaken for genital cancer. Diagnosis of this infection is reportable to the state health department.

TREATMENT

The best treatment for this infection is antibiotics. Doxycycline is the recommended treatment. For someone who can't take doxycycline, alternatives are azithromycin, ciprofloxacin, erythromycin, and trimethoprim-sulfamethoxazole. Treatment is only successful if it is continued until the infection has been cleared—usually in about three weeks. The infection may recur if the antibiotics are stopped sooner.

Scarring may persist despite adequate treatment, but it is usually minimal if medical attention is sought early in the infection. If a secondary bacterial infection develops on top of the donovanosis, this may need to be treated with different antibiotics.

Treatment may not be as successful in a person who has a compromised immune system, such as someone with HIV infection. In this case, the medications are taken for a longer period.

All sexual partners of a person with donovanosis in a period of up to sixty days before the infected person developed symptoms must be treated with antibiotics, even if they are symptom free.

> Donovanosis is completely treatable with antibiotics. Long-term problems from scarring occur when people wait to seek treatment.

EPIDIDYMITIS

incidence: common
cause: bacteria (some sexually transmitted and some not)
symptoms: scrotal pain and swelling, frequent urination, burning with urination
treatment: antibiotics

WHAT IS IT?

Epididymitis can be caused by sexually transmitted bacteria such as those that cause gonorrhea and chlamydia, as well as by bacteria that are not sexually transmitted. Epididymitis can be a complication of urethritis (see the section on nongonococcal urethritis).

Epididymitis is an infection of the epididymis, the structure that sits above each testicle in the scrotum and has a crucial function in the maturation of sperm. Infection of the epididymis usually occurs on only one side of the scrotum.

> Epididymitis has both sexually transmitted and nonsexually transmitted causes.

HOW COMMON IS IT?

There are no reliable statistics about how many men are diagnosed each year with epididymitis, but we do know that it is a common infection. When epididymitis occurs in younger men, it is usually caused by sexually transmitted bacteria, such as chlamydia, gonorrhea, and those that cause nongonococcal urethritis, often acquired through unprotected sex. Epididymitis can occur as a complication of urethritis (1–2 percent of men with chlamydia urethritis develop epididymitis) or without an underlying urethral infection.

In older men without a new sexual partner, epididymitis usually occurs along with a urinary tract infection (UTI), although UTIs are uncommon among men. UTIs may occur in older men because of the noncancerous enlargement of the prostate that many older men experience; this enlargement can lead to incomplete emptying of the bladder and thus predispose a man to UTIs. In these cases it is not clear which comes first, the bladder infection or the epididymal infection.

> **Prompt treatment of bacterial urethritis decreases the likelihood that the infection will progress to epididymitis.**

Men who have recently had a catheter inserted into the urethra or bladder or have been subject to any other invasive procedure in that area may also develop a UTI, epididymitis, or both. In all of these cases, the most common bacterium is *Escherichia coli*, not the sexually transmitted bacteria. Any structural abnormality of the urinary tract system, such as stones or scars (strictures) of the urethra, or any abnormality that causes the bladder to empty incompletely can also lead to UTIs and subsequent epididymitis.

Occasionally, tuberculosis, fungus, and the bacterium that causes syphilis can also cause epididymitis.

WHAT ARE THE SYMPTOMS?

The symptoms of epididymitis are scrotal pain, redness, and swelling, usually on one side. The pain can be severe. There may be symptoms or evidence of urethritis, such as burning with urination and discharge. These symptoms may be subtle or absent, even if urethral infection is present, and they are more common in men whose epididymitis has a sexually transmitted cause. In older men there may be a history of a change in the urinary stream and evidence of a bladder infection, such as pressure in the bladder and burning with urination. The symptoms are usually gradual in onset but can occur suddenly. Acute epididymitis is defined as symptoms lasting less than six weeks; chronic epididymitis as symptoms lasting three months or more.

HOW IS EPIDIDYMITIS TRANSMITTED?

This illness is most often caused by bacteria that can be sexually or nonsexually transmitted. A common myth is that epididymitis is caused by the "back-up" of sperm or urine into the epididymis, which can be caused by straining with urination. This is not true. Although reflux of infected secretions from the urethra or bladder may contribute to epididymitis, it is the underlying infection that is to blame, not the mechanical process of reflux.

The most common bacteria that cause epididymitis—those that cause chlamydia and gonorrhea and the other nonspecific bacteria—are sexually transmitted (see the sections on these infections). These bacteria can be transmitted by unprotected genital, anal, or oral contact with an infected partner. Performing anal sex on a partner increases the risk of infection of the epididymis and urethra, bladder, and prostate with the bacteria commonly found in stool. Condoms—if they are used consistently and correctly and they do not leak or break—prevent the transmission of these bacteria.

As discussed earlier, men can also become infected from UTIs or after surgery of the urinary tract or the insertion of instruments into the urethra and bladder. Any condition that predisposes a man to a bladder infection can also result in epididymitis.

> Condoms, if used correctly, will decrease the likelihood of infection with the sexually transmitted organisms that cause epididymitis.

TESTING FOR EPIDIDYMITIS

The diagnosis of epididymitis is made on examination. A red, swollen, tender testicle on only one side is suggestive of the disorder. An evaluation is usually carried out for urethritis and a bladder infection.

For a urethritis screening test, a man should not have voided for at least four hours prior to the examination, and preferably overnight. A small swab is inserted a short distance into the urethra, and then material from the swab is examined under the microscope for causative bacteria. (See the section on nongonococcal urethritis for more information about these screening procedures). Urine samples can also be screened for gonorrhea and chlamydia (see the sections on these infections). A midstream urine sample is obtained for analysis under the microscope and culturing. Both the screen for urethritis and the screen for white blood cells and bacteria in the urine are important in helping to sort out the cause of the epididymitis.

Other medical conditions can cause testicular pain and swelling. Torsion of the testicle is a medical emergency that occurs when the spermatic cord and blood vessels that lead to a testicle become twisted and cut off the blood supply to the testicle. This condition can lead to the death of the testicle if not quickly corrected surgically. It usually occurs on only one side, so it can be difficult to distinguish from epididymitis. However, torsion of the testicle usually occurs in young men and has a very sudden onset of symptoms, and there usually is no evidence of urethral infection on examination. Epididymitis typically has a more gradual onset of symptoms, but there are exceptions.

If there is difficulty distinguishing between epididymitis and torsion of the testicle, a study such as a Doppler ultrasound can be performed to help make the diagnosis. This test measures blood flow to the testicle and, by bouncing sound waves off the internal structures of the scrotum, allows them to be visualized.

Other testicular problems that can be confused with epididymitis are trauma to the testicle (usually a man will know that this has occurred), testicular cancer, and other infections of the testicle such as tuberculosis, which is rare. An experienced health care provider can sort out these possibilities and order appropriate tests to make the diagnosis. For complicated situations, such as failure of the epididymitis to respond to antibiotic treatment, a urologist should be consulted for further evaluation and treatment.

TREATMENT

Epididymitis is usually treatable with antibiotics. Treatment should be started as soon as possible, even before the results of the tests are known, to decrease the risk of scarring of the epididymis and future infertility. If a sexually transmitted cause of epididymitis (such as gonorrhea or chlamydia) is suspected, the antibiotics generally used are a combination of ceftriaxone and doxycycline. However, if the infection is thought to have resulted from performing anal intercourse, then ofloxacin or levofloxacin is the best antibiotic. If the cause is not thought to be a sexually transmitted bacterium, ofloxacin is again the best choice. If the swelling and pain are significant, bed rest and scrotal elevation are helpful in draining the infection from the testicle. Bed rest should be continued until the scrotum is no longer tender.

If the symptoms are not improved after about three days of treatment, a referral to a urologist is indicated. Rarely hospitalization is necessary to administer intravenous antibiotics. If swelling and tenderness persist after treatment, an evaluation may be performed for other possible causes of testicular pain and swelling, such as testicular cancer, tuberculosis, or fungal causes of epididymitis. These unusual infectious causes may be more common among men with compromised immune systems, such as men with HIV infection. Partners within the past sixty days of men treated for epididymitis must also be evaluated and treated if the cause of infection is known or suspected to be from a sexually transmitted bacterium. Men being treated for a sexually transmitted cause of epididymitis should abstain from sex until they and their partners are treated.

FUNGAL (YEAST) INFECTIONS

incidence: very common
cause: yeast
symptoms: itching, skin redness; discharge in women
treatment: antifungal creams or pills

WHAT IS IT?

Yeast infections of the genital area are caused by fungus; both men and women can have these infections. Yeast infections are not sexually transmitted, because they are not spread from one sexual partner to another, but men and women who are sexually active seem to be infected more often than men and women who are not. Fungal infections are included here because they are a common cause of genital symptoms. Sometimes people assume they have a yeast infection when in reality they have a sexually transmitted infection.

The fungus that most commonly causes yeast infections in women is *Candida albicans*, although there are other species, such as

Candida tropicalis, that are less responsive to the usual treatments. Men can also have *Candida* infections of the penis. Men and (less commonly) women may experience genital rashes caused by a species of fungus known as *Tinea cruris*; this rash, also known as "jock itch," is very common.

HOW COMMON IS IT?

Any person, male or female, whether sexually active or not, can develop a genital yeast infection. There are no reliable statistics on how many people contract such infections because many people self-treat and never see a doctor about a yeast infection. Men probably have yeast infections less often than women, even though they are common in men.

It is estimated that 75 percent of women will develop a symptomatic yeast infection at some point in their lives and that possibly 75 percent of those women will experience another symptomatic infection later. Some women have very frequent recurrent symptoms, with multiple yeast infections each year. It is believed that about 20 percent of women are colonized with yeast in the vagina. This means that even though the yeast is there, it is not causing infection or symptoms, such as itching and discharge. These women may remain symptom free or may develop symptoms later.

The following circumstances make a woman more likely to be a yeast carrier and to develop yeast infections: pregnancy, using oral contraceptive pills (particularly the higher-dose pills), using oral antibiotics (because they eliminate the normal bacteria from the vagina and allow the yeast to overgrow), and having diabetes that is poorly controlled. Douching disrupts the normal environment of the vagina and may make a woman more likely to get a yeast infection. Warm weather, too, makes yeast infection more likely. Yeast likes warm, moist areas of the body, such as the genitals, and wearing clothing that is tight and restrictive tends to make a person more likely to develop a yeast infection. Other vaginal irritation, for example from an allergic reaction to spermicide, may also allow yeast to overgrow.

Suppression of the immune system (through such medications as steroids or such infections as HIV) can also make a woman more susceptible to frequent symptomatic yeast infections. However, just because a woman develops a yeast infection does not mean she has a serious medical problem: as noted previously, some women are simply subject to recurrent symptomatic yeast infections.

Men who are not circumcised tend to have more frequent penile yeast infections than men who are, probably because the area under the foreskin provides a warm, moist area in which yeast can grow. (A fungal infection under the foreskin is called *balanitis*.)

> Genital yeast infections are very common. A yeast infection does not automatically indicate an underlying medical problem, although some medical conditions, such as diabetes, can make a person more likely to develop yeast infections.

WHAT ARE THE SYMPTOMS?

For women, yeast infections usually cause redness and itching of the genital area and a clumped discharge that looks like cottage cheese, though it may be thinner in consistency. The itching can be intense, and it can be internal (in the vagina) or external (on the vulva and anal area). There may be a burning sensation in the genital area, pain with intercourse, and burning with urination when the urine hits the raw skin. There may be a bread-like "yeasty" odor from the genital area. Breaks in the skin may develop if there is significant inflammation; these breaks are sometimes mistaken for other genital infections that cause lesions, such as herpes. The outside of the cervix may appear raw and irritated on examination. The symptoms seem to be especially bothersome before menstruation. Male partners of women with yeast infections may feel a temporary burning or notice redness on the penis after intercourse.

For men, fungal infections in the genital area usually cause itchy red patches of skin, which may occur in the groin area and on the penis and testicles. The red patches are usually flaky in appearance, and they usually (although not always) itch. The lesions of a fungal infection in men can be difficult to distinguish from those caused by other skin conditions, such as herpes and psoriasis.

> Yeast infections may be misdiagnosed as other genital infections such as herpes.

HOW ARE FUNGAL INFECTIONS TRANSMITTED?

It is not clear where yeast comes from or how people become infected. What we do know is that fungal infections are not sexually transmitted, because those who are not sexually active can have fungal infections of the genital area—although, as noted earlier, people who are sexually active seem to get them more frequently. We also know that the bacterium normally found in the vagina, *Lactobacillus*, offers women protection from yeast infections, because when the relative population size of this bacterium is disturbed yeast infection is more likely. And we know that treating the sexual partners of someone who has a yeast infection does not help the person with the infection.

Women who have sex only with women may pass yeast back and forth through the use of sex toys, although there is no scientific evidence for this theory. It has also been suggested that yeast colonization occurs in the gastrointestinal tract in most people and that reinfection of the genital area occurs from this source. However, studies have produced conflicting results: some women with recurrent vaginal yeast infections do not seem to have yeast colonization in the gastrointestinal tract, and treatment of gastrointestinal yeast has not affected the recurrence rate of vaginal yeast infections.

TESTING FOR FUNGAL INFECTIONS

A health care provider diagnoses yeast infection based on the findings of a physical examination and seeing yeast from a swab under the microscope. Sending cultures out to a laboratory is sometimes (but not usually) necessary.

In women, redness of the external and internal genital area is a sign of yeast infection. The acidity of the secretions in the vagina is normal (in the other two common vaginal infections, trichomoniasis and bacterial vaginosis, the pH is high, meaning a lowered acidity). A swab of the vaginal wall will usually reveal yeast under the microscope, although if a woman has self-treated with intravaginal yeast creams within the last few days, no yeast may be seen. If the diagnosis is in doubt and the swab test does not resolve the matter, then a culture may be performed to look for yeast. The Pap smear may reveal yeast, but it is not a sensitive screen and should not be relied upon for diagnosis of yeast infection.

Because treatments for yeast infections are now available over the counter (without a prescription), many women self-treat what they believe to be a yeast infection without seeing a health care provider. Under these circumstances, a woman whose symptoms are due to another genital infection with similar symptoms, such as herpes, may not be properly diagnosed and treated. If she has herpes, she may incorrectly believe that the antifungal medication is responsible for the resolution of the symptoms, when what really happened is that the herpes outbreak resolved on its own. *Any woman experiencing symptoms of a yeast infection for the first time, and especially a woman who frequently has symptoms of yeast infection and has never been diagnosed, should see a health care provider for a definitive diagnosis.* She should be examined when the symptoms are present, because when they have almost cleared up, or after treatment with creams, it may be difficult to determine the cause of the infection.

For men, rubbing the lesions with a cotton swab dipped in normal saline will often show yeast under the microscope, although it is generally more difficult to detect yeast in men than in women by looking under the microscope. If the rash is typical of yeast infection, and other possibilities (such as herpes) have been excluded, sometimes a trial of yeast cream is used as both a therapeutic and a diagnostic tool—that is, if the yeast cream clears up the lesions, then the infection was probably due to yeast.

TREATMENT

For both men and women, antifungal medications provide dependable treatment for yeast infections. Men usually have success with over-the-counter creams applied to the affected area twice a day for two weeks. Treatment with antifungal medication is recommended only for a woman with symptoms, and then only for a woman who has been diagnosed with yeast infection in the past and is certain that yeast is again the cause of her symptoms. For women, there is no reason to treat yeast found on examination if it is not causing symptoms.

Many antifungal creams and vaginal suppositories are available without a prescription, and most of them are well tolerated, except for the rare allergic reaction. Since all over-the-counter creams are equally effective (they cure infection 80–90 percent of the time), using the least expensive cream seems to make sense. Butoconazole cream, clotrimazole cream or vaginal tablet, miconazole cream or vaginal suppository, nystatin vaginal tablets, tioconazole cream or ointment, and terconazole cream or vaginal suppository are all equally effective. Some can be used as a single application, some for three days, and some for a week. Nystatin needs to be used for two weeks and may not be as effective.

Women can use either creams, which are inserted into the vagina with an applicator packaged with the cream, or vaginal suppositories, which are pills that are inserted into the vagina. When using a cream, for best results the medication should be rubbed on the vulva (the outside of the genitals) as well as inserted into the vagina. For women with a history of difficult, recurrent yeast infections, the longer, seven-day course is a better option from the start. Some women experience irritation from the frequent use of the treatments, and in this case an alternative treatment should be used. Because the creams and suppositories are oil based, they may weaken latex condoms and diaphragms.

The antifungal medication fluconazole is available by prescription as oral medication for both men and women. It is as effective as the creams and easier to use, but it has more potential side effects than topical treatments. These include rare allergic reactions and liver toxicity (also rare), so this medication should be used with caution by people with liver problems. Fluconazole is taken as a single oral dose. This medication has adverse interactions with several other commonly taken medications, so it is important that the health care provider know about any other medications a person is taking. Using oral antifungal medication does not seem to encourage the growth of drug-resistant yeast strains.

Most yeast infections are easily treated with topical or newer oral medications, some of which can be taken as a single dose.

Yeast infections can be especially difficult to treat in pregnant women. A longer course of topical treatment (such as a week of one of the creams ending in "azole") is usually necessary to eliminate the infection. Nystatin and fluconazole are not recommended in pregnancy.

Whenever the standard therapies are not effective for a man or woman, taking a culture to make sure that yeast is actually causing the infection is recommended, because the symptoms may be caused by something other than yeast. Occasionally an unusual yeast species—one that is not easily treated by the standard medications—is the cause, and this, too, can be determined by culture.

In addition to using medication, individuals with chronic or recurrent yeast infections must also try to eliminate any underlying factors that may make them susceptible to yeast infections. If a woman is taking birth control pills, she may want to stop taking them or switch to a pill with a lower dose of estrogen to see if this helps. (Another reliable birth control method must be used if the pills are discontinued altogether.) Medications that suppress the immune system, such as steroids, can also cause a yeast infection; if the medications can be stopped, the infection may be easier to cure. Switching to looser-fitting, cotton clothing can help. Douching is discouraged.

Other approaches to treatment that have unproven effectiveness but might help include using yogurt douches and eating yogurt or acidophilus tablets to recolonize the vagina, and decreasing the intake of sweets, bread, and alcohol. Although the *Lactobacillus* in yogurt is different from the *Lactobacillus* in the vagina, and the vagina does not become colonized with the yogurt *Lactobacillus*, some women find relief this way, and the practice is not harmful. Although treating a male partner with antifungal medication while the woman is being treated has not been proven to affect her recovery, if the man has evidence of a yeast infection, he should certainly also be treated.

GENITAL WARTS

incidence: very common
cause: virus (human papillomavirus)
symptoms: painless bumps in the genitals
treatment: topical treatments, freezing with liquid nitrogen

WHAT IS IT?

Genital warts are painless bumps in the genital area that are caused by the human papillomavirus (HPV).

HOW COMMON IS IT?

Human papillomavirus is probably the most common sexually transmitted infection in the United States and the most common problem that brings people to STD clinics. Based on a study in which people without a history of genital warts were tested for the DNA of the virus in the genital area, it is estimated that 75–80 percent of sexually active adults have or have had the genital warts virus. Men and women can be infected regardless of sexual orientation, age, or socioeconomic status. Some people (possibly as many as 60%) who have been infected may "clear the virus" and never have a symptom or know they were infected. The more sexual partners a person has had, the higher the risk of infection; however, even people with only two sexual partners have a 20 percent likelihood of infection; those with four to five partners have a 60 percent likelihood.

There are more than a hundred types of human papillomavirus, and most people have at least one type. In general, the types that cause hand warts are different from those that cause foot warts, which in turn are different from those that cause genital warts, and so on. The different strains generally stay in the area where they cause infection; for example, the hand wart virus is not usually transmitted to the genitals. Genital or anal warts, therefore, are almost always transmitted sexually—that is, a person acquires anal or genital warts by having contact with the anal or genital area of a person who is infected with the virus.

As you will see below, there are still many unanswered questions about HPV in terms of its transmission and detection, which can be frustrating. However, ongoing research will help answer these questions, and provide information on how to prevent transmission. Most promising is a new vaccine, approved by the U.S. Food and Drug Administration (FDA), that has been found to prevent infection with four strains of HPV—the two types that most commonly cause visible warts (HPV 6 and 11) and the two types that cause more than 70 percent of cervical cancers (HPV 16 and 18). This vaccine will be most effective for women and girls who are not yet sexually active, to prevent cervical cancer in the future, and will soon be available in the United States. However, even then, the recommendations about transmission and screening will remain important, since the vaccine does not protect against all strains of the virus that can cause cervical cancer.

WHAT ARE THE SYMPTOMS?

Fewer than 1 percent of people who are infected with HPV develop symptoms. For those who do, the visible symptom is the external genital wart or warts, which look like the warts one might have on the hand: they are usually flesh colored or a little bit darker, and they are harder than the surrounding tissue. They can be raised or flat. The raised warts tend to have a cauliflower-like appearance when looked at closely or with a hand-held lens. Warts may occur singly or in groups, often of varying size, and they may grow together to form larger warts. They do not hurt unless scratched or picked at, in which case they can become irritated. In about 20 percent of people they itch, and in 20 percent of people they disappear on their own. They may remain the same size for some time, or they may continue to enlarge.

> Genital warts are small, flesh-colored bumps that are usually symptom free but may itch.

It can be difficult to know whether or not these "bumps" are warts, because the genital skin is somewhat irregular in appearance in most men and women anyway. Bumps can be a normal part of the genital anatomy—pearly penile papules in men, sebaceous cysts in men and women, or hymen remnants for women. An experienced health care provider can help determine whether the bumps are simply normal anatomy, are caused by HPV infection, or are due to another infection, such as molluscum contagiosum.

Warts can occur anywhere in the anal and genital area, as high up as the lower abdomen and as low down as the upper thighs. A man may have warts in the urethral opening, where they may or may not be noticed. Symptoms include urethral bleeding or discharge, or a change in the stream of urine, although generally warts in the urethra do not cause symptoms.

Women may have warts on the soft surfaces of the inner labia and vagina and on the cervix. Warts on the inner labia and vagina may be raised or flat. Warts on the cervix are usually flat. Internal warts may not be noticed by the woman and may be revealed only on examination by a health care provider. Rarely the virus that causes genital warts can cause warts around the mouth, eyes, and nasal area and on the larynx (voice box), most likely related to oral-genital contact.

There can be a long lag time between infection and the development of visible warts. The usual interval between infection and the first appearance of symptoms is thirty to ninety days, but it may be years. It is not uncommon for people who have not been sexually active for several years to develop visible warts. In this situation, the virus has been dormant (quiet) during those years and then becomes active for some unknown reason.

> Warts viruses may be dormant and cause no symptoms over a person's lifetime, or they may produce symptoms months or years after first exposure.

Most people don't know about this lag time, and it's not uncommon for a couple who have been together for a few years to become very upset when one of them is newly diagnosed with warts, either because the woman has evidence of the virus on a Pap smear or because one of them notices visible warts. This finding often raises great concern that one of them has had sexual contact with another partner. Although this is a possibility, it is also possible that one or both partners had the virus at the beginning of the relationship but didn't know it because they were not having symptoms. Chances are that they both have the virus now, since it is very easy to transmit. It is therefore impossible to say who brought the virus into the relationship—a fact that usually helps relieve concern.

Of the thirty-five or so types of HPV that affect the genital area, the types that have been linked to cervical and skin cancer are usually not the types that cause external genital warts. As noted above, the HPV types that most often cause external, visible warts are types 6 and 11, and the types that most often cause cervical or skin cancer are types 16 and 18. However, other strains of HPV have been linked to cancer as well (for example, strains 31, 33, and 35). And just to make things a bit more confusing, very rarely types 6 and 11 can be associated with cancer, and types 16, 18, 31, 33, and 35 are found in visible warts. In other words, sometimes different types of virus are in the same wart. (See the end of this section on genital warts for more information on HPV and cancer concerns.)

Once a person has been infected with the warts virus, it is unclear whether or not the virus will go away. In the past most researchers thought this was unlikely, but it may be that in some people the virus eventually disappears. As the technology for detecting the quiet (dormant) virus improves, this question may be more accurately answered. The *visible* symptoms may go away either on their own or with treatment. This is true of all types of warts, which tend to recur in the same area of the body where they appeared in the past. When the warts recur, it is usually the same virus reactivating, not a reinfection. Some couples worry that they will keep reinfecting each other through sexual contact, but this does not seem to be the case. Once the virus has been transmitted, it is not transmitted again.

> Once a person has been infected with HPV, the visible warts can be treated, but the virus may persist. There is no known cure for HPV infection. Recurrence usually signals reactivation of the person's own virus, not a reinfection.

For unknown reasons, some people have symptomatic warts that are treated and never recur, whereas others have frequent recurrences. Many people who have compromised immune systems, such as those with AIDS, have warts that are persistent and difficult to treat, but not everyone who has frequently recurring warts has AIDS. One factor that has been linked to frequent recurrences in people with intact immune systems is stress, possibly because stress suppresses the immune system. However, it can be counterproductive to tell someone that frequent outbreaks of warts are due to stress, because this will probably cause the person to experience even *more* stress.

Cigarette smoking has also been linked to frequent recurrences, again probably because the practice suppresses the immune system. One study showed that women who smoke are four times as likely as nonsmoking women to develop visible warts. This finding probably applies to men as well. As discussed later, smoking is also a risk factor for the development of cervical cancer and anal cancer.

A lack of folate in the diet is another apparent cause of frequent recurrences. Folate (or folic acid) can be obtained by eating green, leafy vegetables or by taking a multivitamin daily. Some studies have hinted at the role of antioxidants—such as vitamins A, C, and E, and beta-carotene—in helping to prevent cancer, including cervical cancer due to HPV. Studies have also shown that these nutrients may offer better protection if they are obtained through the diet rather than from a supplement. It is important to remember that for women, having visible genital warts does not mean you have a higher risk of cervical cancer.

HOW IS HPV TRANSMITTED?

Human papillomavirus is transmitted from one person to another through skin-to-skin contact with an infected partner. HPV is not transmitted through blood or genital secretions. The warts viruses may be transmitted even if someone doesn't have visible warts. Condoms may not offer complete protection against transmission, since areas infected with the virus may be outside the areas covered by the condom. The genital types of the virus are most easily transmitted to the thinner skin of the genitals, such as that of the mucous membranes of the vulva, vagina, and cervix for women and of the penis and scrotum for men. The strains of HPV that cause genital warts most often stay in the genital area, although they may rarely be transmitted to the face through oral sex. It is also possible, although very rare, for a person to transmit warts virus to the genitals from another area of the body, in a process called *autoinoculation*. However, most genital warts are transmitted through sexual contact and not through autoinoculation. There is also a small possibility that the virus can be transmitted by inanimate objects, such as towels, although this has not been proved.

> The warts virus can be transmitted even without visible warts being present.

It is difficult, if not impossible, to determine where someone acquired the infection, because of the often long lag time between infection and the development of symptoms, as well as the lack of an adequate screening test for HPV. Transmission can occur whether or not a person infected with HPV has visible warts at the time, and most people don't know that they may be infectious. Whether or not removing the visible warts serves to decrease the likelihood of transmission is not known, but it is assumed that doing so may help to decrease the chance of transmission. Treatment, as described later in this section, is usually performed for cosmetic reasons.

It is generally believed that after several months of sexual contact with an infected partner, the likelihood is high that HPV has been transmitted, whether or not the infected partner was showing symptoms at the time of contact. Studies are under way to provide more information about HPV transmission, but for now there is no test to tell who is or is not contagious. As already discussed, the more sexual partners a person has in his or her lifetime, the higher the chance of becoming infected, whether or not symptoms are present. Because there are no tests available at this time to screen for HPV, it is difficult if not impossible to identify when or from whom infection takes place. This lack of information is, understandably, frustrating for many people. In research studies that have sought to detect the genetic material of the virus, up to 70 percent of the presumably "uninfected" partners of people with a history of HPV were also found to have HPV.

Condom use may help in preventing transmission of the virus. However, as noted above, because the virus is present in the entire genital area, not just the part that a condom covers, the condom may not provide complete protection. Although the effectiveness of both male and female condoms in preventing HPV transmission is not known, using a condom with new partners is still recommended because it may decrease the risk of transmission, and there is evidence that condom use is associated with a decreased risk of cervical cancer in women, increased clearance of the virus in women, and improvement in visible genital warts in men. It is still a good idea not to have sex with a new partner if warts are present (since, with visible warts, there may be a higher risk of passing the virus, although as mentioned above, the virus can be passed even if no visible warts are present) and, again, to use a condom with a new partner.

For couples in long-term relationships in which there is a good chance that the virus has already been transmitted, using condoms to prevent HPV transmission is of uncertain value. Anyone with a history of genital warts should talk with prospective partners about HPV and other STDs (see Chapter 4 on sexual communication). Each couple needs to make decisions about condom use together. It is unlikely that people become reinfected with the same strain of HPV over and over again, and recurrences in one partner are not linked to recurrences (if there are any) in the other partner. However, treatment of visible warts and the use of condoms might decrease infectiousness.

Given that most sexually active people have the virus and that most are completely symptom free (though they can still transmit the virus), the most worrisome outcome from an infection with HPV is the increased risk for skin or anal cancer in men and women and for cervical cancer in women. The number of people who develop these complications is relatively small, and appropriate routine screening, such as Pap smears for women, can detect cancer in its earliest stages, when it can be successfully treated. As mentioned earlier, a new vaccine was recently approved by the FDA and is now available that prevents infection with the most common strains of HPV that cause external warts (about 90% of which are caused by types 6 and 11) and cervical cancer (about 70% caused by types 16 and 18). The study that showed the effectiveness of the vaccine was done in women, and the vaccine will be most effective for women and girls who have not yet become sexually active (and thus not exposed to the virus). The FDA has approved the vaccine for females aged nine to twenty-six. The vaccine will be given in three shots over six months. Whether it will offer lifelong immunity or will require booster shots is not known. Also, it is important to remember that this vaccine does not protect against all strains of warts virus that can cause visible warts or cancer. This means that Pap smears will still be important after this vaccine is available. Research and time will tell whether the vaccine is also beneficial to men. A vaccine that protects against HPV types 16 and 18 alone is also showing promise, and may be available soon. Research is also under way on the development of vaccines to treat symptoms from existing HPV infection.

Another way HPV can be transmitted is from mother to child. Infants may become infected in the womb (possibly through the amniotic fluid) or through contact with the virus at delivery. However, infection via these routes is very rare, especially given how common the virus is.

When a child is diagnosed with genital warts, it does not automatically mean that the child is a victim of sexual abuse, although this possibility must be investigated. Children can be infected at birth by mothers who are themselves carrying HPV, and, as already noted, the infection can take months or years to produce symptoms. Children can be infected through an inanimate object, such as a towel (which, as discussed previously, is possible but unlikely), or through close nonsexual contact with a family member who is infected. Each situation must be addressed individually.

If a mother has visible warts at delivery, she can—although this is rare—pass the virus to her child, causing warts on the larynx (voice box) and occasionally on the eyes or genital area. Laryngeal warts are treatable, although this condition can be serious and recurrent in children. The most common types of HPV found in affected infants are the most common strains that cause visible warts: types 6 and 11. The virus can be passed on to the child even if there are no visible warts at delivery; given the large number of women infected with the virus, it is surprising how rarely this occurs. The virus may be passed to the fetus while in the womb, although this route of transmission is also thought to be very rare.

Mother-to-child transmission of HPV is fortunately very uncommon.

Having the HPV virus does not prevent a woman from becoming pregnant, nor does it increase her risk of a miscarriage or premature labor. However, the virus sometimes becomes more active during pregnancy. If extensive warts are present at delivery, a cesarean delivery may be recommended, especially if the warts are extensive enough to block the birth canal. Cesarean delivery may decrease the risk of HPV transmission to the child, although some babies born by this method still develop warts on the larynx (possibly by transmission through the amniotic fluid in the womb). Therefore, a cesarean delivery is usually not recommended solely for the purpose of preventing transmission of the virus to the newborn. A better approach is to treat warts well before delivery so that they are not present during and cannot interfere with delivery. If the warts are not extensive at delivery, a vaginal delivery is still recommended, because the risk of transmission is low. Talk with your health care provider if you have concerns. The risks and benefits of cesarean deliveries need to be considered, and this is best done one-on-one with your health care provider. Research is under way to determine the best way to prevent laryngeal warts in children born from mothers who have HPV infection.

TESTING FOR HPV

Genital warts have a very characteristic appearance and can generally be recognized by an experienced health care provider. There is a new way to screen for the genetic material of the virus that causes warts (called the Hybrid Capture 2 HPV DNA test). Using samples from the cervix, the test can detect the virus even in women who are otherwise symptom free and determine whether they have the "low-risk" type or the "high-risk" types (types 16 and 18) of HPV. However, this is not a test for screening people who have no symptoms. Its proven use is in helping to clarify abnormal Pap smears (see below).

The health care provider will carefully examine the entire genital and anal area to look for warts. The anal area is often overlooked by health care providers, especially when they are examining heterosexuals, but even without a history of anal sexual contact this is an area where warts can recur. The mouth should also be examined if the person has engaged in oral-genital contact. It is possible, although very uncommon, to see warts in this area.

One of the treatments for warts, freezing them with liquid nitrogen, can also help to diagnose them. Warts tend to "hold" the freeze longer than the surrounding normal skin, so they stay white from the freeze longer. This characteristic can be helpful to distinguish them from skin tags (little pieces of excess skin), which do not react in this way. However, this is not always the case. Applying vinegar (3 percent acetic acid) may also make warts show up more clearly—warts tend to turn white with acetic acid, which normal skin does not do. This is not a specific test, however, and skin bumps that are not warts can also turn white with this test, leading to unnecessary treatment. In addition, the fact that areas of the skin show no white areas when washed with vinegar does not mean that a person is not infected with the virus. It only means that there are no detectable warts present at that time.

For women a procedure called a *colposcopy* is sometimes performed to look for evidence of warts on the cervix that are not easily visible to the naked eye. The *colposcope* is a machine with a large magnifying scope to view the cervix. A colposcopy is most commonly done to look for evidence of warts on the cervix of a woman who has had an abnormal Pap smear, since it is impossible to see the cervix closely without it. It can also be used to examine external skin. Pap smears, which are discussed later in this section, look for the changes that the warts virus can cause on the cervix and that can lead to cervical cancer. The Pap smear is not a reliable screen for the warts virus itself—it is a screen for cervical cancer. Changes in the cells of the

cervix may be reported on a Pap
smear as "suggestive of" or "consistent with" HPV, a finding that
may help make the diagnosis. In
addition, a normal Pap smear

**There is no reliable test to
screen for the warts virus in
people who are symptom free.**

does not mean that a woman is not infected with the warts virus; it
merely means that the virus has not caused a precancerous or cancerous change in the cervix.

It is important to keep in mind that there is no screening for HPV
in people who do not have symptoms. So whether someone's immune
system has gotten rid of the virus, or the virus is just in a "quiet" stage
but may cause symptoms later, is impossible to tell. However, the
new test, mentioned earlier, is being used to look for the genetic material of the virus (the nucleic acid DNA), which may be done on the
same specimen used for a Pap smear, or on a biopsy specimen taken
during a colposcopy. The test may be used during a routine Pap smear,
particularly for women over thirty years old or to help sort out
whether an abnormal Pap smear (called ASCUS—see "The Pap
Smear" later in this section) is likely to be precancerous because the
types of HPV known to pose a risk for cervical cancer are present. Testing for HPV is not a routine part of Pap smears, particularly for women
under thirty who have always had normal Pap smears.

However, even if the types of HPV found on this test are a risk for
cervical cancer, this does not necessarily mean that the woman will
develop cervical cancer at some point in the future. In fact, most
women with these viruses do *not* develop cervical cancer. With appropriate follow-up and monitoring by Pap smears, cervical cancer is
a preventable disease.

TREATMENT

About 20 percent of small warts disappear on their own without treatment. Therefore someone who has a history of warts may want to delay treatment for a few weeks to determine whether a new wart will
resolve on its own. For someone who has difficulty in identifying
warts, a visit to a health care provider is probably a good idea.

The goal of treatment is getting rid of the visible warts, since as
yet there is no way to get rid of the virus once infection has taken

place. Although some people may spontaneously clear the virus once they are infected, no treatment clears the virus completely. Treating the entire genital area using the methods described here—most of which destroy the skin cells in which the virus resides—has not proven effective in eliminating the HPV, and it is extremely painful. If the warts are irritating, uncomfortable, or cosmetically unacceptable, then treatment is recommended.

There is no good evidence that treating the warts eliminates the risk of transmission to others, but it may at least decrease the risk. Treatment of the warts also does not eliminate the possibility of recurrences. In fact, most people who have symptomatic warts will experience recurrences. Warts can be difficult to treat in people who smoke, women who are pregnant, people whose immune systems are suppressed (from drugs such as steroids or from medical conditions such as AIDS), and people with autoimmune diseases such as lupus or skin conditions such as eczema.

> The purpose of treatment is to remove the visible wart. The wart may recur after treatment.

Vaccines are being developed that may prevent people from becoming infected with the warts virus and may possibly aid in the treatment of warts in people who are already infected. Until they become available, however, the following treatments are recommended. You and your health care provider should decide together which treatment is best for you. If one treatment doesn't work, you may want to try another. The treatments described below sometimes cause discoloration of the skin and, rarely, scarring; they are options for the treatment of warts on the external skin, except where noted.

Cryotherapy

Freezing warts with liquid nitrogen is a common treatment for both external warts and warts on the cervix. Cervical warts are always evaluated first by colposcopy and biopsied to make sure they are not cancer before they are treated with cryotherapy. This treatment destroys the skin cells where the virus is located. It is not recommended for vaginal warts, however, since freezing this fragile tissue may damage the walls of the vagina and cause a fistula (a track or tunnel leading to deeper tissues). The same goes for warts inside the anus and rectum, which must be treated by an expert such as a proctologist or gastro-intestinal surgeon.

Using a Q-tip or a liquid nitrogen spray gun, the health care provider applies liquid nitrogen to, or sprays liquid nitrogen on, each wart for 10–20 seconds—long enough to freeze the wart but not long enough to cause scarring. The liquid nitrogen treatment itself is slightly painful, and the wart usually becomes red and irritated over the next few days. A small blister may form. If the wart is not gone in a week or two, retreatment may be necessary. Retreatment is in fact often necessary, especially if the warts were large when first treated. This method has a clearance rate of 68 percent and a recurrence rate of 21–39 percent. It is an acceptable treatment during pregnancy.

Topical Treatments

In topical treatments, either podophyllin (10–25% solution) or trichloracetic acid (TCA; 80–90% solution) is painted on external warts on the genitals and near the anus, either alone or in combination with liquid nitrogen. The treatments are applied only to the warts and not to the surrounding, normal skin, since they can be irritating to normal tissue. These treatments destroy the skin cells where the virus is located, and podophyllin also prevents wart cells from dividing.

Podophyllin, which has been used as a treatment for warts for half a century, is applied only to visible external warts. It is not used on warts on the mucosal skin (as in the inner labia, vagina, or urethra), because it can be absorbed into the system and cause side effects. Application of podophyllin is usually not painful, although it must be washed off four to six hours after application in order to avoid irritation of the skin. A follow-up visit for repeat treatment is recommended in one or two weeks if the wart does not clear up. This method of treatment has a clearance rate of 32–79 percent and a recurrence rate of 27–65 percent. It should not be used during pregnancy, and should be used only on small areas of warts, without open skin.

Milder-strength podophyllin is available by prescription as either a solution or a gel. Called podofilox (0.5% podophyllin), it is used primarily to treat external genital warts and is most effective for small warts. Podofilox is applied to the warts twice a day for three days (without washing it off), followed by a four-day period of no treatment. This cycle can be repeated for up to a total of four weeks. If the warts are not gone by then, stronger treatment must be obtained from a health care provider. (For larger warts, stronger treatment may be necessary from the start.) Podofilox is not recommended for warts that are difficult to reach.

Podofilox is a treatment option for people who are traveling or are otherwise unable to get to a health care provider easily. Although it is expensive, it may nevertheless be economical if a person does not have to visit a health care provider for treatment. It has a clearance rate of 45–88 percent and a recurrence rate of 33–60 percent. It should not be used during pregnancy.

TCA stings when applied and may cause more scarring than podophyllin. It can be used safely on warts on the mucosal surfaces of the body, such as the inner labia and the vagina, as well as on external warts on the genitals and around the anus. It can be used for urethral opening ("meatus") warts. TCA is applied only to visible warts. After treatment with TCA, a follow-up visit is recommended in about a week, when the irritation from the first treatment has healed, to determine whether the wart has persisted. TCA has about a 70–81 percent success rate in clearing the visible wart after treatment and a recurrence rate of 36 percent. It is safe to use during pregnancy.

Electrosurgery

In electrosurgery, an electrified blade or wire is used to cut out a wart, usually after the area has been numbed with a local anesthetic. It can be used to treat oral warts, external genital warts, and warts around the anus. This is one of the more expensive treatments, and although it may be slightly more effective than topical treatments, the success rate depends to a large extent on the skill of the health care provider performing the procedure. It has a clearance rate of 35–94 percent and a recurrence rate of 22 percent.

Surgery

Surgery on warts is usually performed with a scalpel after the area to be treated has first been numbed with a local anesthetic. Surgery is often the treatment of choice for very extensive warts, either in the external genital area or in the anal area, and it can be used for oral warts as well. After the procedure stitches may be used to close the area. This is another more expensive treatment. It has a clearance rate of 93 percent and a recurrence rate of 29 percent.

Laser Surgery

In laser surgery, a high-intensity beam of light is focused on the affected tissue, usually with the aid of a microscope, in order to remove it. The procedure is primarily recommended for extensive external genital or anal warts. The success of the procedure depends on the skill of the health care provider performing the surgery. Because it is expensive and usually involves an outpatient visit to a hospital and general anesthesia, it is most often recommended for warts that are difficult to treat or extensive. It has a clearance rate of 27–82 percent and a recurrence rate of 95 percent. Podophyllin, podofilox, imiquimod (see below), TCA, and cryotherapy are preferred over laser surgery.

The entire genital area should not be treated with the laser in an attempt to rid the genitals of the virus; this treatment method has been shown to cause precancerous changes in the vagina from the extensive tissue destruction.

Imiquimod

Imiquimod is a topical cream that triggers the body's own immune response in the treatment of external warts (it is not to be used for warts of the vagina, cervix, or inner anal area). It is less painful than some of the other treatments. Imiquimod is applied in a thin layer three times a week on alternating nights, at home, for up to sixteen weeks (though many people clear their warts in much less than sixteen weeks). It is washed off in the morning, six to ten hours after application. The advantages of this treatment, despite the sometimes lengthy treatment time, are that the recurrence rate is lower and that, like podofilox, it can be used at home. It seems to work better for women than men. Women have a clearance rate of 72–84 percent; men have a clearance rate of 33–59 percent. The recurrence rate is 5–19 percent in women and 6–23 percent in men.

Imiquimod is an option for people who are traveling or who for any other reason cannot visit their health care provider for treatments.

It is expensive and should not be used with barrier methods of birth control, such as condoms and diaphragms, because it makes them more likely to break or leak. It can cause redness and irritation of the skin as well as skin ulcerations, but there is usually less pain than with the other topical treatments. The safety of imiquimod in pregnancy is not known. It is approved for use by people aged twelve and older.

REGARDLESS of which treatment procedure is used, follow-up treatments are often necessary to get rid of a wart completely, depending on its size when first treated and its location. Talk with your provider about which treatment would be best for you.

If warts do not respond after several attempts at treatment, then the diagnosis or treatment should be reconsidered. Warts that are unusual looking should be biopsied to rule out the possibility of cancer.

Finally, there are two treatments that are *not* recommended. Injection of the medication alpha-interferon into the base of the wart is a painful treatment for warts and usually does not produce better results than the medications and procedures described above. It is not recommended for the treatment of warts and is unsafe during pregnancy. Similarly, topical treatment with 5-fluorouracil cream is not recommended at this time, although clinical trials are under way that may ultimately prove the usefulness of this treatment.

THE RISK OF CANCER

As mentioned earlier, some strains of HPV cause cervical cancer and also make people more likely to develop skin cancer in the genital area, particularly anal cancer and penile cancer in men and vulvar cancer in women. *The percentage of people who have the genital warts virus and go on to develop cancer is very small,* considering that 40–70 percent of the population may be infected with HPV.

Cancer of the vulva in women and the penis in men and anal carcinoma in men and women are most commonly caused by HPV types 16 and 18, which are not the most common types that cause external warts. On the other hand, if warts in these areas of the body have an unusual appearance, a biopsy should be performed to screen for cancer. A health care provider who has experience in treating warts should be consulted. There is no good way to screen for these types of cancer other than through visual examination. Use of Pap smear techniques to screen for anal cancer is being considered, but is not yet routine.

Each year in the United States, approximately 12,000 women develop cervical cancer, and about 4000 women die each year from the disease. Types 16 and 18 of the warts virus have the strongest connection with cervical cancer, but some of the other strains have also been linked to cancer. HPV types 16 and 18 are the most common types of warts virus found in sexually active adults, and when cervical cancer lesions are studied, types 16 and 18 are found in the lesions about 90 percent of the time. However, these are not the types that usually cause external warts; those are types 6 and 11.

Cervical cancer is not the most common cancer among women; lung cancer is, which is a good reason to quit smoking! Another good reason to quit is that there seems to be a link between HPV, cervical cancer, and smoking. Smoking causes damage to the immune system. In women who have HPV and cervical dysplasia and who smoke, the dysplasia is more likely to progress to more serious stages of cancer. Also, people with HPV and visible genital warts are more likely to have recurrences if they smoke.

> A very small percentage of the millions of women infected with HPV develop cervical cancer. A yearly Pap smear and pelvic examination will usually detect the changes that the warts virus can cause on the cervix and that may lead to cervical cancer, while it is in the early, treatable, and curable stages.

Cervical cancer occurs among both young women and older women. Women who have sex with men as well as women who have sex with other women are susceptible to infection with the warts viruses and therefore are at risk for cervical cancer. *Cervical cancer is completely curable if it is detected early enough.* In fact the number of women who develop cervical cancer has decreased dramatically over the years because of screening by means of the Pap smear, which is effective at detecting abnormal changes in the cells of the cervix, called *cervical dysplasia*, that can lead to cervical cancer. Women who do not understand the importance of this yearly screen, along with a pelvic examination, or who for one reason or another decide not to follow up on the results, miss an important opportunity to protect their health.

It is not clear why some women develop cervical cancer from HPV infection and others do not, although it is likely that when a woman with HPV develops cervical cancer it is the result of a combination of risk factors. Some possible risk factors are:

—Smoking (and possibly even second-hand smoke)
—Having first sexual intercourse at a young age
—Having multiple sexual partners
—Having a compromised immune system
—Lack of folic acid, vitamins D or C, and beta-carotene in the diet
—Having a history of other sexually transmitted infections
—Having a sexual partner with a history of multiple sexual partners
—Long-term use of oral contraceptives (according to some but not all studies)

Although the use of oral contraceptive pills may be a potential risk factor for the development of cervical dysplasia in women with HPV (possibly because of the mild suppression of the immune system caused by the hormones in the pills), it is not recommended that women with HPV discontinue taking birth control pills for this reason.

Anal cancer is rare in the United States. The types of HPV (types 17 and 18) that increase the risk for cervical cancer also increase the risk for anal cancer. As in cervical cancer, precancerous changes in the anal area, called "dysplasia," if left untreated, can progress to cancer. However, not everyone who has anal cancer has evidence of HPV infection. Although a history of receiving anal sex is a risk for anal cancer, 85 percent of people who develop anal cancer report they have never received anal sex. Other risks for anal cancer include smoking and age over fifty. Also, women who have cervical dysplasia may have a higher risk of developing anal dysplasia, and possibly cancer. People who have a compromised immune system, such as those with HIV infection, are also at a much greater risk for anal cancer. However, many people with anal cancer do not have any obvious risk factors; much remains unknown. Symptoms of anal cancer may be very nonspecific: anal itching, bleeding, irritation (all of which could also be caused by benign, common problems such as hemorrhoids), and difficulty in having bowel movements.

Pap smears of the anal area and genetic testing for the virus are not yet standard health care procedures. Research is being carried out to determine whether this routine testing may be of benefit. Some have proposed that testing should be done for people at high risk (such as HIV-positive homosexual or bisexual men who receive anal intercourse, and HIV-positive women who receive anal intercourse). The best way to diagnose anal cancer is by visual inspection, *anoscopy* (the health care provider inserts a small scope into the anal area to visualize the inner tissues), and biopsy of any suspicious areas. For couples engaging in anal intercourse, condom use may decrease, but not eliminate, the risk for anal cancer again, because a condom does not protect the entire area where HPV may be present.

Talk with your health care provider about screening and prevention for anal cancer, particularly if you are at high risk (you have received anal sex or are HIV positive). There is no defined role for the HPV DNA test in screening for anal cancer or skin cancers in men or women.

For men, another risk associated with HPV is skin cancers of the genitals, such as Bowen's disease and bowenoid papulosis, as well as the rare cancer of the penis. All of these are squamous cell cancers of the genital skin. About a third of men with penile cancer show evidence of HPV infection (meaning that other factors, unknown at this time, are a risk for this type of cancer). Being uncircumcised may be a risk for acquiring genital warts, as well as a risk for penile cancer. One theory is that men who are uncircumcised and who do not routinely clean under the foreskin (lack of routine cleaning may cause chronic inflammation) may be at higher risk for penile cancer. Another is that uncircumcised men have a larger amount of "mucosal" skin on the penis, which may be more vulnerable to infection with the virus. There is no current evidence that HPV infection is a risk for prostate cancer. Again, the vast majority of men with HPV infection never develop cancer of any kind.

Women may develop lesions on the vulva and vagina from HPV, which in very rare cases can lead to cancer. This is most common among older women or women who have compromised immune systems (such as women with HIV infection), but younger women may also develop these conditions. However, the presence of these lesions does not mean a woman has HIV infection! Risks for cancer of the vulva and vagina are similar to those for cervical cancer (see above). Evaluation is done by visual inspection of the genitals and of internal vaginal areas during a speculum exam; treatment of HPV lesions in the vaginal canal is usually done with TCA. The health care provider will take a biopsy of any lesions on the vulva or vagina that look suspicious.

THE PAP SMEAR

The Pap smear is one of medical history's success stories for preventing a disease, cervical cancer. The test is named after the man who developed it, George Papanicolaou. Over the forty years since the use of Pap smears began, there has been a 70 percent reduction in the number of women diagnosed with invasive cervical cancer. However, about 12,000 women in the United States are diagnosed each year with cervical cancer; and almost 4000 women die of the disease each year. A Pap smear is an important test because it provides early evidence of cancer, and many women with cervical cancer have no symptoms in the early, treatable stages.

The Pap smear is recommended as a screen for all women over the age of eighteen, or earlier if a woman becomes sexually active at a younger age. *All* women, not just young women, need to be screened for cervical cancer. In fact, as many as one of every four women in the United States who are diagnosed with cervical cancer is over the age of sixty-five. Not just women who have sex with men, but also women who have sex with other women need to get yearly Pap smears, because HPV can be passed through genital contact, not just by intercourse.

Even if a woman has delayed having a Pap smear for several years, she should have this very important health screen as soon as possible, because it can detect precancerous changes early, so that treatment can be initiated that will prevent or cure cervical cancer. For women who have a history of external warts (or women who have partners with a history of external warts) and a normal Pap smear, the recommended schedule for Pap smears is no different than for any sexually active woman, because most sexually active women have the warts virus even if they have never had symptoms.

There are two ways to examine cells from the cervix. One is to rub cells onto a glass slide, which is then preserved with a fixative and sent to the laboratory for review. The other, newer method involves placing the cells in a liquid; this technique may provide better accuracy, because it allows the cells to maintain their shape better than does the older method. Women under age thirty should have a Pap smear every year if the traditional glass slide technique is used, every two years if the liquid-based Pap test is used. At age thirty and after, if a woman has had three consecutively normal Pap smears, she can switch to every other year (no matter which method is used to evaluate the sample), or every third year, if she has had three normal Pap tests in combination with the HPV DNA test. Why the cut-off at age thirty? Many sexually active people under the age of thirty have HPV infection, and it is thought that many of them (possibly as many as 80%) clear the infection at some point. So a positive HPV DNA test does not predict whether a woman under the age of thirty will have a problem later in life. A woman over thirty found to be positive for HPV has a greater chance of having had the infection for a long time, and therefore of being at higher risk for problems resulting from the infection. However, again, even women over thirty who have HPV are not destined to get cervical cancer; considering how common the virus is, cancer is an extremely rare event.

Not all Pap smears that come back as "abnormal" are abnormal because of precancer or cancer. As discussed below, some abnormal Pap smears result from conditions that are not serious, or are reversible or easily treated. Also, cervical cancer usually doesn't happen overnight. It typically takes years for changes to occur that become cancer; so, getting Pap smears at the recommended intervals makes cervical cancer, in most cases, a preventable disease. And, if detected in its earliest, or precancerous, stages, cervical cancer is curable.

In menstruating women, the best time for a Pap smear is between one and two weeks after a menstrual period. Results are not as reliable if the test is performed during menstruation. For best results, a woman should not have intercourse or douche and should not use intravaginal creams or tampons within two days of having the test.

A woman who has had a hysterectomy that involved the removal of the cervix for a reason other than cervical or uterine cancer does not need to get yearly Pap smears. If her ovaries were not removed, then a yearly examination to determine the size of the ovaries is still recommended. If a woman had a hysterectomy because of cervical cancer or "precancerous lesions," then follow-up Pap smears are recommended. Women who have had a normal Pap smear three times in a row may not need to get the test as frequently. Talk with your health care provider about how often you should have a Pap smear. Women over the age of seventy who have an intact cervix, who have had three or more documented and consecutive normal Pap smears, and who did not have an abnormal smear within the past ten years, can stop having Pap smears.

Women whose immune systems are compromised, such as those infected with HIV, should have more frequent Pap smears, since they risk having a more rapid progression to cervical cancer. A Pap smear is generally recommended every six months for HIV-positive women, but can be done yearly thereafter if the result is good. The test should be done more frequently if abnormalities are noted, and colposcopy is often recommended right away, rather than a "watch and wait" approach. New tests for the genetic material of HPV may allow HIV-positive women to have less frequent Pap smears; stay tuned.

Health care providers must take an adequate specimen, so that there are enough cells for an accurate evaluation. This step is essential, and a woman should feel entirely free to ask her health care provider about it. This will be indicated on the result of the Pap smear that the laboratory issues. If an adequate specimen was not obtained, a repeat smear will be necessary.

Two types of cells are seen on the cervix: the *columnar cells* line the inside of the cervix and are also found in the uterus; the *squamous cells* are on the outside of the cervix and are also found in the vagina. They meet on the cervix in an area called the *transformation zone* or *squamocolumnar junction*, which may be inside the cervix in a woman over the age of thirty or on the outside of the cervix in a younger woman or a woman taking birth control pills. Cells for the Pap smear are taken from this area, since these rapidly dividing cells have the highest risk for changes that can lead to cervical cancer.

Pap smear results are reported in four ways, known as the class system, the Bethesda system, the CIN (cervical intraepithelial neoplasia) system, and the descriptive system. Which system is used depends on the laboratory to which the specimen was sent. The Bethesda system is now used by most laboratories. The results are reported as follows:

1. Class I
   Bethesda system: within normal limits
   CIN system: normal
   Return at regularly scheduled interval for next Pap screening

2. Class II
   Bethesda system: infection, reactive or reparative changes seen, or atypical squamous cells of unknown significance (ASCUS) or atypical glandular cells of undetermined significance (AGUS). Although this is still considered a "negative" Pap smear in terms of cancer screening, either infection or "atypical cells" may be seen, and these may or may not be precancerous. Many things that can cause an ASCUS Pap smear are not cancer. These include menstrual blood, vaginal creams or gels, recent intercourse or use of a tampon, yeast infections, atrophy (thinning) of the tissues (as seen in postmenopausal women), and use of an intrauterine device. Other terms that may be used for this Pap result are "benign cellular changes," possibly indicating the presence of an infection that needs to be treated, and "reactive cellular changes," which often means temporary inflammation or irritation and usually does not require treatment. Your health care provider can provide guidance about the need for treatment.

   Traditionally, any infection that is found is treated and a follow-up Pap smear done, usually in four to six months. If no abnormality is present on the follow-up smear, another one is recommended in four to six months, and then another four to six months later. If this last one is normal, then a woman can resume her normal schedule of Pap smears. If a persistent abnormality is seen on any of the follow-up Pap smears, a colposcopy is recommended. (Sometimes, however, a health care provider is concerned about the initial Pap smear finding and performs a colposcopy right away.) This is how all ASCUS Pap smears were handled before 1999, and many abnormalities resolved on their own, without intervention.

   Now, the new test that looks for the genetic material of HPV helps to distinguish the worrisome (i.e., precancerous) ASCUS smears from the less concerning (those caused by infection or inflammation). The sample for HPV testing is collected at the same time as the Pap smear, as long as the liquid-based Pap is done; if the slide method is used, you may need to come back for an HPV test if your health care provider decides this is necessary. The test helps to determine whether the worrisome types of HPV (types 16 and 18) are present. If they are, your health care provider will probably recommend a colposcopy rather than the older "watch and wait" approach over a period of eighteen months. Although neither approach is 100 percent accurate, the HPV test done with the Pap smear is more sensitive in accurately detecting abnormalities than the repeat Pap smear method.

An AGUS Pap smear (atypical glandular cells of undetermined significance) may indicate a rarer problem with the glandular cells of the cervix. As with an ASCUS Pap smear, this problem is usually not cancer, but to make sure, colposcopy is recommended. Cancer of the glandular cells of the cervix accounts for 10–15 percent of cervical cancers and is much less common than cancer of the squamous cells (85–95%).

3. Class III
   Bethesda system: squamous intraepithelial lesion (low- to high-grade squamous intraepithelial lesion, or SIL)
   CIN system: CIN 1–3
   Descriptive system: dysplasia (mild to severe)
   This category encompasses a wide range of possible Pap smear results. In general, the lower the grade or number, the lower the need for concern, although close follow-up is recommended for all women whose Pap results fall into this category. About two-thirds of the lower-grade lesions resolve without treatment.

   For the lower-grade lesions (low-grade SIL, CIN 1, or mild dysplasia), a colposcopy and biopsy of suspicious areas is recommended.

   If the Pap smear comes back as a higher-grade lesion (high-grade SIL, CIN 2 or 3, or moderate or severe dysplasia), then a colposcopy is recommended, with a biopsy of any abnormal areas and treatment as appropriate. About a third of the changes in this category progress to cancer if not treated. Close follow-up is essential.

4. Class IV

Bethesda system: high-grade SIL

CIN system: CIN 4

Descriptive system: carcinoma in situ (CIS)

Although this is not a finding of cancer, it indicates more worrisome changes than those described previously and has a higher chance to progress to cancer. A colposcopy should be performed, and treatment is indicated if any malignant changes are found.

5. Class V

Bethesda system: squamous cell carcinoma or adenocarcinoma

CIN system: invasive squamous cell carcinoma or adenocarcinoma

Descriptive system: positive for malignant cells

This finding indicates invasive cervical cancer—either *squamous cell carcinoma,* which results from malignant changes in the outer cells of the cervix, or *adenocarcinoma,* which results from malignant changes in the inner cells of the cervix. A colposcopy must be performed, and treatment is indicated.

When a woman has her yearly examination, she should speak with her health care provider about her Pap smear results and understand what they mean. She may also want to ask for a copy of the results for her own files. If you don't hear about your Pap smear result, don't assume that everything is O.K. If your health care provider doesn't contact you, make sure you get in touch with your health care provider to find out the result.

When the Pap smear result indicates an abnormality of dysplasia or cancer, there are several options for treatment. They can be treated by cryotherapy, removal of part of the cervix, laser surgery, loop electrosurgical excision procedure (LEEP), or surgical excision, including *cervical conization* (in which a cone of tissue is removed from the cervix). Even advanced lesions may be cured with these procedures.

The progression from precancerous changes to cervical cancer is very slow. Many women with HPV are concerned about the risk of cervical cancer, fearing that they have a ticking time bomb inside them. This is simply not true for the majority of women with HPV. If a woman follows the recommendations given here, having routine Pap smears and appropriate follow-up and treatment of any visible external warts, then she need not worry unduly about the risk of cancer. Certainly most of the millions of women infected with HPV do not develop these complications.

A final note: The Pap smear is not a test for STDs, such as chlamydia and gonorrhea, although many people mistakenly think that it does provide a screen for all STDs. Specific tests must be performed for these infections. Sexually transmitted infections such as herpes (if there are lesions on the cervix) and mucopurulent cervicitis can cause inflammation on the cervix, which also may result in an abnormal Pap smear. It is often better to defer the Pap smear until these infections have been treated and have resolved, so that the Pap smear can accurately perform its intended function: identifying problems caused by the warts virus.

GONORRHEA

incidence: common
cause: bacterium (*Neisseria gonorrhoeae*)
symptoms: burning with urination, discharge, pelvic pain, spotting between periods
treatment: antibiotics

WHAT IS IT?

Gonorrhea is a sexually transmitted infection caused by the bacterium *Neisseria gonorrhoeae*. This bacterium can cause a number of genital infections: infection of the urethra, cervix, and pelvic organs (causing pelvic inflammatory disease, or PID) in women, and the urethra, epididymis, and prostate in men. Women who have had a hysterectomy can contract a gonorrheal infection in the urethra and genital glands. The bacterium can also cause infection of the throat, conjunctiva, and rectum; joint infection; and meningitis. People who become infected with gonorrhea may be at increased risk of acquiring and transmitting other sexually transmitted diseases, including HIV infection.

HOW COMMON IS IT?

Anyone can become infected with gonorrhea, and although the overall number of people infected in the United States each year is decreasing, among young people the number is increasing. The reported rates of gonorrhea are highest among women aged fifteen to nineteen. More than 600,000 people are infected each year in this country, more commonly young, sexually active persons and those with multiple sexual partners. Also at higher risk are women who do not use a barrier method of birth control and who use oral contraceptives (the pill), since this practice makes the cervix more vulnerable to infections. Some women erroneously believe that the pill offers protection against STDs (this is *not* true) and so they do not use condoms; this practice puts them at higher risk for infection.

The rate of gonorrheal infection is increasing among young, sexually active adults.

Women who have sexual contact only with other women are unlikely to become infected with gonorrhea, since there is usually no contact with the cervix. However, if sex toys are used, there may be a possibility of transmitting gonorrhea.

WHAT ARE THE SYMPTOMS?

Men are more likely to be symptomatic than women: 90 percent of men have symptoms; 60–80 percent of women have symptoms. If a person infected with gonorrhea experiences symptoms, the symptoms usually appear within a few days of infection, but they may develop at any time from one day to a few weeks afterward.

Although many people with gonorrhea experience symptoms, both men and women can have a gonorrheal infection and be symptom free.

Women

Symptoms of cervical infection with gonorrhea are discharge (often yellow) from the vagina and spotting between periods or after sexual intercourse. Between 10 and 20 percent of women who are infected with gonorrhea develop PID. With PID, the infection moves from the cervix up into the uterus, Fallopian tubes, and ovaries, and there can be pain in the pelvis, pain with intercourse, and fever in addition to discharge and bleeding. There is a risk of infertility caused by the scarring that can occur; this scarring also puts women at increased risk of an ectopic pregnancy (a pregnancy outside the womb, such as in the Fallopian tubes). Pelvic pain from the scarring caused by an untreated gonorrheal infection can be chronic—lasting a lifetime for some women.

A woman can also acquire a gonorrheal infection of the Bartholin's glands; located inside the vaginal opening, these glands provide lubrication for the vagina. Gonorrheal infection of these glands causes a painful, noticeable swelling at the vaginal opening. The urethra can also become infected by gonorrhea in women, causing painful urination which may feel like that experienced with a common bladder infection. Finally, the gonorrheal infection can move to the abdominal area and cause infection around the liver (a condition called Fitz-Hugh Curtis syndrome), producing pain in the upper right part of the abdomen.

Women with gonorrheal infection in the cervix can also experience it in the rectum, even if they have not received anal sex. Most likely this co-infection results from secretions from the genital area reaching the anal area and causing infection.

Men

The most common symptom of a gonorrheal infection in a male is discharge from the penis, along with burning with urination or just an irritated feeling in the penis. If there is discharge, it is usually copious and yellow—though it may be scant and clear, like the discharge caused by a chlamydial infection. Occasionally the penis becomes slightly swollen, and the urethral opening can become inflamed.

If gonorrhea is not treated, the urethral symptoms may eventually disappear, but epididymitis can occur as a complication. In epididymitis, the scrotum becomes inflamed and tender, usually on only one side. This infection can cause scarring that may interfere with a man's fertility. Epididymitis has become less common as a complication of gonorrhea since the introduction of antibiotics, but it may still occur if treatment is delayed. (See the section on epididymitis.)

> Gonorrheal infection can cause scarring in the genital area, which can lead to fertility problems in both women and men.

Men and Women

For men and women, gonorrheal infection in the anal area acquired through receptive anal intercourse can cause rectal pain, itching, discharge, bleeding, and pain with a bowel movement. However, infection in the rectal area frequently causes no symptoms at all.

Gonorrhea in the throat can be acquired if a person performs oral sex on a partner who has gonorrhea in the genital area, particularly on a male partner. Ninety percent of people who acquire gonorrheal infection in the throat have no symptoms; those who do have symptoms generally experience a sore throat.

Gonorrheal eye infection is usually severe, with redness, a thick yellow discharge, and difficulty seeing.

Rarely gonorrhea can also cause skin lesions (which appear as painful pimples) and joint infection (redness, swelling, and pain in a joint) after spreading through the bloodstream from the site of the initial genital infection.

Very rarely gonorrhea may settle in the heart valves, causing an infection called *endocarditis,* or in the lining of the brain and spinal cord, causing *meningitis.* People who have experienced suppression of the immune system for one reason or another, such as those who are infected with HIV, may be more vulnerable to endocarditis and meningitis caused by gonorrheal infection.

> **Gonorrhea can also infect the eyes, joints, heart valves, and lining of the brain and spinal cord, and it can cause sores on the skin.**

Women who acquire gonorrhea while they are pregnant run an increased risk of losing the child (spontaneous abortion) and premature delivery, as well as passing the infection to the child's eyes and throat during delivery.

HOW IS GONORRHEA TRANSMITTED?

Gonorrhea is transmitted through sexual contact with a person who is infected, whether or not the infected person has symptoms. The throat, genital area, and rectal area can become infected. Gonorrhea is very easy to transmit through sexual contact. Women are more vulnerable than men to acquiring the infection.

> **Gonorrhea is very easy to transmit through sexual contact.**

Gonorrhea is also easily transmitted through anal intercourse, and the rates of transmission for oral sex are similarly high, especially for a man or woman performing oral sex on a man who has gonorrhea. Similarly, if a man or woman has gonorrhea in the throat and performs oral sex on a man, the man receiving oral sex has a high risk of becoming infected in the urethra. However, a man or woman with gonorrhea in the throat performing oral sex on a woman has a lower risk of transmitting gonorrhea to the woman, because the area of the gonorrheal infection (the throat) is not contacted during oral sex with a woman. If the woman who was receiving oral sex from the man or woman had gonorrhea in the genital area, there would be a low risk of transmission as well, because the throat would not come into contact with the genitals or cervix.

Transmission does not occur through inanimate objects, such as towels or toilet seats, but the infection may be passed through sex toys. Condoms, if they are used consistently and correctly and do not break or leak, will prevent transmission of gonorrhea. Other barrier methods, such as diaphragms and cervical caps, may help decrease transmission to women, but they are not as effective as condoms in preventing infection.

Condoms offer protection against gonorrhea and other STDs.

TESTING FOR GONORRHEA

Testing for gonorrhea involves an examination during which cultures are taken from any area that was exposed to a partner and therefore is a potential site of infection. These areas include the urethra for men, the cervix and urethra for women, and the throat and anal area for men and women, if these areas have been exposed.

For men, a swab of the discharge from the urethra is taken, examined under the microscope, and tested. The bacterium can often (but not always) be seen under the microscope. As with tests for nongonococcal urethritis (NGU) and chlamydia, the examination is most accurate if the man does not urinate beforehand. To culture for gonorrhea, the urethral swab is brushed across a plate that contains substances on which *Neisseria gonorrhoeae* grows; it can take up to forty-eight hours for the growth to be evident. For women, a pelvic examination must be performed to diagnose genital gonorrhea. Swabs are taken from the cervix, the urethra, or both, and these are sent for culture. It is unlikely that the bacteria will be seen on a sample from the cervix, throat, or anal area.

A newer test, called the nucleic acid hybridization test, looks for the bacterial DNA. This test can be used on swabs of the cervix or vagina from women, urethral swabs from men, and urine from men and women. However, it is not recommended for testing the throat or anal area for gonorrhea. A culture is still the best test for these areas.

> Testing for gonorrhea involves swabbing exposed areas and identifying the gonorrhea bacterium or its DNA.

Your health care provider will usually do a complete screen for sexually transmitted infections if you are suspected of having gonorrhea, since people exposed to gonorrhea have often been exposed to other STDs as well.

TREATMENT

Several medications are now recommended as first-line choices for treating gonorrhea of the genital and anal areas. A person who is diagnosed with gonorrhea is usually treated for NGU and chlamydia as well, because the likelihood of co-infection with the bacteria that cause these infections is high. Some gonorrhea treatments are given as an injection, some are available as a week-long course of oral medication, and some are available as a single pill—which is the easiest way to treat any infection.

A shot of ceftriaxone or an oral medication, such as cefixime or a quinolone (ciprofloxacin, levofloxacin, or ofloxacin), will successfully treat gonorrhea. Recently however, in some places in the world, including the United States (particularly Hawaii and California), and in some populations (men who have sex with other men), gonorrhea has been found to be resistant to the quinolones. If you have a gonorrhea infection, talk with your health care provider about the best treatment for you—the options other than the quinolones will probably be prescribed.

If more extensive infection—such as epididymitis or PID—is suspected, then a longer course of antibiotics is necessary (see the sections on epididymitis and on pelvic inflammatory disease). Early diagnosis and treatment are necessary to prevent such complications as scarring and infertility. Again, quinolones (such as ciprofloxacin) are not recommended if you are a man who has sex with men or if you travel to or live in an area where resistance to this antibiotic is high.

Gonorrhea can also cause infection of the eyes (conjunctivitis), which requires treatment from an ophthalmologist (eye doctor). Gonorrhea sometimes spreads through the blood to other areas or organs, such as the joints (causing arthritis), skin, heart valves (endocarditis), and rarely the lining of the brain (meningitis). These serious complications require treatment with intravenous (through the vein) antibiotics and hospitalization.

If symptoms persist after treatment with medications, it is important to see your health care provider for a follow-up examination, because these treatments are sometimes not fully effective. As with any treatment for an STD, you should abstain from sex while you are being treated, and continue to abstain and seek help if you still have symptoms after treatment. Having gonorrhea once makes you more vulnerable to getting it again if you are exposed. See Chapter 5, "What Is 'Safer Sex'?" to learn about ways to become safer.

Sexual partners must be treated for gonorrhea as well. This means everyone who has had sexual contact with an infected person in the last sixty days, even if they have no symptoms or evidence of infection on examination. Or, if it has been more than sixty days since the person diagnosed with gonorrhea had a sexual contact, then the last person he or she had sex with should be tested and, if necessary, treated. In most states, if a person is diagnosed with gonorrhea, this is reported to the state health department. The health department can help in contacting partners anonymously so they can receive treatment.

HEPATITIS A, B, AND C

Hepatitis is an inflammation of the liver. Alcohol, medications, and autoimmune diseases can all cause the liver to become inflamed, as can some inherited medical conditions (for example, Wilson's disease and alpha$_1$-antitrypsin deficiency) and certain viruses. Of the many viruses that can cause liver damage, this section focuses on three that can be transmitted through sexual contact as well as in other ways: hepatitis A, hepatitis B, and hepatitis C. Also discussed here is hepatitis D, which can occur in people who are infected with hepatitis B. Other hepatitis viruses—types E, F, and G—are currently under investigation, but they are not at this time thought to be sexually transmitted. How hepatitis A, B, and C viruses cause damage to the liver is not yet known, although it may be that the body's immune response to the infection causes the liver damage.

HEPATITIS A

incidence: common
cause: virus (hepatitis A)
symptoms: nausea, yellowing of the skin, diarrhea
treatment: none (usually resolves on its own)

WHAT IS IT?

Hepatitis A is a virus that causes infection and inflammation of the liver. It has been recognized since the 1940s as a virus distinct from hepatitis B, and was finally identified in 1973. One often hears of outbreaks of hepatitis A associated with improper food handling in restaurants, but, less commonly, hepatitis A can be transmitted sexually, especially through oral-anal contact. Hepatitis A and hepatitis B are sexually transmitted infections that can be prevented with a vaccination.

HOW COMMON IS IT?

Approximately 30,000 people are diagnosed with hepatitis A each year in the United States, but the Centers for Disease Control estimates that over 100,000 new cases may occur each year in this country. Most of these cases are not the result of sexual transmission. Many people are symptom free or do not seek care for their symptoms. With the hepatitis A vaccination that became available in 1996, there has been a decline in new infections in the United States.

It is estimated that by the time they reach young adulthood, 15–25 percent of the people in the United States have been infected with hepatitis A, usually by consuming contaminated food or water. As people age, the likelihood that they have acquired hepatitis A increases, with blood tests of more than 75 percent of adults over age seventy showing past infection. In the industrialized world, improvements in sanitation have decreased the number of people infected in childhood, whereas in developing countries, where sanitation and water quality may be inadequate, childhood infection is still very common. In many countries, more than 90 percent of children are infected by age five. Infection in childhood may not be a bad thing: most children who become infected with hepatitis A are symptom free, whereas most adults are symptomatic, and although fatalities are rare from hepatitis A, most of the deaths that do occur are in newly infected adults. People who have not been vaccinated or received immune globulin (see the discussion on transmission below) before travel to areas of the world where hepatitis A is very common are at increased risk of infection as well.

> Most children who become infected with hepatitis A are symptom free; most adults who are infected have symptoms.

WHAT ARE THE SYMPTOMS?

Symptoms usually take about four weeks (with a range of fifteen to fifty days) to appear after infection with hepatitis A. Fewer than one in ten children below the age of three develops symptoms, whereas most adults become symptomatic. Symptoms usually start abruptly with muscle aches, headache, fatigue, malaise, loss of appetite, nausea, and vomiting, Occasionally a period of fever and muscle aches occurs before the onset of acute infection. Diarrhea usually follows. Jaundice, darkening of the urine, and lightening of the color of the stools usually come later in the course of the illness. Liver swelling leading to abdominal pain is also common. Some experience a sore throat. Most people resolve the infection within several weeks to two months after becoming symptomatic. On rare occasions symptoms may briefly recur a short time after the initial infection and then resolve completely.

The symptoms are very similar when a person becomes infected with and symptomatic from other types of viral hepatitis, such as hepatitis B and C. Fatalities are less common for hepatitis A than B during this acute phase, however, with less than 0.2 percent of those infected dying from hepatitis A. Fatalities are more common among people older than fifty years; especially vulnerable are people with underlying liver problems or other medical problems. Because of this, it is especially important for people with liver problems from other causes to receive a hepatitis A vaccine. Hepatitis A, unlike hepatitis B or C, never causes chronic infection or chronic liver disease, although some people have a "relapse" of symptoms within the first year of infection. A person who has been infected with hepatitis A is protected from ever getting it again.

HOW IS HEPATITIS A TRANSMITTED?

Transmission usually occurs through the fecal-oral route—that is, a person becomes infected by ingesting infected fecal material. The stool of an infected person has high quantities of the virus, and very little of the virus is required to transmit infection. Unfortunately the highest risk of transmission of the virus via the stool occurs some two weeks before a person becomes symptomatic (if indeed he or she is going to become symptomatic) and knows that he or she is infected. By the time someone develops jaundice (yellowing of the skin), the quantity of virus shed in the stool has decreased, although people can continue to shed virus for one week after the onset of illness. Most people cannot recall when or where they became infected.

Infected people who improperly wash their hands after a bowel movement and have fecal material on their hands when preparing food can easily transmit the virus to those who eat the contaminated food. The virus is very hearty and can live outside the body, such as in bodies of water, for long periods—possibly up to several months. Shellfish, which concentrate impurities such as the hepatitis A virus, can cause infection if they are eaten raw or are not cooked adequately. Because of this risk, and the risk of other potentially harmful infections that can be transmitted in the same way, it is not a good idea to eat raw seafood. Heating foods for one minute at temperatures greater than 185° Fahrenheit kills the virus in food, and using disinfectant with a dilute solution of bleach in water kills the virus on surfaces such as countertops.

Infected children who are not toilet trained and are around other children—for example, in a daycare center—can spread the infection to other children and adults. Family and household contacts of those who are infected frequently become infected themselves. In addition, institutional staffs, such as nursing home employees, may also be at higher risk.

Sexual transmission can also occur via the fecal-oral route, although this is rare. A person can become infected with hepatitis A through oral-anal contact (called *analingus* or *rimming*) or by stimulating a partner's anus with the fingers and then not washing the hands before placing them in the mouth or preparing food. Occasionally outbreaks of hepatitis A occur among men who have sex with other men in urban settings. Other types of sexual contact are not thought to be a method of transmission. Studies of men who have sex with other men have shown that the more sexual partners a man has, the more likely he is to become infected with hepatitis A. This is true for any person, regardless of gender or sexual orientation, who practices oral-anal contact with multiple partners. Outbreaks are sometimes seen among people who use illegal drugs, whether injection or non-injection drugs.

> Hepatitis A can be transmitted sexually through oral-anal contact.

At various times during infection, the saliva and blood of an infected person may also contain the virus, but it is very rare that transmission takes place through contact with saliva or blood. Although occasional outbreaks among persons who use intravenous drugs may be due to blood transmission, the more common method of transmission, via the fecal-oral route, may actually be the cause in these cases as well. Blood banks screen for all types of hepatitis, so transmission through blood transfusion is very rare.

Thorough washing of the hands after using the restroom and avoiding anal-oral contact with an infected person generally prevent transmission of hepatitis A. In addition, in 1996 a breakthrough in the prevention of hepatitis A became available: a vaccine that offers protection against acquiring the infection. This vaccine is composed of whole hepatitis A virus that has been inactivated and therefore cannot cause infection. It is given in two doses as a shot in the deltoid muscle of the arm, waiting six to twelve months between doses. Adults older than age seventeen are given a higher dose than children two to seventeen years of age.

The first vaccine becomes effective about two weeks after it is given and offers a 94–100 percent protection rate against acquiring hepatitis A. The second vaccine provides protection greater than 99 percent and is thought to last more than twenty years. A person who does contract hepatitis A after receiving the vaccine will experience milder symptoms than someone who has not been vaccinated. Children younger than two years of age should not receive the vaccine, nor should pregnant or nursing mothers. Most people tolerate the vaccine well; allergic reactions are rare, and mild discomfort where the vaccine was given is the most common side effect.

Elderly people and any person older than forty who grew up in an area presenting a high risk of infection probably should be tested for the presence of immunity before receiving the vaccine. Giving the vaccine to someone who has already had the infection (and thus cleared it, providing lifelong immunity to reinfection) would not be harmful, but it would be unnecessary.

The vaccine is recommended for persons traveling to an area where hepatitis A is very common, including Africa, Asia except Japan, the Mediterranean basin, Eastern Europe, the Middle East, Central and South America, Mexico, and parts of the Caribbean. The Centers for Disease Control (see this book's appendix) offers free travel information and recommendations about vaccines for people traveling to specific areas of the world. The vaccine is also recommended for men who have sex with men and for users of illegal drugs, both injection and non-injection drugs. Daycare and institutional workers may also benefit. People with chronic liver problems also benefit from the vaccine, since they may experience more serious illness if infected.

Within the United States, Native American and Alaskan Native populations are at higher risk for becoming infected with hepatitis A, so vaccination is recommended for these groups, as well as for people in areas of the country where the risk of infection is high.

This vaccine is only effective against hepatitis A; it offers no protection against other types of viral hepatitis. Of note, a combined hepatitis A and B vaccination is now available.

If a person has been exposed to someone who has been infected with hepatitis A and may have been infected but has not yet shown symptoms, there is something that can be done. This person can receive the hepatitis A vaccine for future protection and also receive an immune globulin shot, which will provide shorter-term protection against infection about 80–90 percent of the time. (Immune globulin is composed of antibodies to the hepatitis A virus as well as to other infections, which can help fight off the infection before the person's own immune system kicks in to combat it.) *To be effective, an immune globulin injection must be given within two weeks following the exposure.*

The immune globulin injection can also be given to persons traveling to areas where hepatitis A is common and who have not received the vaccine, or in whom the vaccine has not had sufficient time to work. Since the vaccine takes more than two weeks to be effective, immune globulin is the choice for a person who within two weeks will be traveling to a country with a high risk for infection. Immune globulin has "time-limited" effectiveness, however, probably losing its ability to offer protection within three months of the injection.

There is a low risk of problems, such as allergic reactions, from the immune globulin injection. It is usually more painful than the hepatitis A vaccine. Immune globulin is pooled from donated blood; it is screened for hepatitis B and C and HIV infection and is routinely treated with chemicals to kill these viruses. It presents a very low risk of transmission of these infections: no cases of transmission of hepatitis B or C or HIV have been reported to date from the immune globulin shot. It is as safe for pregnant and nursing women, children, and immunosuppressed individuals as for the rest of the population.

> **People at high risk of infection should be vaccinated against hepatitis A.**

TESTING FOR HEPATITIS A

There is a simple blood test to screen for hepatitis A. This test can distinguish between someone who is newly infected (less than six months ago) and someone who was infected more than six months ago. By the time symptoms develop, people generally show evidence of the infection on a blood test. The test looks for antibodies, the immune system's response to the infection. These antibodies usually take about a month after infection to develop, and once infected with hepatitis A, a person has antibodies as evidence of the infection in his or her blood for life; the antibodies also confer protection against acquiring the infection a second time. If the blood test for hepatitis A is negative but infection is still suspected, a repeat test should be performed in a few weeks. If the blood test remains negative, hepatitis A infection may be excluded, and alternative reasons for the symptoms—such as other forms of viral hepatitis or a reaction to medications—should be sought.

A person who has been infected with hepatitis A and resolved the infection, and a person who has received the vaccine for hepatitis A, each show the same positive blood test result. Neither will become infected with hepatitis A again.

TREATMENT

The treatment for hepatitis A is supportive, meaning that the symptoms are treated with rest, fluids, and antinausea medications. It is important to avoid placing stress on the liver, to avoid any medications that can cause further damage, and, most of all, to avoid all alcohol. There is no specific diet to follow. Most people recover from symptoms in about six weeks, although it can take up to three months for a person to feel completely back to normal. Hospitalization is occasionally necessary.

HEPATITIS B

incidence: common
cause: virus (hepatitis B)
symptoms: nausea, yellowing of the skin, diarrhea; can become chronic
treatment: none for acute infection, interferon for chronic infection

WHAT IS IT?

Hepatitis B is a virus that causes liver inflammation and damage. Recognized since the 1960s, it is a serious health concern in the United States and worldwide. The virus can cause acute as well as chronic infection, which increases the risk of later complications. Hepatitis B infection can be prevented with a vaccination.

HOW COMMON IS IT?

Approximately 100,000 people are infected with hepatitis B every year in the United States, and each year approximately 5000 people die as a result of the infection. Approximately 10 percent of the population in the United States shows evidence of (past or current) infection on blood testing. Even in the era of HIV and safer sex, the number of people newly infected is continuing to increase. In the United States, over 50 percent of hepatitis B transmission is from sexual contact. Heterosexual transmission is on the rise; homosexual transmission is decreasing, probably because of the safer sex practices adopted to prevent HIV transmission.

Sexual contact with an infected person and injection drug use with needle sharing are the two most common ways in which hepatitis B is transmitted.

The risk of becoming infected with hepatitis B increases with the number of sexual contacts a person has. People who have sex in exchange for money are at very high risk. Anyone who has been diagnosed with another sexually transmitted disease is also at higher risk of being infected with hepatitis B, through unsafe sexual practices. In one study of 2000 people who were patients at an STD clinic, 28 percent of those twenty-five and older showed evidence of hepatitis B infection, whereas 7 percent of those younger than twenty-five showed evidence of infection. About 5 percent of those infected in the United States become carriers of the infection, as discussed later in this section.

There are some geographic differences in patterns of hepatitis B infection. In most Southeast Asian and some African countries, the rate of infection is high. About 90 percent of people in these countries have evidence in their blood of previous or current infection with hepatitis B, and approximately 10–20 percent of them are carriers of the infection.

Mothers who are chronically infected with hepatitis B have a greater than 90 percent chance of infecting their unborn children while in the womb and during delivery. If a child is infected, there is a high probability that he or she will become a carrier of hepatitis B as well; however, steps can be taken to help protect against infection of the newborn (see the discussion later in this section).

WHAT ARE THE SYMPTOMS?

Many people are surprised to learn that most of those who are infected with hepatitis B do not manifest any symptoms. In fact, only about one-third of those who show evidence of past infection with hepatitis B on blood testing recall being sick. Older people and those in poor health generally have a higher risk of becoming sicker with infection.

Most people with hepatitis B infection have few or no symptoms.

Symptoms, if they do occur, usually arise within six weeks to six months after infection, most often within about two months. Fewer than half of those infected develop symptoms. Symptoms can occur sooner (if a person was exposed to a large amount of virus at infection) or later (if a person received immune globulin soon after being infected). (Immune globulin, described in more detail shortly, is an injection that provides some protection against acquiring the infection after someone has been exposed.)

Before they become sick with the more classic symptoms of hepatitis, about 15–20 percent of those infected develop joint aches and a flat to slightly raised rash that may itch. This occurs as the body is developing an immune response to the infection and is a result of the large quantity of antibody produced. An infected person may next develop jaundice (yellowing of the skin), abdominal pain, nausea and vomiting, lightening of the color of the stool to a so-called clay color, and darkening of the urine to a brownish color.

These symptoms, which can be severe, usually last about one to two months, although the fatigue can sometimes last longer. A small percentage of infected people go on to develop what is called *fulminant hepatitis*, with severe liver damage that can lead to death. About 1 percent of people who develop symptoms of acute hepatitis progress to liver failure, and about 75 percent of them die from this severe illness. Remember, however, that most people do not show any symptoms that they have even been infected.

Carriers. Although 95 percent of adults who are infected with hepatitis B go on to clear the infection and then have lifelong protection against ever becoming infected again, about 2–6 percent of them become carriers. Unfortunately, infants who are infected have a much higher rate of becoming carriers, up to 90 percent. Children who acquire the infection have about a 20–60 percent likelihood of becoming carriers. A *carrier* is a person whose immune system was not able to clear the infection from the body, so the virus persists and the carrier remains chronically infected and infectious to others throughout his or her lifetime. People with impaired immune systems, such as those with HIV infection, are more likely than others to be carriers. Those who develop symptoms of hepatitis B infection are also more likely to become carriers than those who do not. As noted above, people infected at an early age are much more likely to become carriers than people infected later in life (90% of infected infants, 60% of infected children under the age of five, and only 2–6% of infected adults). People with chronic hepatitis B infection are at risk for developing scarring of the liver (cirrhosis) and liver cancer (hepatocellular carcinoma).

> About 5 percent of people infected with hepatitis B cannot clear the infection and become carriers, which means they are infectious to others.

Carriers can occasionally clear the virus from their systems and cure themselves of hepatitis B. How and why some people clear the infection while others do not is unclear. For those who remain carriers, routine monitoring by a health care provider for complications from the disease is essential.

People with chronic hepatitis B infection may sustain damage to organs other than the liver, similar to that seen with hepatitis C infection (discussed subsequently). Such symptoms include disorders of the skin (*polyarteritis nodosa*), kidneys (*glomerulonephritis*), and blood cells (*cryoglobulinemias*). A specialist in diseases of the liver (a hepatologist) should be consulted if you have chronic infection with hepatitis B.

HOW IS HEPATITIS B TRANSMITTED?

People who become infected with hepatitis B are contagious to others during the weeks before they become symptomatic and for up to several months following infection. Those who become chronically infected are potentially infectious to others throughout their lifetimes.

People with acute hepatitis B infection should be considered infectious to others until their blood work shows they have cleared the infection, which may take up to three to six months after infection.

Hepatitis B is transmitted by infected body fluids, including blood, semen, vaginal secretions, fluid from wounds, and saliva if contaminated by blood. It is possible that any body fluid from an infected person may carry enough virus to infect another person. Hepatitis B most commonly is transmitted through blood exposure, via sexual contact, and from mother to child. Household contacts (members of the household not sexually intimate with the infected person) should not be at risk of infection, unless they are exposed to body fluids such as blood. Because this can happen unknowingly, it's a good idea for household contacts of someone with chronic hepatitis B infection to be vaccinated.

Blood Exposure. The risk behaviors in this category include sharing equipment for injection drug use, tattooing, or body piercing; receiving a needle-stick injury (as a health care worker might); and receiving a transfusion with infected blood or blood products. The hepatitis virus can last quite a long time outside the body, so household contacts should not share razors, toothbrushes, and so on, with someone who has a hepatitis B infection. Since the blood supply in the United States has been screened for hepatitis B since 1975, the risk of becoming infected from a transfusion is very low.

Sexual Contact. Hepatitis B can be passed through anal, vaginal, and oral sex, and possibly even through kissing. The risk of infection with hepatitis B increases with the number of sexual partners a person has. The fastest-growing group of infected people is heterosexuals. In one study, 21 percent of heterosexuals with more than five sexual partners in the past four months had hepatitis B, whereas those with fewer than five partners had a lifetime risk of infection of 6 percent. Sexual partners of people who are infected have a high risk of becoming infected themselves. *People who know their partners are infected should be immunized.* In fact, any sexually active adult should be immunized.

Mother-to-Child Transmission. If a woman is infected during her pregnancy, particularly during the last trimester of pregnancy, or if she is a carrier for hepatitis B infection, she has a high risk of infecting her child. Infection can occur while the child is in the womb, but it most often occurs during delivery, possibly from mixing of maternal and fetal blood. Children who are infected at birth more often than not become carriers themselves. Infected mothers may also inadvertently infect their infants after birth, through contact with infected body fluids; breast milk, however, seems to be safe. A baby born to a mother who is infected with hepatitis B may show some evidence of infection in the blood at birth, but the baby may not be truly infected, because it may be the mother's antibody that is being seen in the blood. However, a baby who persists in showing evidence of infection in the blood about four months after delivery can be assumed to be truly infected. Immunizing at-risk babies at delivery offers a good possibility of preventing these babies from becoming infected.

How Can You Protect Yourself from Becoming Infected with Hepatitis B? A safe and effective vaccine against hepatitis B has been available for over twenty years. This vaccine is manufactured from proteins from the surface of the hepatitis B virus. Vaccination is given in three doses over a period of six months. Unfortunately the cost prevents many at-risk people from receiving the vaccine. Those who are at risk for hepatitis B may want to be screened before receiving the vaccine series, since they may have already been infected and therefore would not need the vaccine. (However, no harm is done if a person who already has hepatitis B receives the vaccine.) The most common side effects from the vaccine are arm pain and mild, flu-like symptoms. Approximately 95 percent of people who receive the three shots acquire lifelong protection from infection. Poor response to the vaccine may be due to advanced age, obesity, or smoking. There is also a newer vaccine that combines protection against hepatitis A *and* B. You can be checked after immunization to make sure that you have had an adequate response to the vaccine.

In the past, efforts were made to immunize only those who were thought to be at high risk for hepatitis B. This did not stem the tide of new infections, so a new approach is now advocated, which, since 1991, includes universal vaccination of all infants. The following groups of people should consider receiving the vaccination, as long as there is no contraindication or history of previous infection:

1. Sexually active men who have sex with other men
2. Men and women who have been recently diagnosed with an STD
3. All unvaccinated people being evaluated for an STD
4. Anyone who has had more than one sexual partner in the past six months
5. Any child aged eleven to twelve years who has not already received three shots
6. Any person with multiple sexual partners
7. Sexual partners or household contacts of anyone with chronic hepatitis B infection
8. Users of illegal drugs (both injection and non-injection)
9. Health care workers who may be exposed to body fluids
10. Dialysis patients or people who receive blood products
11. People who travel to areas of the world where there is a high level of infection
12. Residents of correctional facilities
13. Prostitutes

Certain people immunized against hepatitis B should be tested for immunity, particularly if they are HIV positive (because HIV-positive individuals may not show a good response to the vaccination), are on dialysis, have sex with or share needles with people who are carriers of hepatitis B, or are infants born to infected mothers. Testing should be done about one to two months after the last shot. If the test doesn't confirm that the immunization series was effective, the entire series of shots should be given again.

If a person who has not been immunized has been exposed to someone who is infectious with hepatitis B, the exposed person should receive the vaccination series as well as a dose of immune globulin specifically directed against hepatitis B within fourteen days of exposure. The vaccination itself, if given after exposure, offers some protection against acquiring the infection. Adding a shot of immune globulin improves the outcome. Immune globulin is a collection of antibodies that help to protect against infection on an acute basis; it provides a "boost" for the immune system, but only for a short time, so the vaccination series is given at the same time to offer long-term immunity as well. The immune globulin provides three to six months of immunity.

Vaccination plus immune globulin is a good idea after sustaining a needle-stick injury, receiving a bite from someone who is a carrier of hepatitis B or newly infected with hepatitis B, or sexual exposure to a person who is either a carrier or newly infected. If a person has sex with an infected partner, this vaccine–immune globulin combination can be given within fourteen days of the contact, but it offers the most protection if given within forty-eight hours of exposure. If there is a significant exposure from a needle-stick injury or from an exposure on a mucosal surface (such as the eyes or mouth), then this combination should be given within twenty-four to forty-eight hours after the exposure. In both of these scenarios, the follow-up vaccinations must be given at one- and six-month intervals.

For a child born to a mother who is infected with hepatitis B, the same combination of vaccine series and immune globulin is given, usually within twelve hours of birth. This treatment has a high rate of success in preventing the child from becoming infected with hepatitis B, decreasing the likelihood of infection from 80 percent to 5–15 percent. All pregnant women should be tested to determine their hepatitis B status, so that their newborns can be tested and treated if they have been exposed.

Besides vaccination, the other method to help prevent the transmission of hepatitis B through sexual contacts is to use condoms or other barriers for oral, anal, and genital intercourse if a partner's status for hepatitis B (and other STDs) is not known (see Chapter 5 on safer sex). Women who have sex with other women can transmit the virus through oral sex and exchange of vaginal secretions. Dental dams or plastic wrap may decrease the risk of infection in such cases. All partners of those found to be infected with hepatitis B should be immunized. Of note, a combination hepatitis A and B vaccination is now available.

TESTING FOR HEPATITIS B

There are specific blood tests for hepatitis B. Early in the infection the blood tests may be negative in a person who is actually infected; later blood tests will show evidence of the infection in such a person. Ask your health care provider what your test results mean and whether or not you need additional tests to rule out infection.

The tests that are most helpful to diagnose hepatitis look for the

body's immune response to the
virus (antibodies), particles of the
virus itself, or the genetic material of the virus, in the "polymerase chain reaction," or PCR,
test. The blood tests can distin-

Blood tests can detect infection with hepatitis B. A person who tests negative and is at high risk should consider being vaccinated.

guish among people who are newly infected, people who have been infected and have cleared the infection, people who have been infected
and are carriers, and people who have been vaccinated—although
follow-up tests may be necessary to make these distinctions. To determine the stage of infection, it may be necessary to perform a liver
biopsy, which involves taking a piece of liver tissue (with the person
under anesthesia) and examining the sample under a microscope.

Tests that measure how well the liver is working, called *liver enzyme tests* or *liver injury tests*, are not an adequate screen for hepatitis B. Although results of these tests are often elevated in acute and
chronic hepatitis, normal liver enzyme results cannot be interpreted
as ruling out viral hepatitis infection.

When a person is found to be a carrier of hepatitis B, it is recommended that a blood test also be performed for hepatitis D, or *delta
hepatitis*. This is an infection that can occur only in individuals who
have hepatitis B infection, since the delta virus needs the hepatitis B
virus to survive. Hepatitis D can be sexually transmitted but has a
higher risk of transmission from blood exposure, such as through injection drug use or receiving transfusions with infected blood. (The
U.S. blood supply has been screened for hepatitis D since the 1970s.)
A person can be infected with hepatitis D at the same time that infection with hepatitis B occurs, or he or she can become superinfected
with hepatitis D while a carrier for hepatitis B. In either situation, severe liver damage and death can result, or the person is likely to become a carrier for hepatitis D as
well as B, which can hasten the
progression of liver disease to cirrhosis. The diagnosis of hepatitis
B and D, in both the acute and
chronic forms, is reportable in
most states to the health department.

Hepatitis D, also known as delta hepatitis, is an infection that can occur only in people already infected with hepatitis B.

TREATMENT

Most people infected with hepatitis B have few or no symptoms associated with infection. Those who do have symptoms can usually improve with rest and treatment of the symptoms. Most people do not need to be hospitalized, and in fact unnecessary hospitalization may do more harm than good, because it puts others at risk of becoming infected. For anyone with severe infection, or anyone in a situation that puts him or her at increased risk for complications as a result of infection—such as those with other medical problems or over the age of forty—hospitalization may be necessary to provide monitoring and supportive care.

People who are newly infected are usually watched for three to six months to see whether their bodies are able to clear the infection on their own. For people with chronic hepatitis B infection, there are several options for treatment. These include medications such as interferon (alpha or pegylated), lamivudine, adefovir, dipivoxil, and entecavir. Interferon has a lot of side effects, including fatigue. There is much ongoing research in this field to find the best treatment options. If you have hepatitis B, a hepatologist (liver specialist) can help you decide which of these options is best for you.

A liver transplant remains an option for people with liver failure, although there is a strong likelihood that the new liver will also become infected with hepatitis B. Studies are under way to find ways to prevent such reinfection.

Anyone who has hepatitis B (either acute or chronic infection) should be careful to avoid other things that can harm the liver. Any alcohol may further damage the liver and increase the risk of developing liver cancer. Use of all medications needs to be checked with the health care provider in case they cause harm to the liver. And immunization against hepatitis A should be given to everyone who has not already been infected.

HEPATITIS C

incidence: common
cause: virus (hepatitis C)

symptoms: fatigue, nausea, yellowing of the skin, diarrhea; often
              becomes chronic
treatment: none for acute infection, interferon for chronic infection

WHAT IS IT?

The hepatitis C virus is the most common cause of what was once
called "non-A, non-B" hepatitis, a term formerly used to describe viral hepatitis that was not caused by hepatitis A or B. Hepatitis C is a
major health concern in the United States and around the world, and
it is the most common cause of chronic liver disease in the United
States. Hepatitis C was discovered in the late 1980s, and blood tests
for this virus have been available since 1990.

Several types of hepatitis C virus have been recognized so far, each
with a slightly different genetic makeup. A person may have infection with one or several types. Although the symptoms the viruses
cause are similar, their response to treatment with medication (alpha-
interferon) differs, and their degree of infectiousness may also differ.
The most common types in the United States are hepatitis C types 1
(a and b), 2, and 3. Type 4 is more common in northern and central
Africa and the Middle East, whereas type 5 is seen in South Africa and
types 7, 8, and 9 in Vietnam.

HOW COMMON IS IT?

Approximately 150,000 people are diagnosed with hepatitis C infection each year in the United States, and it is estimated that 2.7 million people in this country are infected. Since hepatitis C is not reportable to the health department in many states, this probably is a
low estimate. Approximately 38 percent of those infected have a current or past history of injection drug use; more than 50 percent of injection drug users who share needles are positive for hepatitis C. In
addition, 10–20 percent were infected by sexual or household contact,
4 percent by blood or blood product transfusions (mostly acquired before screening was put in place; the risk of infection from a transfusion today is less than 0.03%), and 2 percent by occupational exposure
such as accidental needle-stick injuries. Some people who are diagnosed and deny any high-risk activity may be embarrassed to admit
to the behavior, but, even taking that into account, there are infected
people who do not have any obvious risk factor.

WHAT ARE THE SYMPTOMS?

About 70 percent of people who contract hepatitis C do not develop symptoms, so they would not know they had been infected unless they were tested. If symptoms do develop, they are usually mild and occur one to two months after infection. They include jaundice (yellowing of the skin) in about 25 percent of those who develop symptoms, nausea and abdominal pain, loss of appetite, fatigue, and fever. Occasionally the initial symptoms of new infection can be severe and even fatal, but this is rare for hepatitis C. If symptoms do occur, they usually last two to twelve weeks. Fatigue is the most common symptom.

Sixty to eighty percent of people infected with hepatitis C develop chronic hepatitis, often evidenced by abnormal findings on liver enzyme tests. Possibly 20 percent of people infected with hepatitis C "clear" the virus from their system, meaning their body is free from infection. If this is going to happen, it usually happens in the first three to five months after infection. Sometimes the results of standard liver tests (looking at liver enzymes, for example) are normal in people with hepatitis C infection, so these tests are not a screen for new or persistent infection.

The amount of liver destruction varies from person to person, and it can be made worse by such other potential causes of liver damage as medications, alcohol, or infection with hepatitis A or B. A person who drinks alcohol and has hepatitis C, for example, has a chance of developing cirrhosis (scarring of the liver) ten times greater than that of someone who is infected with hepatitis C and does not drink alcohol.

Once infection has been shown to persist in the blood for more than six months, it is unlikely that the body will be able to get rid of the virus on its own. Some people, however, do clear the virus—possibly as many as 20 percent (meaning their liver tests return to normal, and virus cannot be detected in their blood by the polymerase chain reaction, or PCR, test, described below).

Why most people become chronically infected, and some do not, is unclear. The virus may be able to mutate, or change itself, so that it can escape detection by the body's immune system. Still, some populations seem less likely to become chronically infected. Children, for instance, are less likely than adults to develop chronic infection, whereas people who acquire infection after the age of forty are more likely to experience a rapid progression of liver injury.

Years after first infection (twenty years on average), persons who have chronic infection of the liver due to hepatitis C may develop such serious problems as cirrhosis (which occurs in about 20–30% of those infected with hepatitis C). In people with hepatitis C who develop cirrhosis, hepatocellular carcinoma (cancer of the liver) can also occur. The risk of developing hepatocellular carcinoma is thought to be less than 3 percent per year of infection. Also, in people with hepatitis C infection and cirrhosis, the likelihood of complications such as ascites (fluid in the abdomen), variceal bleeding (bleeding in dilated vessels in the esophagus), jaundice, and mental confusion (due to encephalopathy) is about 4 percent per year. Once these problems have occurred, the only cure for the infection is a liver transplant. All of these problems are more common among people who have sustained other liver damage during that time, such as that caused by alcoholism.

It also seems that some types of hepatitis C are more likely to progress to cirrhosis and cancer than other types. Unfortunately, one of the most common types of hepatitis C (that caused by type 1b of the virus) is also the most common type to progress. In addition men and older people are more likely to develop these complications. A liver biopsy (which involves taking a piece of liver from a person under anesthesia and then examining the sample under a microscope) can determine much more accurately than can blood tests how much liver damage has occurred from infection.

About 20 percent of people who develop cirrhosis also develop liver failure. Hepatitis C infection is the most common reason for liver transplantation in the United States: about 30 percent of the liver transplants are in people with hepatitis C infection, and in many of these recipients other factors, such as alcohol abuse, caused liver damage.

Although serious complications are possible in those infected with hepatitis C, many people who are infected do not have these problems, and they remain symptom free. Being aware of the importance of taking precautions to protect against further liver damage—by, for example, not drinking alcohol, avoiding reinfection, and avoiding medications that can cause liver damage—will help protect against complications. Not only is the liver more susceptible to damage from alcohol, but alcohol increases the replication of the virus and accelerates the damage it causes. Daily marijuana use has also been associated with rapid progression of liver damage.

Some other conditions can be caused by chronic infection with hepatitis C. These include problems of the blood, kidneys, skin, and thyroid, to name just a few. People with hepatitis C infection should receive close medical follow-up, preferably by a liver specialist (hepatologist).

HOW IS HEPATITIS C TRANSMITTED?

Hepatitis C is most often transmitted through contact with infected blood. Persons at especially high risk for hepatitis C infection are injection drug users, hemodialysis patients, and anyone who received blood transfusions or a solid organ transplant before July 1992 or clotting factor transfusions before 1987. About 90 percent of posttransfusion hepatitis was caused by hepatitis C before screening of the blood supply began. It is estimated that up to one of every ten individuals who received a transfusion in the 1970s and 1980s was infected with hepatitis C. Since screening has been in place transfusion-related hepatitis has become rare.

Sharing needles in injection drug use poses a high risk of transmission. It is estimated that over 60 percent of people who are diagnosed with hepatitis C acquired the infection by sharing works for injection drug use. Likewise, over 50 percent of injection drug users who are screened are found to be hepatitis C positive. Tattooing with an unclean needle can also transmit hepatitis C. The chances of becoming infected from a needle-stick injury from an infected person are estimated to be between 3.5 and 10 percent. Other, less common causes are scarification, as part of religious ritual, or receiving a piercing from an unclean needle.

There is some debate about how easily hepatitis C can be transmitted sexually. Hepatitis B and HIV are almost certainly easier to transmit sexually than hepatitis C. Studies have shown that hepatitis C can be transmitted through sexual contact; however, on average, only 1.5 percent of long-term spouses of people who are infected with hepatitis C, who themselves have no other risk for infection, are found to be infected. Hepatitis C infection rates seem to be higher among people at risk for other sexually transmitted diseases, such as people with multiple sex partners, people infected with other STDs, people who don't use condoms, and people who have sex with partners who use injection drugs. Men who have sex with men seem to be at the same risk as heterosexual partners; no studies have looked at women who have sex with women. Studies are under way to further clarify the risk of acquiring hepatitis C infection from sexual contact.

Hepatitis C can be transmitted from mother to child during pregnancy, although not as easily as hepatitis B. About 5 percent of children born to mothers who are infected with hepatitis C are infected at birth. It may also be possible for the mother to infect the child after delivery through close contact (about 3% of children who were not infected at birth, but whose mothers have hepatitis C, also develop infection), although hepatitis C does not seem to be transmitted through breast milk. So far we do not know how to prevent transmission from mother to child.

Clearly, to avoid acquiring hepatitis C it is essential to avoid needle sharing among injection drug users and to avoid exposure to infected blood. Even less-invasive activities, such as sharing straws to snort cocaine, have been linked to the transmission of hepatitis C. If you are using injection drugs, get help to stop. If you can't stop, don't share needles or works with other people. As for sexual contact with someone who is infected with hepatitis C, condoms can be used to decrease the risk of infection, but this is a decision couples must make for themselves after being counseled about the risks. Each couple must decide which precautions they wish to take, depending on the level of risk with which they are comfortable. The risk of acquiring infection through sexual transmission from an infected partner may be less than 1 percent for each year that sexual contact continues. Condoms may decrease the risk. If an uninfected partner has genital herpes, it may be easier for him or her to acquire hepatitis C. Furthermore, if the partner with hepatitis C is

> Hepatitis C can be transmitted through sexual contact, although the risk seems to be much lower than for hepatitis B. Persons infected with hepatitis C should use condoms with new sexual partners. Couples who have been together a long time before one of them is diagnosed with hepatitis C may choose not to change their sexual practices.

also infected with HIV, there seems to be an even greater risk of his or her sexual partner becoming infected with hepatitis C.

Hepatitis C does not seem to be transmitted through the kind of casual contact that normally takes place in households and in the workplace. Neither does saliva seem to pose a risk, unless it is contaminated with blood, in which case transmission may be possible. Breast milk is also safe. Hepatitis C does not seem to be transmitted through food or water, as is hepatitis A. Nevertheless, a person with hepatitis C should try to avoid having any contact with others in the household that could result in transmission, such as sharing razors, toothbrushes, or nail-clipping equipment. Hugging, kissing (if there is no exposure to blood), casual contact (such as in a work situation), sneezing or coughing, and sharing eating utensils are not risks for transmitting hepatitis C.

Not everyone who is exposed to hepatitis C becomes infected. After an exposure there are currently no steps that can be taken to absolutely prevent infection, although prompt treatment with interferon has shown good results, as discussed later in this section. Injections with immune globulins (proteins in the body that fight infection) have not been shown to provide any protection before or after exposure.

No vaccine is available to prevent infection from hepatitis C, and there probably will not be one in the near future. Vaccines stimulate antibody response to an infection, and the antibody must be protective for the vaccine to work. The antibody that is stimulated from natural infection with hepatitis C does not offer any protection against reinfection, unlike the antibodies to hepatitis A and hepatitis B. In addition, the hepatitis C virus tends to mutate, changing the proteins on its surface rapidly, so a vaccine that is made to the proteins at one time may not offer protection at a later time. This characteristic of the virus also means that once a person is infected with hepatitis C, he or she could become reinfected with the virus again. A person infected with hepatitis C should therefore avoid any activity that poses a risk of reinfection. Such a person should also be vaccinated against hepatitis A and B, if he or she has never been infected with these viruses, because infection with these other types of viral hepatitis could cause severe illness and possibly even death.

TESTING FOR HEPATITIS C

People should consider getting tested if they have ever used injection drugs, received blood clotting factors (such as for treatment of hemophilia) before 1987, or a blood transfusion or organ transplant before 1992, have undergone hemodialysis, or have evidence of liver disease. People who work in health care settings and have been exposed to a needle stick or to body fluids splashed onto mucosal membranes, and children born to mothers who have hepatitis C, should also be tested. Other people who may be at risk are those who have received tattoos or body piercings, have had sex with someone infected with hepatitis C, have had many sexual partners, are spouses or household contacts of people with hepatitis C, or have shared straws for intranasal cocaine. People in any of these situations should consider testing.

People often find out they are positive for hepatitis C when they are donating blood or after routine testing reveals mild abnormalities in their liver blood tests. To many this information is a great surprise. Some may have engaged in high-risk activity (such as injection drug use with equipment sharing) perhaps twenty or more years ago and breathed a sigh of relief when they tested negative for hepatitis B and HIV, not realizing there was another virus to be concerned about. Not everyone with hepatitis C has elevated liver enzyme tests, however. In fact, up to a third of infected people may have normal liver tests, or test results that fluctuate between normal and slightly abnormal over time.

If you test positive for hepatitis C, you may feel overwhelmed and possibly depressed. Make sure you seek out emotional support if you need it, as well as counseling about treatment, transmission, and so forth. That support may come from a close friend, a support group, or a counselor.

A person can have a small amount of blood drawn to test for hepatitis C. The test, called the enzyme immunoassay (EIA), looks for antibodies that the body makes in response to the hepatitis C virus. When this test was first introduced in 1990, its results were found to be not very accurate. Many people showed a positive test when they were not infected, and some showed a negative result even though they were infected. More sensitive versions of the test became available in 1993. Anyone who was told in the late 1980s or early 1990s that he or she had hepatitis C, especially if there were no obvious risk factors for the disease, should now have another, more sensitive, blood test performed. The new EIA test, now standard for screening, is about 95 percent sensitive (meaning it detects infection in 95% of people who have an infection). A new, home version of the test has been approved by the FDA—"Hepatitis C Check" (made by the Home Access Health Corporation; see this book's appendix). The same company also produces an at-home test for HIV.

Recent infection with hepatitis C may not be detected on a blood test, even if the person is having hepatitis symptoms, because 40–50 percent of people with symptomatic acute hepatitis C infection have not yet developed antibody. When a person is diagnosed with acute hepatitis and the blood test is negative for hepatitis C, the test should be repeated in two to three months to confirm that the symptoms were not caused by hepatitis C. Most people test positive on the blood test ten weeks after infection, although it may take up to six months, and in some cases longer.

> There are several tests for hepatitis C. Those who tested positive before the early 1990s may want to have a new test performed, because the old tests resulted in many false positive results.

If there is concern about a new infection and the blood tests are "negative," a test to look for the genetic material of the virus (such as the PCR test—see below) may be a good idea, since it may detect a new infection before the body has time to develop antibodies (which are what the EIA detects). The PCR test may show as "positive" within days to eight weeks of infection. It is not clear, however, how long after a possible infection one can be certain that a "negative" PCR result truly means someone has not been infected. The standard EIA test is still the best test for screening.

A positive result on the EIA test does not distinguish between individuals who were infected but have cleared the virus and those who are still infected. Rarely, an EIA becomes "negative" after being "positive" for people who have been infected for a long time.

Two tests are commonly used to determine whether the EIA test results are accurately positive. The first is the recombinant immunoblot assay (RIBA), which also looks for antibody to the virus but is more sensitive than the EIA. The second test looks for the genetic material of the virus, which can be done with a PCR test or a branched DNA (bDNA) test, with the PCR test being more common because it is slightly more sensitive. Neither of these tests is recommended as a first test for screening; both are used as confirmatory tests. Neither is 100 percent accurate, however. If you have this test, it is best to discuss the results with your health care provider.

The test for the genetic material is the best confirmatory test, since it looks directly for the genetic material of the virus, and the RIBA may continue to be positive in a person who had hepatitis C infection in the past but has cleared the infection. However, if the RIBA is used, and if the person tested positive on the EIA and negative on the RIBA, she or he is considered not to have infection (a follow-up PCR should be done three to six months later just to make sure). If the RIBA result is positive or "indeterminate" (meaning unclear), then the person should be tested for the genetic material of the virus (the nucleic acid RNA).

Similarly, if the EIA is positive and the test for the genetic material (such as the PCR) is negative, a follow-up is still recommended in a few months, just to be sure. The test that looks for the genetic material of the virus can be used not only to confirm a positive EIA test, but to check on the response of the infection to treatment. Your health care provider may also do a test to see which of the six types of hepatitis C virus are present, because treatment may vary depending on the type.

If a person tests positive on the EIA and negative on the confirmatory tests, there are several possible explanations: the test may have been inaccurate, or perhaps the person had an infection in the past and has cleared the infection. There is still the possibility of infection, but the level of virus is too low to be detected. This is uncommon, however.

People with compromised immune systems (such as those with AIDS or those undergoing dialysis) may not show antibodies to the hepatitis C infection, and therefore the traditional screening test, the EIA, would not reveal the infection. For these people, the test for the genetic material (such as the PCR) may be a better first screen.

As you can see, interpreting these tests can be challenging.

The interpretation of all these tests is best done in consultation with a hepatologist (liver specialist) because of the potentially confusing results. A liver biopsy may be performed to help determine the progression of the infection. As noted previously, a biopsy is the best way to determine whether a person is experiencing continuous damage to the liver. A liver biopsy may identify someone with advanced liver disease even if he or she is symptom free.

Tests of liver function or status (liver enzyme tests) such as those carried out as part of a routine blood test are not an adequate screen for hepatitis C. These tests can often be normal even when someone is infected. For most people with hepatitis C, the results of liver enzyme tests fluctuate from normal to slightly elevated over time. For those who are exposed to someone with hepatitis C and wish to be tested for infection, it is recommended that they receive PCR, EIA, and liver enzyme tests as soon as possible, and four and twelve weeks later.

TREATMENT

Many studies are currently under way to find effective treatments for hepatitis C. As mentioned earlier, some people spontaneously clear the virus and do not need treatment. When to treat, and which treatment is best, is a decision to be made with the hepatologist. Research is under way to determine the best treatments and when to treat. The mainstay of treatment of acute and chronic infection is interferon. Interferon is a protein normally made by cells of the immune system in response to viruses. Alpha-, beta-, and pegylated interferon have shown some success in the treatment of acute hepatitis C; ribavirin is also sometimes used in combination with the interferon.

Sometimes the hepatologist may wait for three months after symptoms start following acute infection, to see whether the body clears the virus on its own. Waiting for this time period does not seem to adversely affect later success with treatment, although people who do develop symptoms with acute infection and people infected by a blood transfusion (which is rare today) are often treated right away, because they may have a higher risk of developing chronic infection. When treatment is shown to rid a person of the virus, follow-up at three-month intervals is usual to check that the virus is really gone; this check-up uses the test that looks for the genetic material of the virus.

If you have a chronic hepatitis C infection, talk with your hepatologist about when and if you should receive treatment. Factors that influence whether or not to treat include other medical conditions, the stage and severity of infection, the likelihood that you will have problems with the treatment, and the type of hepatitis C virus. A liver biopsy will probably be performed before starting treatment. Pegylated interferon, with or without ribavirin, is the standard treatment for chronic hepatitis C; therapy is continued for six to twelve months. The most common side effect is fatigue; fever, chills, and muscle aches are also common.

Once again a reminder: anyone who has chronic infection with hepatitis C should make every effort to prevent damage to their liver from other causes. Vaccination against hepatitis A and B is very important, as is not drinking alcohol, using drugs, or taking medications that may harm the liver. Talk with your health care provider about these and other measures you can take to keep your liver healthy.

HERPES

incidence: very common
cause: virus (herpes simplex virus)
symptoms: painful sores on the skin, with many variations
treatment: no cure; antivirals to treat and prevent symptoms

WHAT IS IT?

Herpes is a viral infection caused by the *herpes simplex virus* (HSV), of which there are two types: herpes simplex 1 (HSV-1) and herpes simplex 2 (HSV-2). Although HSV-1 and HSV-2 are distinctly different viruses, they cause similar symptoms. HSV-1 usually occurs around the mouth (where it causes cold sores), and HSV-2 usually occurs in the genital and anal areas. However, infection with these viruses can occur anywhere on the body. Mucosal skin surfaces—such as those around the mouth, genitals, and eyes—are most vulnerable, as are areas of broken skin. People infected with either HSV-1 or HSV-2 never get rid of the infection; however, as discussed below, the symptoms are usually intermittent and manageable.

The Greek word *herpes* means "to creep," referring to the way in which the virus moves along nerves from the root bodies out to the surface of the skin. Genital herpes was first recognized as an STD in the 1700s, but the virus itself was not identified until the early 1960s. The herpes simplex viruses are only two of the viruses in the herpes virus family, which also includes the *varicella-zoster virus*, which causes chicken pox and shingles, and *Epstein-Barr virus*, which causes mononucleosis.

A 1982 *Time* magazine cover story was headlined "Herpes: Today's Scarlet H"—a title derived from Nathaniel Hawthorne's novel *The Scarlet Letter*, in which a scarlet "A" was sewn onto the clothing of adulterous Puritans to brand them as promiscuous. The *Time* article seemed to imply that if you had herpes, you were labeled for life as promiscuous or unclean. This stigma is undeserved, but many people still believe it.

Even as recently as 1982, when that *Time* article appeared, many health care professionals believed that relatively few people had herpes and that, if they did, they usually suffered from very painful genital sores and therefore knew that they had an infection. Now we know much more than we did in 1982. It is clear, for example, that many people who become infected with herpes viruses are not promiscuous; that most people are infected with either type 1 or type 2 or both; and that many people are unaware that they are infected, because they have no symptoms or very mild symptoms, which they would not recognize as resulting from herpes infection.

HOW COMMON IS IT?

Approximately 70 percent of adults have oral herpes by the time they reach the age of forty, although there is some thought that HSV-1 infection—the usual cause of oral herpes—is becoming less common in childhood now than in the past. Most people acquire oral herpes through nonsexual transmission before the age of five, such as from an adult with oral HSV-1 who kisses them or from other children. Many people are not even aware that they have oral herpes, because about two-thirds of those with HSV-1 infection around the mouth are completely symptom free. They may remember having had cold sores as children, but they have not had recurrences as adults. Still others continue to have cold sores into adulthood.

HSV-2 infections can also occur around the mouth, but this is not common, and people who have oral infection with type 1 herpes rarely contract a second infection around the mouth with type 2 herpes.

When people do get infected with type 2 herpes in the mouth, they are usually completely symptom free. People usually acquire oral HSV-2 by performing oral sex on a person who has genital HSV-2 infection.

> **Approximately 70 percent of adults have oral herpes. Fewer than one-third of them ever get symptoms.**

Genital herpes is also very common: about fifty million adults in the United States over the age of fifteen have genital type 2 herpes, and about half a million new infections occur each year in this country. It is estimated that about one in five adults has genital herpes caused by either type 1 or type 2 virus. Genital herpes is almost always sexually transmitted. Those who are newly sexually active—people in their teens and twenties—have a high risk of acquiring genital herpes.

About 50–70 percent of first infections with genital herpes in the United States are caused by HSV-2, and about 30–50 percent are caused by HSV-1. Just as with oral herpes, the term *genital herpes* does not refer to a specific type of herpes—it can be caused by either type 1 or type 2 herpes viruses. And also as with oral herpes, most people who have genital herpes are unaware that they have been infected, because either they have no symptoms or they have symptoms they don't recognize as being those of herpes. Most people still think that herpes always causes painful blisters and ulcers, but the symptoms can be, and often are, more subtle (see the discussion of symptoms below).

> **About fifty million Americans are infected with genital herpes, making it one of the most common sexually transmitted infections.**

Even though genital herpes is very common, a great deal of misinformation is being circulated about it. People often label type 1 herpes as the "good" herpes and type 2 herpes as the "bad" herpes. Actually neither one is good or bad. It's just that one most commonly causes cold sores of the mouth, and the other most commonly causes genital sores. The artificial good-bad distinction arose because genital herpes is usually caused by sexual contact, and our society has mixed feelings about sex and sexuality.

WHAT ARE THE SYMPTOMS?

The symptoms of herpes usually last for a short time and go away for long stretches of time, so many people put the symptoms out of their mind and don't seek medical attention. When people do seek medical help, they may find that some health care providers are not very well informed about herpes. This is a rapidly expanding area of research, and many health care providers probably rely on out-of-date information. For this reason, if possible, those with herpes should obtain care for the infection from an STD specialist or from an infectious disease specialist if they feel that their questions are not being satisfactorily answered.

When a person becomes infected with oral or genital herpes, he or she may or may not know it. About 40 percent of people infected with genital herpes are completely symptom free with their first infection, and nearly 70 percent of people with oral herpes never notice cold sores. It is estimated that 20 percent of people with genital herpes will never have symptoms in their lifetimes and that 80 percent will—although most of them will not realize that their symptoms are from herpes.

Outbreaks and Asymptomatic Shedding of the Virus

As discussed previously, the classic symptoms of blisters and ulcers do not occur in everyone who has herpes. If symptoms do develop, however, they usually do so within two to twenty days of first infection. After infection with herpes, whether or not a person develops symptoms, the virus moves from the skin into the nerve endings that supply the area of the skin that was infected. It migrates along the nerve endings to the nerve root body, or ganglion, which is near the spinal cord. Here the virus remains quiet, or dormant, and then periodically migrates back out to the surface of the skin.

When the virus migrates back to the surface of the skin, a person may develop symptoms, such as a sore or itching or tingling on the skin, or he or she may remain completely symptom free. The condition in which there are symptoms is called an *outbreak*; when the virus comes to the surface of the skin and doesn't cause

Both oral herpes and genital herpes viruses can move to the surface of the skin and fail to cause symptoms.

symptoms, the condition is referred to as *asymptomatic* or *subclinical shedding of the virus.* Sometimes there is a warning that the virus is reactivating; this warning, called a *prodrome,* may consist of itching, tingling, or pain in the area where the outbreak takes place, but before there is any evidence on the skin. However, not everyone experiences prodromes.

Everyone who has oral or genital herpes, whether type 1 or type 2, will shed without symptoms at some point. How often this occurs varies from person to person, but on average it occurs for about 4 percent of the days in a year; asymptomatic shedding is more common in people with HSV-2 than with HSV-1. Why some people shed more than others, and why some people have more outbreaks than others, is not clear.

Two things are clear, however: people who are newly infected (for less than a year) have more asymptomatic shedding than those who have been infected for a longer time, and people who experience more frequent symptomatic outbreaks also tend to shed the virus more often without symptoms than those who rarely have outbreaks. (This characteristic of the disease is discussed in more detail later in this section.)

Herpes symptoms from the *recurrent* outbreaks are usually much less severe than those from the initial infection. Thus, for the person who is subject to a very severe first outbreak, there is some consolation in knowing that this will most likely be the worst outbreak ever to occur. As the body becomes adjusted to the virus and begins to build up some immunity, the episodic outbreaks become milder in most people.

If a person has symptoms that persist continuously for months or years, then a cause for the symptoms other than herpes should be considered. In addition, when someone has been diagnosed with herpes, he or she may assume that *any* genital symptom is caused by this virus and therefore may not seek medical attention. People with herpes should be aware that such assumptions can lead to problems, and they should seek medical attention whenever they experience new or unusual symptoms. Men tend to experience recurrences of herpes more frequently than women. In addition, the longer a first infection with herpes lasts, the more likely a person is to have frequent recurrences. If a first outbreak with HSV-2 lasts more than thirty-five days, a person can expect an average of eight outbreaks a year. A person whose first outbreak of HSV-2 lasts less than thirty-five days can expect about four outbreaks a year. Most people with genital HSV-1 experience only about one outbreak a year.

Various factors can trigger an outbreak. Some people, for example, believe that emotional or physical stress brings on oral and genital outbreaks. Others find that outbreaks are brought on by certain foods (nuts, chocolate), trauma to the skin, menstruation, fatigue, poor nutrition, illness, and exposure to sunlight (particularly for cold sores). Keeping track of potential triggers, possibly in a diary, is a good idea; then the triggers can be avoided in the future. Sometimes, despite "doing everything right," people still have outbreaks. Why the virus goes from inactive to active in some individuals but not in others is not understood, but researchers are actively investigating this question.

The virus does not usually spread to other areas of the skin in people infected with herpes who are otherwise healthy. An exception to this finding is a phenomenon called *autoinoculation*. Especially during the first few weeks of an initial infection, before the body has built up immunity to the virus, a person may spread the virus to other areas of the body by touching the area of infection and then immediately touching another area of the body. This is uncommon and generally can be prevented by washing the hands thoroughly after touching any infected area.

In individuals who are not healthy, such as those with compromised immune systems (people with AIDS or people undergoing chemotherapy), the virus can spread on its own to other areas of the body. This process, called *dissemination of the virus*, is uncommon. Herpes symptoms also tend to be more prolonged, and are usually more severe in general, in people with compromised immune systems.

> As with most STDs, the lack of symptoms does not indicate the lack of infection with herpes.

Where Symptoms Occur

When the virus comes out to the skin after the initial infection, it may cause symptoms or shed from any area on the skin supplied by the nerve that is infected. For example, a person with oral herpes infection can experience a cold sore or shedding of the virus in any area on the face, but most commonly between the nose and the chin, and usually around the mouth. Although oral herpes may (rarely) cause symptoms on the gums and hard palate, sores inside the mouth are usually not the result of herpes infection. Aphthous ulcers, the painful ulcers that occur *inside* the mouth, are not cold sores; it is not clear what causes them, but they are very common and not serious.

Genital herpes infections can occur in any part of the body supplied (reached) by the infected nerve, but they most commonly occur in the genital area, including the pubic hair region, the groin, and (for men) the penis, scrotum, and urethra, and (for women) the labia, urethra, vagina, and cervix. Genital herpes outbreaks can also occur on the anal area and part of the buttocks. If someone has always had outbreaks in one area of the genitals, such as on the labia, and then has a recurrence on the buttocks, she may worry that she has somehow "spread" the infection herself. What has actually happened is that the virus took a different path along a nerve root during that outbreak, causing symptoms to appear in a different spot. Furthermore, people may shed the virus from any of these regions during an outbreak. A lesion on the penis, for example, is obviously shedding virus, but virus may also be found on the testicles and anal area at that time. Asymptomatic shedding can occur from any skin area that the nerve supplies.

> **Herpes symptoms can occur on any area of skin that the infected nerve supplies.**

The Range of Symptoms

Herpes symptoms range from no symptoms at all in some people to painful ulcers or blisters (the classic symptoms) in others. More subtle symptoms include red, itchy, or tingling areas; red bumps or pimple-like bumps; and tiny slits or "scratches." First infections with herpes tend to cause more severe symptoms than recurrences, but as mentioned previously, some people have no symptoms when they become infected, so there are exceptions to this generalization.

Lesions on skin surfaces—such as the face; the penis, pubic area, buttocks, and scrotum for men; and the outer labia, buttocks, or pubic area for women—usually form a scab as they heal. However, lesions that are on mucosal surfaces—such as the anal area, inner labia, vagina, or urethra—do not form a scab as they heal. These lesions usually do not leave a scar. Symptoms usually last for a few days and then clear up.

Other symptoms may accompany the sores, or the sores may be the only symptoms of an outbreak. Lymph nodes in the groin may swell and be painful when a person has a genital herpes recurrence, or those in the neck may enlarge during an oral herpes recurrence. Other possible symptoms are headache, back pain, leg pain, stiff neck, sore throat, heightened sensitivity of the eyes to light, and a feeling of being tired and achy all over, similar to the experience of having the flu.

Some unusual symptoms that can occur in the genital area are numbness or increased sensation in the genital area or lower back, weakness or tingling in the legs, and constipation. These symptoms tend to be more common with the first infection, but they may also occur in future outbreaks. With genital herpes, a woman may experience a vaginal discharge or pain with urination. A man with a herpes infection may feel burning during urination, with or without discharge, and without lesions.

Some symptoms make it hard to distinguish herpes from other infections or problems in the genital area. For example, allergic reactions to soaps or spermicides can cause itching and breaks in the skin of the genital area that can mimic herpes. Genital fungal infections in men can cause red, itchy areas. Many women mistake their herpes symptoms for yeast infections, and since yeast medications are now available without a prescription, women may think they are successfully treating a yeast infection when in fact they are experiencing herpes symptoms that resolve, over time, on their own.

Women may also mistake herpes symptoms for a bladder infection. A herpes lesion that is located near or inside the urethra, or urinary opening, may cause burning with urination, which may feel like a bacterial bladder infection. Taking an antibiotic will seem to make the symptoms resolve, when what really happens is that the herpes lesion heals on its own. Some other STDs also cause sores in the genital area and burning with urination.

> Herpes symptoms can be varied and may differ from person to person. They may be mistaken for a yeast or bladder infection in both men and women.

An initial herpes infection can occur in the anal and rectal area, most often after receiving anal sex. This infection usually causes rectal pain and discharge, which may be bloody, and it can also cause fever, muscle aches, and changes in bowel movements. (See the section on proctocolitis, proctitis, and enteritis.) Recurrences of outbreaks can occur in the rectal area. Although HSV outbreaks inside the rectum usually occur as a result of receptive anal intercourse, herpes outbreaks can occur around the anal area even in someone who has never received anal sex, because the nerve that supplies that area also supplies the genital area.

Herpes infections can cause more serious symptoms. For example, genital herpes outbreaks can cause inflammation of the lining of the spinal cord, called *meningitis*. Meningitis caused by herpes is a type of viral meningitis, which is different from the often life-threatening bacterial meningitis. Symptoms of viral meningitis are a stiff neck and pain in the eyes when looking at light. Most people who have a first infection with genital herpes have some inflammation of the spinal fluid, since the virus is in a nerve, but only a small percentage develop *symptoms* from this inflammation. For a very few people, the only symptom of recurrent herpes outbreaks is viral meningitis. Meningitis from herpes infections seldom causes any permanent problems, but it may recur, either with or without subsequent outbreaks. This is, fortunately, not common.

Very rarely, oral herpes infections can cause inflammation of the tissues of the brain, called *encephalitis*. Signs of this infection are headache, fever, confusion, seizures, and neurological impairment, depending on which area of the brain is affected. Encephalitis can result in permanent neurological symptoms. However, considering how common oral herpes infections are, this is an extremely rare complication.

How Long Do Symptoms Last?

First infections generally take longer to heal than recurrences, for both oral and genital herpes. First outbreaks with herpes in the genital area, whether type 1 or type 2, last about ten to fourteen days on average, although they can last for as long as six weeks if not treated. The outbreak may last even longer if a person is taking oral steroids (which decrease the body's ability to fight the infection) for other medical conditions or is mistakenly applying topical steroids in efforts to treat the sores. It is not uncommon for new lesions to erupt within a few days of each other during first infections. Treatment with oral antiviral medications will shorten both the first episode and recurrent infections (see the discussion of treatment).

The first symptoms that a person may recognize may actually be a recurrent outbreak from a prior infection; recurrent outbreaks usually last about five to seven days. As noted earlier, some people with herpes are unaware of it when they first become infected and only notice symptoms later, during a recurrence.

The symptoms that are caused by HSV-1 or HSV-2 in the oral or genital area are exactly the same. The only difference is that type 2 herpes tends to recur less frequently than type 1 in the oral area, and type 1 tends to recur less frequently than type 2 in the genital area.

> Type 1 and type 2 herpes cause exactly the same symptoms; the only difference is the frequency of outbreaks they cause in different areas of the body.

The bottom line for most people is that herpes is simply an occasional physical annoyance that can be treated with medication. For many people, herpes doesn't even cause symptoms. Herpes doesn't cause cancer (there used to be a worry about herpes putting women at risk for cervical cancer, but this does not seem to be the case), and in otherwise healthy individuals it doesn't spread to other areas of the body. It is often the emotional issues that are harder to deal with, as discussed later.

HOW IS HERPES TRANSMITTED?

Both types of herpes simplex virus are transmitted by skin contact with an area of a partner that is infected, or with secretions that are infected with the virus, such as semen, vaginal secretions, and saliva. The most vulnerable areas for acquiring herpes infections are mucosal surfaces, such as the mouth and throat, genital skin, or conjunctiva of the eye. Women acquire genital herpes more easily than men, probably because women have a larger area of mucosal skin surface in the genital area than men, which means there is a larger area vulnerable to infection. Anywhere on the body where the skin is broken is also a vulnerable area.

Herpes is not transmitted through inanimate objects such as towels, drinking glasses, and toilet seats, but there is the possibility (although unproven) that it may be transmitted through the use of shared sex toys, if they are immediately exchanged between partners. The virus is inactivated when secretions dry, and it doesn't last long outside the body. (Theoretically, if someone with a genital lesion or oral lesion had direct contact

> **Herpes is not transmitted by inanimate objects.**

with an object, such as a towel, which was then immediately put into contact with a vulnerable area of another person, such as the genitals, eyes, or mouth, then transmission could take place. But the likelihood of this actually happening is very remote, and there are no documented cases of herpes being transmitted in this way.) Herpes cannot be transmitted through the water or surfaces of a hot tub or a swimming pool. The only way to get herpes in a hot tub is to have sex with an infected partner in a hot tub.

When to Abstain from Sex

It used to be thought that in order to transmit herpes, the infected person must have a sore or another symptom of a herpes outbreak, such as itching, tingling, or leg pain. In other words, the message was "If you're having an outbreak, abstain from sex, but if you're not having symptoms, then you can safely have unprotected sex and not transmit the virus." We now know that the first part of this statement is true, but the second part is not. *Herpes can be transmitted when someone is not having symptoms.* This is new information for most people, including health care providers.

This had been suspected for a while, because many couples with one partner infected with genital herpes and the other partner uninfected found that the virus had been transmitted, even though they had been careful during outbreaks. Research has shown that the virus can be detected in the mouths of people with oral herpes, or the genital areas of people with genital herpes, even when they are not experiencing symptoms. Although we don't know how much virus is necessary for

> **Most herpes transmission occurs from people who are not aware that they are infectious.**

transmission, this research shows that herpes can be transmitted by an infected person who has no symptoms. It is estimated that most transmission of oral and genital herpes occurs when people are unaware that they are infectious.

Because it is important to abstain from sex during a herpes outbreak, it's important to know when outbreaks are occurring. Some people with herpes infections believe that they can tell when they are having an outbreak, that they always have some warning sign that lets them know ahead of time. However, this is not always true. In the case of asymptomatic shedding, unfortunately, no one knows for sure when shedding days occur. Some people shed as infrequently as a few days out of the year, whereas others may be shedding as often as several days per month. People seem to shed the virus more frequently around the time of symptomatic outbreaks, such as during the week before and after an outbreak, but it's possible to shed at any time. However, it is important to keep in mind that people with herpes are not always shedding virus.

If one partner is not infected and the couple is trying to prevent transmission, it's a good idea to abstain from sex when symptoms are present. People should consider themselves as "having an outbreak" from the appearance of the first symptom until the lesion is replaced by normal-appearing skin. *Even if you are not sure whether the symptoms are from an outbreak, play it safe.* Using a condom for genital sex at this time does not necessarily offer full protection, because a person may be shedding virus outside the area that a condom protects; but a condom will probably decrease transmission.

Symptoms that may indicate that the virus is active are tingling; itching; a red area or bump that may or may not be painful; a slit in the skin; an ulcer, blister, or pustule; or leg pain. These are warning signs that the virus may be on the surface of the skin and that the person may therefore transmit the virus to others.

What Is the Likelihood of Infection?

Many people want to know the likelihood of getting herpes from a partner who is infected with genital herpes. For couples who abstain from sex during an outbreak but have sex without a condom between outbreaks, the average risk is *10 percent for the uninfected person to acquire herpes from the infected partner over the course of a year.* In other words, ten people out of a hundred in such a relationship will, after a year, have contracted herpes from their partner via asymptomatic shedding, but ninety people out of a hundred will remain uninfected.

> An uninfected partner has on average a 10 percent chance of acquiring herpes from an infected partner after a year if the couple is not regularly using a barrier method during sexual intercourse.

As noted earlier, women have a higher risk of becoming infected. An uninfected man having unprotected sex with an infected female partner in the above scenario has about a 4 percent risk of getting genital herpes after a year, whereas a woman having unprotected sex with an infected male partner has about a 10 percent chance of getting herpes after a year if she already has HSV-1 orally, but about a 32 percent chance of getting herpes after a year if she is completely negative for herpes. These statistics are derived from studies of discordant couples (one person has herpes and the other doesn't) over a specified period of time. Whether these statistics hold for every year a couple has been together, or whether they change with time, is not yet known. Usually the longer a person has herpes, the less active that person's virus becomes, so for any specific couple these numbers may decrease over time. Studies are under way to evaluate further the risk of infection.

For a woman having unprotected sex with a female partner, the risk is probably lower overall than the risk of having sex with an infected male partner, although transmission may still take place between women through genital rubbing and through oral sex.

Clearly, it is not inevitable that a person who is sexually active with a partner who has herpes will contract herpes. For some couples, even after years of unprotected sexual contact only one of the partners has herpes. Then there are those who are sexually intimate with a person with herpes just once or only a couple of times and acquire herpes from that contact.

A few truths seem to hold for most people regarding transmission of the herpes viruses. First, a person who has had a past infection with one type of herpes virus will not get reinfected in that area of the body with the same strain of the virus. For example, a person with genital HSV-2 will not be repeatedly infected with genital HSV-2 on reexposure. Therefore *couples in which both partners are infected with genital type 2 herpes, for example, do not need to worry about transmission to one another*. They will not reinfect one another through genital sexual contact. Furthermore, the likelihood of acquiring a new infection with HSV-2 in another area of the body is low, because the antibody that is produced following the initial infection, which circulates through the body, offers protection at other sites.

People with type 2 herpes will almost never acquire a new type 1 infection, because the antibody to type 2 offers nearly complete protection against a new type 1 infection. Therefore, neither oral nor genital sex for a couple with both partners having HSV-2 poses a risk of reinfection. Although HSV-1 offers some protection against acquiring HSV-2, the protection is not as complete, and someone with type 1 can acquire a type 2 infection if exposed. However, as discussed later, it is unlikely that a person will acquire HSV-2 in the same area where he or she has the HSV-1 infection.

Similarly, two people who are infected with oral type 1 herpes will not reinfect one another through kissing. However, there is a risk that they could infect one another through oral sex, although this risk seems to be low. If only one partner has oral HSV-1, then the uninfected partner can more easily acquire genital HSV-1 through oral sex, especially if it is performed while the infected partner has a cold sore.

Generally people who have one type of herpes infection in one area of the body are unlikely to acquire a different strain of herpes infection in the same area of the body. For example, if a person who has oral HSV-1 performs oral sex on a person who has genital HSV-2, it is unlikely (although still possible) that the first person will become infected with oral type 2 herpes in addition to the existing type 1 infection. A person who does not have oral or genital herpes and performs oral sex on a person with HSV-2 can acquire the infection in the mouth, but this person would not be likely to develop symptoms, and it would be very unusual if he or she shed this virus asymptomatically—oral HSV-2 infection is usually completely symptom free and does not seem to shed frequently. As mentioned previously, the partner with type 2 herpes

> **People generally do not acquire type 1 and type 2 herpes in the same area of the body.**

genitally runs little or no risk of acquiring type 1 herpes in the genital area, since the antibody to HSV-2 offers almost complete protection against acquiring a new HSV-1 infection.

Tools for Preventing Transmission of Herpes

Since it is likely that everyone with herpes infections, whether oral or genital, type 1 or type 2, sheds when they are symptom free at some time or another, one might think, "Since practically everyone has herpes, and it's not clear when it's safe to have sex, it's inevitable that I'll get it if I have a partner who has herpes!" or "I'm going to get herpes anyway, so I might as well give up trying not to get it." Other people want to do everything they can to prevent transmission of herpes. Couples who have been together a while and are planning to remain together might not be as worried about transmitting the virus. In my opinion, it is always a good idea to discuss the question of herpes early in a relationship, before becoming sexually active, so that you can decide together how you want to approach this issue. (See Chapter 4 on sexual communication for more details.)

Everyone, and every couple, approaches the issue differently. It is best to make decisions based on accurate, current information, not on myths. Likewise decisions must be made together, as a team. Sometimes the person with herpes thinks it is entirely his or her responsibility, but this is not the case. Facing the question of herpes is often the first difficult decision that a couple makes, and working through· this issue can be the first step toward real closeness. Remember: being in a relationship involves confronting thousands of issues over time. Herpes is just one of them. The initial emotions when you're diagnosed with herpes can be overwhelming, but give yourself time and don't beat yourself up. Herpes is a very common virus, not a punishment. Remember that millions of people with herpes form loving, lasting relationships with partners, and over time herpes often becomes more of a manageable, periodic nuisance than something that defines one's life.

Here I present some tools for couples who want to take steps to prevent the transmission of herpes. What can you do to protect yourself from getting herpes, or how can you keep from transmitting herpes to your partner? The first thing is to know your herpes status. Getting a blood test will tell you about your status for both type 1 and type 2 herpes (see the discussion of testing later in this section); you don't need to be experiencing symptoms to be tested. Couples who know partners' individual statuses for herpes infections can then make informed decisions about what type of sexual contact is safe and what type is risky. If you or your partner have not had this test performed and thus don't know whether one of you has herpes, then use a condom to help protect against transmission until you can be tested. As noted earlier, if both partners have the same kind of genital herpes (both have type 1 or both have type 2), then they will not reinfect one another, nor will they trigger outbreaks in one another.

Couples in which one partner has herpes and the other does not should abstain from sex during outbreaks, since the risk of transmission is greater at this time. Between outbreaks, condoms help reduce the chance of transmission of virus by about 50 percent (as noted earlier, this protection is not total because shedding in an area outside that covered by the condom can transmit virus). For nonpenetrative intercourse for which a

Condom use helps decrease the risk of herpes transmission.

condom can't be used, another barrier method, such as a dental dam, could be used. The spermicide nonoxynol-9 should not be used. New studies have shown that it may cause irritation to the skin, which can make transmission of herpes easier.

A promising development has occurred in herpes research in the last few years. Studies have shown that taking a herpes medication suppressively (every day) decreases asymptomatic shedding of the virus by more than 90 percent. Furthermore, a 2004 study showed that taking 500 mg of valacyclovir every day decreased transmission to uninfected partners by about 50 percent. Therefore, suppressive therapy for the infected partner is now an option for couples who want to "take every precaution" against an uninfected partner becoming infected. There are no data suggesting that the person who *does not* have herpes can prevent infection by taking an antiviral medication (since the medications work only in people already infected with the virus).

Extensive research is being performed to find a vaccine to prevent people from ever becoming infected with herpes viruses. Although some vaccines initially showed promise in studies in the 1990s, none has been found 100 percent effective in preventing transmission of herpes from partner to partner. One vaccine that is the focus of research may help reduce symptoms, and may reduce (although not completely prevent) trans-

> **In the near future, there may be new options for preventing herpes transmission.**

mission in women who are newly infected with herpes and have never been infected with either type of herpes before. However, this vaccine does not seem to prevent infection in women who are already infected with HSV-1, or prevent infection in men. Other vaccines are under study as well. Stay tuned!

Transmission from Mother to Child

Millions of women with herpes have normal, healthy babies every year, and *generally herpes is a problem in pregnancy only when there is a lack of understanding about how herpes can be transmitted during pregnancy, or when the parents are not aware of their herpes status.* If you and your partner, as well as your obstetrician or nurse midwife, know your herpes status, and if your obstetrician or nurse midwife is well informed about herpes and pregnancy, then precautions can usually be taken to prevent transmission to the child. First, the facts.

Herpes can be transmitted to the fetus (particularly if the mother becomes infected while she is pregnant), to the newborn during delivery (if the mother has virus present in the genital area at the time of delivery), and to the infant (if he or she is kissed by someone who has a cold sore). About 5 percent of infants who are infected with HSV are infected while in the womb, 85 percent are infected by passing through an infected birth canal at delivery, and about 10 percent are infected after birth. Women with a history of herpes have a low risk of transmitting the virus to their newborn infant. The greatest risk of transmitting the virus to the newborn is posed by a mother who becomes infected during the pregnancy. In the United States, about 1 in 4500 live newborn infants is infected with herpes (called *neonatal herpes*). Between 20 and 30 percent of neonatal herpes cases are caused by HSV-1, and between 70 and 80 percent by HSV-2. Infants infected with herpes at birth have symptoms ranging from mild skin, eye, and mouth infections to disseminated infection with permanent neurological symptoms to death. Children who do survive are at risk for developmental delay, even if they had only mild symptoms at birth. Prompt treatment of the infant with herpes medications can help subdue the symptoms, but the medications may not work as well in advanced cases.

A woman who is infected with herpes *before pregnancy* has antibodies in her bloodstream, which are the body's immune response to infection and offer protection against new herpes infection. These antibodies (and the immunity they convey) are transmitted to the fetus in the womb, so there is a low risk of the fetus becoming infected in the womb if the mother had herpes before she became pregnant. The greatest risk of infection in this situation occurs during delivery, when the newborn may be exposed to a large quantity of virus, especially if the woman is experiencing an outbreak. If a woman with herpes is having an outbreak or prodrome (warning signs that an outbreak is coming, such as tingling, itching, burning, etc.) at the time of delivery, then a cesarean delivery is recommended to prevent passage of the baby through the infected birth canal. (Rarely, babies born by cesarean delivery are nevertheless infected with HSV, probably because they were infected in the womb or during premature rupture of the membranes.) If the mother is not having an outbreak, there is a very small chance (less than 1%) that she will be shedding virus through the birth canal at delivery; if she is shedding, there is a small chance (also less than 1%) that the child will become infected. So, for women who have herpes and who give birth vaginally, the overall risk is less than 1 percent that the baby will become infected.

> The risk of transmission to a fetus or newborn is small when a woman acquired genital herpes infection before the pregnancy began.

The decision whether or not to have a cesarean delivery is an individual one, and it must be discussed with one's health care provider. Cesarean deliveries are not routine for all pregnant women with herpes, since this procedure is not in itself without risk, and the risk of transmission to the baby when there is not an outbreak is very low in a woman who acquired the infection before the pregnancy. A woman who knows she has herpes can prepare for this decision well in advance.

It is recommended that, during labor, infants whose mothers are infected with herpes should not be connected to fetal scalp monitors (which rely on electrodes that create tiny cuts in the scalp) or delivered with the use of forceps unless absolutely necessary, since the trauma that occurs from these instruments may allow entry of the herpes virus and thus increase the risk of infection.

When a woman and her health care provider are unaware that she has herpes, no discussion of options will have taken place, and precautions will not have been taken to prevent transmission. In this case, if the woman is having an outbreak when she goes into labor, decisions must be made during the delivery. Blood tests for herpes earlier in the pregnancy should be considered for all women, so that planning can be done in advance.

Testing later in the pregnancy is also a good idea, to make sure that a woman has not acquired herpes *during the pregnancy. Both the pregnant woman and her partner should be tested.* A woman who acquires a herpes infection during her pregnancy, especially during the last trimester, runs the highest risk of transmitting the infection to the fetus. To clarify why an infection during pregnancy, particularly in the last trimester, is so concerning: when a mother experiences a first infection, the fetus may become infected in the uterus. A woman who is newly infected is also more likely to shed the virus at delivery, so the newborn has a higher chance of being exposed to virus during passage through the birth canal. If the infection occurs earlier in the pregnancy, there is a possibility that the mother will develop antibody and transmit it to the fetus, so that by the time the baby is born he or she will have some protection against infection. However, if a new infection of the mother occurs later in the pregnancy, such as during the last trimester, it is not likely that there will have been time for the mother to develop antibody and pass it to the fetus, so the baby will be at higher risk of becoming infected if exposed to virus at delivery.

Any woman who is thinking about starting a pregnancy should discuss herpes and herpes testing with her health care provider.

A woman who experiences a true first-episode infection (meaning it is the first time she has been infected with genital herpes) and is shedding virus at delivery has a 30–50 percent chance of transmitting the virus to her infant. As already noted, the later in the pregnancy that a woman contracts herpes, the higher the risk that she will have an outbreak or be shedding virus at delivery. This is why infections later in pregnancy cause the greatest concern. *If a pregnant woman does not have herpes but her partner does, the couple should use condoms during the pregnancy and should consider abstaining from sex during the last trimester, since this is the riskiest time for the baby.* Couples should be aware that herpes can also be transmitted through oral sex. If the pregnant woman does not have a history of cold sores in the mouth or genital herpes, and the partner has a history of cold sores, oral sex (partner performing oral sex on the pregnant woman) should be avoided during the third trimester. If a male partner has herpes and the pregnant woman does not, the man may also want to consider using suppressive therapy (see the discussion of treatments) with antiviral medication during the pregnancy. Most neonatal herpes is preventable if both the woman and her partner are aware of their herpes status and take precautions during pregnancy.

> If both partners are tested for herpes before the pregnancy (and possibly during the pregnancy as well) and take precautions during the pregnancy, most problems can be averted.

Cultures performed on the mother at delivery, or even the polymerase chain reaction (PCR) test (discussed below), usually take at least several days to show a positive result if virus is present, and tests to detect shedding that are performed several days before delivery do not reveal anything about shedding at the time of delivery. The only benefit of performing these tests at delivery is to help guide therapy should the infant become ill; that is, a positive test for herpes may help diagnose the infant's symptoms as being caused by herpes, and treatment may be started more quickly. A test may show up as positive even before the infant becomes symptomatic, and in that situation herpes medication should be started for the baby right away. Even though the presence of virus in the mother's test doesn't necessarily mean that the baby has been infected, it is probably better to be safe. Symptoms indicating that the infant may be infected include lack of appetite, skin lesions such as blisters, fever, and sluggishness. These symptoms may take up to a month to develop in an infected infant.

Two studies have looked at whether using antiviral medication (acyclovir) suppressively during the last two weeks of pregnancy might decrease the need for cesarean deliveries by decreasing the frequency of shedding and outbreaks during delivery, and results have shown that this could be the case. Although none of the antiviral medications has been approved by the FDA for use during pregnancy, some obstetricians are prescribing acyclovir during the last two weeks of pregnancy for women with a history of herpes, to suppress shedding at the time of delivery. Most obstetricians would recommend acyclovir during pregnancy for a first infection or a severe recurrence. For women who acquire a new infection in the third trimester, the decision is whether or not to use acyclovir and/or have a cesarean delivery. It is best to make this decision in conjunction with your obstetrician. The makers of acyclovir have a registry of women who inadvertently used acyclovir during their first trimester, and a higher risk of birth defects is not evident. However, because of concerns about possible harm to the fetus, the FDA has not approved antiviral medication for this purpose. Talk with your health care provider about the risks and benefits to decide what is best for you.

A final word about herpes and other STDs. Any genital ulcer disease, such as herpes, makes transmission of other sexually transmitted infections, such as HIV, easier, because breaks in the skin can provide a way for the HIV virus to enter. So it is very important that people with herpes be concerned with protecting partners from acquiring infection (see Chapter 4 on sexual communication and Chapter 5 on "safer sex") and that they take precautions and be safe with new partners, to avoid becoming infected with other STDs themselves.

TESTING FOR HERPES

A definitive diagnosis of herpes cannot be made without testing. A lesion may look like a herpes lesion, but a test must be performed to determine if it is in fact herpes. Anyone with symptoms suggestive of herpes (as discussed previously) should be seen by a health care provider as soon as possible, because delay can make accurate diagnosis more difficult. Furthermore, the type of herpes a person has (HSV-1 or HSV-2) should also be determined, since the risk of transmission and prediction of future outbreaks depend on the virus type.

There are several ways to diagnose herpes. Some, such as culture and Tzanck prep, involve testing during outbreaks, whereas others, such as the blood tests, can be carried out even when a person is not having herpes symptoms. Skin tests for herpes can be inaccurate, re-sulting in a false negative up to 50 percent of the time for recurrent lesions, meaning that the test doesn't detect herpes, even though it is the cause of the symptoms. Therefore if the results of a skin test are negative, additional testing should be done—either a test of another lesion or a blood test, as described below.

A note on having a positive test result for herpes: For most peo-ple, the emotional issues surrounding a diagnosis of herpes are more difficult than the physical symptoms. It is normal to have strong emo-tions when receiving this diagnosis. Most people learn to cope well and, with education and time, begin to see herpes as an occasional physical annoyance, not a life-defining illness. Several excellent re-sources for support and information about herpes, as well as other chronic STDs, are listed in the appendix of this book. Support groups, help from organizations such as ASHA (American Social Health As-sociation), a close friend to confide in—all may be helpful as you are adjusting to the diagnosis.

See Chapter 4, "Sexual Communication," for a discussion about broaching the topic with sexual partners. Although talking with part-ners can be difficult, being honest and upfront can save heartache later. *Not* talking about herpes before becoming intimate can break trust in a relationship. When you tell a new partner, be informed about herpes and have literature available. How you present this informa-tion will most likely affect how your partner responds. And remem-ber, since one in five people in the United States is infected, if you break the ice on this topic your partner may be able to talk openly if she or he is also infected.

Viral Culture

This is the best test if a "lesion" (a change in the skin) is present. To culture a lesion, a swab of the area of the skin that is symptomatic is taken and placed into culture medium. This fluid is taken to a labo-ratory, where it is placed in contact with animal cells in culture. In seven to ten days, certain changes, consistent with herpes, occur in the animal cells if the virus is present. Additional tests can then be performed to determine what type of herpes—type 1 or type 2—is present.

Cultures are performed as soon as possible after a lesion occurs, because the longer the wait, the less likely a culture is to provide an accurate result. *For this reason a positive culture of a lesion is helpful, but a negative culture does not mean the person does not have herpes.* If the lesion has already progressed to the scab stage, then it may be too late to

When a culture result comes back as positive, the type of herpes (type 1 or 2) will often be reported. A negative culture does not mean a person is not infected with herpes; it simply means that no virus was present in that sample.

do a culture, since little virus is present. Viral cultures are the recommended test if there is a visible change on the skin. However, even when someone has herpes, he or she may show no virus about 50 percent of the time.

Tzanck Prep Test

The Tzanck prep test is not performed today as often as in the past, because it is less sensitive than viral culture in the diagnosis of herpes. This test is performed by scraping a lesion, putting the sample on a slide, staining it, and looking under the microscope for characteristic cell changes. It cannot distinguish between HSV-1 and HSV-2. If a lesion is present, the preferred test is a culture, not a Tzanck prep.

Antigen Detection

Antigen detection is performed on a sampling of a lesion and can usually provide results more quickly than culture because nothing needs to "grow." The test is designed to detect the antigens or proteins that are on the surface of the virus. Even in the scab stage, a lesion may have antigen present, so this test may be more sensitive than a culture in testing an older lesion. It cannot distinguish between the types of herpes, however, and a negative test does not rule out herpes. This test is not routinely available.

Polymerase Chain Reaction Test

The PCR test is newer. It is intended to detect the genetic material of the herpes virus and is much more sensitive than viral culture tests. It is also much more expensive than culture tests and is not offered in all areas of the country. It can be used to test a lesion or spinal fluid to evaluate for herpes. The PCR test is not FDA approved for testing lesions, however. It can distinguish between HSV-1 and HSV-2.

Pap Smear

Sometimes a Pap smear shows changes consistent with herpes if there is an outbreak on the cervix at the time the smear is performed, but the test is not a reliable screen for herpes. (See the section on genital warts for more information on the Pap smear.) In one study, in which women had active cervical inflammation from herpes that was confirmed by culture, the Pap smear detected the herpes virus only about 60 percent of the time. It also cannot distinguish between HSV-1 and HSV-2.

Blood Tests

In the past ten years, many new blood tests for herpes have become widely available. All of these blood tests can distinguish between HSV-1 and HSV-2. However, unlike a test that uses a swab from a lesion, blood tests don't reveal *where* a person has infection. For example, someone who tests positive for HSV-1 most likely has infection in the mouth area, but could have infection in the genital area; without symptoms, it's impossible to tell. Blood tests also take time to become positive following the infection, because they look for the body's immune response to the infection, not the infection itself. Antibodies are proteins made by the body's immune system in response to infection; once they are present, they remain for life. Therefore, a positive test for antibodies doesn't indicate when or where someone became infected.

Some of the antibody tests developed before 1999 did not clearly distinguish between HSV-1 and HSV-2. In fact, if you had oral infection with HSV-1, there was a good chance that you would also test positive for HSV-2, and vice versa. Unfortunately, these older tests are sometimes still used to test for herpes, often in settings where testing for STDs is not routinely done. The newer, more accurate, blood tests look for antibodies to a specific protein on the surface of the virus, called "glycoprotein G" (or "gG"). People infected with HSV-1 show antibodies to the "G1" protein, and people infected with HSV-2 show antibodies to the "G2" protein. Ask your health care provider if the blood test to be used distinguishes between these proteins. The tests are reasonably accurate, but not 100 percent. There are two such tests that can even be done in the health care provider's office to look for antibodies to HSV-2 (but not HSV-1) by testing blood from a finger stick.

These blood tests may take up to six months to show a positive result after someone has been newly infected, so, particularly in the early stages of infection, a negative result doesn't rule out infection. Again, even though these tests are very good, they are not 100 percent accurate, and in rare situations tests may miss an infection or give a false positive result.

If you decide to have a blood test for herpes, ask your health care provider for one of the tests that specifically looks for the "G" proteins. There is a very sensitive blood test called the "Western blot." This test is not commonly available, however; it is used mostly in research settings.

The blood tests cost, on average, between $20 and $140. When are these blood tests useful? Some of the following scenarios are situations in which a person may want to get screened for herpes:

> The herpes Western blot assay is a reliable way to test for herpes even if a person doesn't have symptoms. However, it is rarely used except in research.

—A person has symptoms, but other testing (like a culture) is negative.
—A person has had symptoms suggestive of herpes, but no symptoms right now.
—A person has a partner who has herpes and wants to know if he or she is at risk for acquiring infection.
—A person is at risk for other STDs or already has another STD, such as HIV.
—A person wants a "full screen for sexually transmitted infections."

When genital sores or ulcers are present, other possible diagnoses must be considered. Syphilis, lymphogranuloma venereum, and chancroid are additional STDs that can cause genital ulcers. In addition, certain medical conditions, such as the inflammatory bowel disorder called Crohn's disease, can cause genital sores. The autoimmune disease Behçet's syndrome can cause genital ulcers as well as oral ulcers and conjunctivitis.

> **Not all genital ulcers are the result of herpes infection, although herpes is by far the most common cause of genital sores in the United States.**

TREATMENT AND PREVENTION OF OUTBREAKS

There is no cure for herpes, but there are very good medications that can prevent symptoms and can treat symptoms when they do occur. Some of these medications are useful for both type 1 and type 2 herpes. Some people are concerned that, "If I take this medication now, it won't work in the future," or "If I take this medication now to suppress my outbreaks, when I stop taking it they'll be really bad." This is not true. Taking these medications does not alter how often or how severe your outbreaks will be in the future. The medications are available only by prescription in the United States, and they are expensive. Acyclovir, valacyclovir, and famciclovir are all available in pill form to be taken by mouth; acyclovir is also available as a cream; and penciclovir, the active ingredient of famciclovir, is available as a cream as well. Acyclovir has been available by prescription since 1982; valacyclovir and famciclovir became available in 1996. These medications do not prevent infection if an uninfected person takes them. They only benefit people who have herpes. *Steroids should not be used to treat herpes, because they can make the infection worse.*

Acyclovir, valacyclovir, and famciclovir are converted into their active forms by an enzyme present in the herpes virus but not in the human body. These antiviral medications act by interrupting the virus's ability to replicate itself. They do not remove the virus from the body, but by stopping its replication they shorten the duration of an outbreak and decrease the severity of the symptoms (if taken *episodically*, that is, during an outbreak). To help prevent outbreaks in an infected individual, these medications can also be taken daily (*suppressively*). All three medications are useful for both the prevention and treatment of genital herpes outbreaks, whether caused by HSV-1 or HSV-2.

The cream form of acyclovir has not been proven effective in preventing or treating outbreaks of oral or genital herpes. A newer cream

form of famciclovir has recently
been approved for the treatment
of recurrent cold sores (but not
genital herpes). It shortens the
duration of outbreaks and diminishes their symptoms. Someone

> Safe and effective medi-
> cations are available to
> treat herpes symptoms and
> help prevent outbreaks.

with a history of recurrent oral herpes who wishes to treat symptoms
episodically can choose either acyclovir or the penciclovir cream.

Another treatment for cold sores that doesn't require a prescription is the cream docosanol. This acts in a different way from the medications listed above. It prevents the herpes virus from entering skin
cells after the virus reactivates. Docosanol is not approved for treatment of genital herpes.

Before you begin taking any medication, you and your health care
provider should carefully discuss the benefits and the possible side
effects, as well as how to take the medication correctly. Deciding
whether to take the medication at all, or whether to take it only during an outbreak or daily to prevent outbreaks, is up to you. Some individuals may find one medication more effective than another. Because first outbreaks are often the most severe, however, it is usually
a good idea to take medication for the first outbreak. Sometimes, if
the outbreak is particularly severe and is taking longer than ten days
to heal, the medications may be used for a longer time than for recurrences.

The medications discussed here are most effective for episodic
treatment when started within twenty-four hours of the beginning of
an outbreak, or even during the "prodrome" (symptoms such as burning, tingling, itching, and so on, that may herald the outbreak is coming). The sooner treatment is begun, the better. Because there is no
reason to visit a health care provider's office for every outbreak, anyone who decides to use one of the medications episodically should ask
his or her provider for an *unlimited use prescription* for this purpose;
such prescriptions are usually valid for a year.

Acyclovir, valacyclovir, and famciclovir have also been approved
for the *suppression* of genital outbreaks. When taken daily, they decrease the frequency of genital outbreaks in about 70–80 percent of
those taking them, and they completely prevent outbreaks in about
50 percent.

RECOMMENDED DOSAGES
FOR THE TREATMENT OF HERPES OUTBREAKS

	MEDICATION	DOSAGE
FIRST EPISODE OF GENITAL INFECTION	Acyclovir	400 mg by mouth three times a day for seven to ten days, or 200 mg by mouth five times a day for seven to ten days
	Valacyclovir	1000 mg by mouth twice a day for seven to ten days
	Famciclovir	250 mg by mouth three times a day for seven to ten days
RECURRENT EPISODIC GENITAL INFECTION	Acyclovir	400 mg by mouth three times a day for five days, or 800 mg by mouth twice a day for five days or three times a day for two days
	Valacyclovir	500 mg by mouth twice a day for three days, or 1000 mg once a day for five days
	Famciclovir	125 mg by mouth twice a day for five days, or 1000 mg twice a day for one day
SUPPRESSION OF GENITAL INFECTIONS	Acyclovir	400 mg by mouth twice a day
	Valacyclovir	500 mg by mouth once a day, or 1000 mg once a day for those with ten or more outbreaks a year
	Famciclovir	250 mg by mouth twice a day
TREATMENT OF COLD SORES	Acyclovir	400 mg by mouth three times a day for five days, or 200 mg by mouth five times a day for five days
	Penciclovir cream	Applied every two hours while awake, for four days
	Valacyclovir	2 g twice a day by mouth within twenty-four hours of the start of a cold sore
	Acyclovir cream	Applied to the cold sore every three hours while awake, for seven days
	Docosanol cream	Applied to cold sore five times a day
SUPPRESSION OF COLD SORES	Acyclovir	400 mg by mouth twice a day
REDUCTION OF RISK OF TRANSMISSION	Valacyclovir	500 mg by mouth once a day (as well as safer sex practices; see text)

For the prevention of oral outbreaks, oral acyclovir has proved effective. When a person is planning to be in the type of situation that usually brings on a cold sore, such as a skiing vacation with its attendant exposure to sunlight, he or she may want to take acyclovir suppressively for a week or two before the start of exposure and during the trip, to prevent an outbreak, or have penciclovir cream on hand to treat an outbreak if one occurs. Using a sunscreen lip balm may also help prevent cold sores.

The efficacy of the oral medications valacyclovir and famciclovir in the treatment and suppression of cold sores has not yet been established. Acyclovir is the treatment of choice for infected newborns and also for those with herpes encephalitis, a severe infection of the brain, which fortunately is uncommon.

Otherwise healthy people who take these medications experience few side effects. In those who do develop side effects, the most common are headache, nausea, and dizziness. When valacyclovir was taken in dosages much higher than usual, people with serious immunodeficiency (such as those with an advanced stage of HIV infection or those taking drugs to suppress an immune reaction to a transplanted organ) developed a rare kidney and blood disorder called hemolytic uremic syndrome. If you have HIV infection and want treatment for herpes, talk with your health care provider. The treatment recommendations are slightly different for people with HIV and often involve higher doses and a longer course of medication for outbreaks and suppression of outbreaks.

The first year of infection is the worst for most people, because they have more frequent outbreaks. Until the virus becomes less active, taking the medication on a suppressive basis can be very helpful. Of course, certain people won't need to do this, because they won't have frequent outbreaks or their outbreaks will be manageable. A person who decides to take medication suppressively for a time may want to try stopping it at some point to see if the virus is still as active. If, after stopping the medication, that person continues to have very frequent outbreaks, then he or she will probably want to resume suppressive treatment. Otherwise, using the medication only to treat outbreaks might be the best approach. Taking these antiviral medications suppressively does not seem to cause the herpes virus to become resistant to them. Such resistance occurs only very rarely, in immunocompromised persons. Studies have shown that suppressive use of acyclovir for six years or valacyclovir or famciclovir for one year has not been associated with either resistance or adverse side effects. There are no known effects on sperm production in men or on fertility in men or women. And again, it is important to emphasize that the future frequency of outbreaks is not affected by the use of these medications.

The cost of the medications can be a problem if they are not covered by insurance. Several drug companies have begun manufacturing acyclovir at a reduced cost. It is much less expensive and probably just as effective as the original medication (although it should be noted that the studies cited for this section in this book's references were performed with the original acyclovir). Talk with your health care provider about this option if cost is a major deterrent to treatment.

If treatment is unsuccessful with the dosages and schedules listed earlier, then you may take certain steps to obtain relief from symptoms:

—Make sure that other medications you are taking do not interfere with the antiviral ones (probenecid, for example, can interfere with antiviral medications) and are not suppressing your immune system.

—Keep lesions as dry as possible; this will speed healing.

—Have yourself tested for other health problems that could be causing suppression of the immune system.

—If one of the antiviral medications doesn't work, try a different one.

—Make sure that you are taking the appropriate dosage.

—Consider trying alternative therapies (described below).

—Keep track of triggers in your environment that may be causing your outbreaks (such as stress, specific foods, or lack of sleep) and try to modify them.

—As a last resort, have the virus tested for acyclovir resistance (this is rare in otherwise healthy people).

Herpes infections of the eye—which occur, rarely, through autoinoculation by touching a genital infection and then touching the eye, and more often occur through reactivation of facial HSV-1— should be managed by an ophthalmologist. Almost all herpes in the eye results from infection with type 1 herpes. Effective medications for treating herpes infections of the eye include topical trifluorothymidine, vidarabine, idoxuridine, acyclovir, and interferon.

As mentioned earlier, vaccines are currently being tested as a way to prevent symptoms in already infected persons, and this treatment may hold some promise for the future. Vaccines initially developed for other diseases—such as smallpox, influenza, and polio—have not proven effective in preventing infection with or treating herpes.

Although resistance to these medications is rare, people with compromised immune systems (such as those with HIV infection) have a higher risk. For people who are immunocompromised and have herpes that is resistant to acyclovir, the medication foscarnet has proven effective. If you have HIV and herpes, it is best to seek advice from an HIV specialist about treatment for your herpes. The recommendations for treatment and suppression differ from those for non-HIV-infected people.

ALTERNATIVE APPROACHES TO HERPES MANAGEMENT

Of the many nontraditional approaches to the management of herpes symptoms, most have not been adequately studied. No nontraditional treatment has proved as effective as the antiviral medications described above (acyclovir, valacyclovir, and famciclovir). Furthermore, when studied as rigorously as these medications, no nontraditional treatments have proved more effective than placebo. Some therapies not found to be effective are *Echinacea,* Siberian ginseng, and zinc. Most of the following therapies work best as complementary medicine—that is, they should be used *along with* standard medical treatment. Be aware that *there are no cures for herpes yet:* Avoid anyone claiming to offer a cure. Do not pay a lot of money for treatment whose safety and effectiveness have not yet been studied, especially if doing so means that you will not be able to afford antiviral medications, whose safety and effectiveness *have* been proven.

Here are several nontraditional approaches to the management of herpes that may help and that (based on all that we know) will not hurt:

Ice. Applying ice directly to the area of an outbreak may help to lessen the severity of symptoms, and may help prevent an outbreak altogether if applied when prodrome or warning symptoms occur. Placing the ice in a plastic bag and then wrapping it in a thin towel may make this treatment more tolerable. It can be used for both oral and genital herpes.

Drying Agents. Agents that dry the skin, such as cornstarch and alcohol, may promote healing, because the drier the lesions are, the more quickly they heal. However, alcohol may cause pain when it comes into contact with lesions. In addition, wearing loose cotton underwear can promote healing of genital lesions by allowing them to dry.

Nutrition and Diet. A large body of medical research supports the role of a nutritious diet in keeping the immune system strong. The immune system is a complex network of cells, organs, and tissues that defend the body against infections. Malnourishment weakens it and renders the body more susceptible to viral, bacterial, and parasitic infections.

There has been much discussion about the relationship between diet (and specifically the amino acids L-lysine and arginine) and the frequency and severity of herpes outbreaks. L-lysine is an amino acid found in eggs, meat, and milk as well as other foods. Its effectiveness in controlling and treating herpes outbreaks has had mixed results, and L-lysine is at this time not generally thought to be effective for the treatment of herpes simplex infections.

In the late 1970s, studies showed that L-lysine suppressed recurrent infection and hastened recovery from infection when taken in doses of 800–1200 mg per day. However, these studies were performed with small numbers of participants, and the results may have been due to a placebo effect. Many earlier studies of L-lysine were similarly flawed, and the question of whether or not the amino acid really works has not yet been satisfactorily answered. Many people believe that taking L-lysine supplements (found in most health food stores) or eating foods rich in L-lysine helps them manage their herpes better. No harmful side effects have been noted with its use in dosages less than 4000 mg per day, although, once again, there has not been a sufficient number of long-term studies.

Some researchers believe that the amino acid arginine stimulates the growth of the virus and that the reason lysine works is that it blocks the metabolism of arginine. On the other hand, arginine supplementation has been proven to boost the body's ability to fight off bacterial infections in burn patients and people who have undergone surgery. In many of the studies of L-lysine, arginine intake was not monitored, and this may be why the various studies have yielded conflicting results.

Some foods, such as nuts and chocolate, which many people associate with herpes outbreaks, are high in arginine. For certain people, caffeine, alcohol, and smoking are additional triggers for outbreaks. If you find that a specific food stimulates outbreaks, by all means limit your intake of it.

Stress Reduction. There is no doubt that emotional and physical stress can have negative effects on the immune system, and many people believe that stress triggers outbreaks of their herpes. Studies have shown that stress does not in fact *cause* frequent outbreaks; instead, those with herpes may become stressed as the virus is reactivating, possibly even before they notice symptoms. Then, when an outbreak occurs, they believe it was the stress that triggered the outbreak. However, it is often difficult to draw such fine distinctions between cause and effect, and techniques to lower stress do make herpes more manageable for most people.

Counseling may be helpful to deal with the emotional issues that many face when dealing with herpes. Regular exercise can reduce stress as well as provide other benefits. Setting aside adequate time for sleep and taking a break every day for relaxation (even as little as fifteen minutes) can also be helpful. Meditation practices, such as yoga and tai chi, have been beneficial for some people, not only in controlling herpes, but also in maintaining overall well-being. Techniques such as respiration-based relaxation, guided imagery, and cognitive stress management may help decrease the tension resulting from herpes outbreaks.

Topical Anesthetic Creams. Again, keeping the lesions dry will promote healing. However, when lesions are particularly painful, some have found that applying a topical anesthetic sparingly and for a short time, until the antiviral medications begin to provide pain relief, can be helpful.

Warm Baths. Warm baths can be soothing to genital sores. If urination over the lesions causes a lot of discomfort, urinating while sitting in a tub of warm water makes the process less painful.

Acupuncture. Although there are no studies proving that acupuncture reduces the frequency of outbreaks, some people claim that acupuncture decreases the pain associated with outbreaks.

HIV INFECTION AND AIDS

  incidence: common
      cause: virus (human immunodeficiency virus)
   symptoms: sometimes viral illness after infection, but often none initially;
             later, weight loss, fever, lymph node swelling, recurrent
             infections
  treatment: no cure, but medications can slow disease process

WHAT IS IT?

The human immunodeficiency virus (HIV) is the virus that causes the acquired immunodeficiency syndrome (AIDS). AIDS is the final stage of HIV infection, when the virus has caused sufficient damage to the immune system to make a person vulnerable to other infections. There is no cure for HIV. The first reports of people dying from AIDS emerged in the early 1980s, and the understanding that HIV was the cause of AIDS came soon after. No one knows exactly how, when, or where HIV originated, but tissue and blood samples from people who lived on the African continent in the 1950s have shown evidence of HIV.

Two types of HIV are recognized: HIV-1 and HIV-2. There are also some variations among the HIV-1 types; nine have so far been recognized. HIV-1 is the primary strain seen in all areas of the world except West Africa, where HIV-2 predominates. Only about a hundred cases of HIV-2 have been reported in the United States, and all of these were among people who had traveled to West Africa, or had had sexual contact with someone from West Africa, or had received a blood transfusion, or an injection from a needle that was not sterile, in West Africa. Nevertheless, in most areas of the United States, testing for HIV usually includes testing for both types of the virus.

The virus infects certain cells of the immune system, which is the body's defense system against infections and the development of cancer, specifically those that have a particular protein, the CD4 protein, on their surface. One cell type, CD4 lymphocytes or T helper cells, is an important part of the immune system. HIV is a type of virus called a *retrovirus*, a term used to describe the process by which it infects a target cell. When the virus attaches to a cell, its genetic material is incorporated into the genetic material of the cell. The infected cell then makes new HIV, which can go on to infect other cells. When HIV attacks CD4 cells, it causes them to die. This then leads to a weakened immune system, which means the infected person becomes susceptible to other infections.

When a person is first infected, a large amount of virus circulates in the system, and initially the number of CD4 cells declines; however, the body's immune system then regains control and suppresses the virus for a period of about ten years. Eventually, however, the virus somehow "outsmarts" the body's immune system and starts destroying the cells it has infected, a process that makes the infected person very vulnerable to other infections and malignancies. At this point, a person is considered to have AIDS. Why this happens, and why it occurs at different times for different people, is not clear, although genetic differences may determine a person's susceptibility to infection with AIDS as well as how long it will take the person to develop AIDS if he or she becomes infected.

Many people do not seek HIV testing out of fear of stigma. From the beginning, HIV infection was politicized to an extent seen for few other diseases. People infected with HIV were denied access to insurance and health care, lost jobs and housing, became targets of social stigma, and were often "blamed" for their illness. Many people did not seek—and some still do not seek—testing for fear of these real consequences. As we begin the twenty-first century, there are signs of positive change in people's attitudes toward HIV and individuals infected with HIV. There are now people who have lived a long time with the virus, because of advances in medications—so that some draw parallels between living with HIV and living with other "chronic" diseases. But there is still a lot of work to be done. If you have HIV and feel you have been discriminated against, contact the Centers for Disease Control's STD and HIV/AIDS Hotline to file a complaint and find out about your rights.

On the medical front, as we gain a clearer understanding of how HIV works and how we can better prevent and treat HIV infection, hope grows that the new century will bring further breakthroughs and a cure. As of this moment, there is no cure, although recent advances with medications to treat HIV infection are very promising. Through the continued efforts of the medical community, governmental bodies, and citizens' groups to keep HIV research a top priority, and through education and the teaching of safer sex practices, there is hope of stemming the tide of this epidemic throughout the world.

Because recommendations for treatment are constantly evolving, I provide here just a brief overview. For specific recommendations about treatment, it is best to consult an HIV specialist.

HOW COMMON IS IT?

Worldwide, more than twenty-five million people have died in the AIDS epidemic, and more than forty million people are thought to be infected with HIV. The developing world, where cost prohibits access to medications and where testing and counseling are not readily available, is especially hard hit. In the United States, more than 700,000 people are infected, and more than 450,000 have died since 1981. Although the first reports of AIDS in the United States were among men who have sex with men, worldwide, heterosexual sexual contact is the most common route of transmission. People who are infected with HIV are frequently symptom free and therefore may not know they are infected, and thus they can unknowingly pass the virus to others.

> Most people infected with HIV are symptom free and would not know they were infected unless they were tested. However, they can still transmit the virus to others.

In the United States, the group with the largest proportional increase in the number of people infected is heterosexuals, although at present most AIDS patients are men who acquired HIV through sexual contact with other men. The heterosexual groups most at risk are those who share injection drug works (and thus may pass infected blood) or have partners who do; adolescents, irrespective of sexual orientation; and people of color. African Americans and Hispanics are disproportionately represented among those infected, in the United States and throughout the world. For example, although African Americans and Hispanics each make up only about 13 percent of the population of the United States, more than half of new HIV diagnoses are among people of color.

Women of color, in particular, are a vulnerable group. However, it is important to understand that people of *any* sexual orientation or economic or racial background can become infected with HIV.

> People who share injection drug works, and their partners, are a fast-growing group of those newly infected in the United States.

WHAT ARE THE SYMPTOMS?

Most people who are infected with HIV have no symptoms: they feel fine, they look fine, and they would not know they were infected unless they were tested. However, between 30 and 70 percent of *newly infected people* develop a flu-like illness within two to six weeks of becoming infected. Symptoms usually last one or two weeks and include a sore throat, fever, night sweats, lymph node swelling throughout the body, muscle aches, and a diffuse flat, red rash over the entire body. The symptoms resolve on their own.

It is during this time that most people develop antibodies to the infection, a process called *seroconversion.* Antibodies are proteins that the immune system makes in response to infections. It is also at this time that people have a large amount of the virus circulating in their systems, and there can also be a temporary drop in the number of circulating CD4 cells (the specific type of cell of the immune system that the virus infects), owing to direct damage by the virus. Because these symptoms are so vague, those experiencing them may seek no medical care at this time. If they do seek medical care, they may be diagnosed with HIV infection or misdiagnosed with one of the many of the viral infections that can cause similar symptoms. Again, not everyone has these symptoms, and, certainly, not every cold or flu signals HIV in-

> Some people experience flu-like symptoms after infection with HIV, but these can often be confused with the symptoms of other viral illnesses.

fection. Early in their infection, people may not test positive by the conventional tests (which look for antibodies); a test that looks for the genetic material of the virus (called an HIV plasma RNA, or "viral load," test) may show evidence of infection. However, this result always needs to be confirmed by another test, such as the test for antibodies, over the next weeks to months.

Soon after initial infection the body begins to succeed in keeping the virus in check, and a person remains symptom free, on average, for ten years, although the time may range from months up to seventeen years for a person who is not taking HIV medication. During this time, it is not uncommon for infected people to notice lymph node enlargement throughout the body. Lymph nodes, which are found in many locations in the body (see Chapter 1), may swell as a result of infections and malignancies, both of which stimulate the immune system. Because HIV infection involves constant stimulation of the immune system, the nodes are often swollen, even early in an infection. Indeed this may be the only symptom of HIV infection at this time. People become sicker as the virus causes their CD4 count to fall, making them more susceptible to certain infections (called opportunistic infections) and malignancies. It is assumed that everyone with HIV infection will eventually develop AIDS.

AIDS is defined in an HIV-positive person as a syndrome comprising various clinical conditions, a fall in the CD4 count to below 200 (meaning 200 cells per cubic millimeter), or both criteria. A person with AIDS is usually monitored by measuring the level of his or her CD4 cells. A healthy person typically has a count of more than 500 cells; as this number declines, the body becomes vulnerable to outside infections and also to malignancies.

> AIDS takes, on average, ten years to develop after initial infection with HIV. It is at this time that the body becomes vulnerable to outside infections and malignancies.

Some infections are more likely to occur at certain times during a person's illness, depending on what the CD4 count is. The only symptoms that a person with a CD4 count greater than 500 may have are lymph node swelling and, for women, recurrent vaginal yeast infections. Many people in this category, however, experience no symptoms. When the CD4 count drops into the 200–500 range, infected persons are more likely to be vulnerable to pneumococcal pneumonia, pulmonary tuberculosis, herpes zoster (shingles), oral candida (yeast) infection, cervical cancer, anemia, Kaposi's sarcoma, and non-Hodgkin's lymphoma, among other diseases. Persons with CD4 counts that fall within the 100–200 range are more vulnerable to *Pneumocystis carinii* pneumonia, AIDS dementia, and wasting syndrome (the inability to maintain a normal body weight). Symptoms that may indicate the infection is causing problems with the immune system include weight loss, fever, cough, shortness of breath, diarrhea, and a white rash in the mouth called "thrush," which is a type of fungal infection.

People with CD4 counts between 50 and 100 are more likely to develop cytomegalovirus retinitis, toxoplasmosis, and cryptococcosis. And those with CD4 counts less than 50 may develop *Mycobacterium avium* complex infection, cryptosporidiosis, progressive multifocal leukencephalopathy, and primary central nervous system lymphoma. As described in the discussion of treatment below, careful monitoring of the CD4 counts makes it possible to take prophylactic medications at the appropriate time to help protect against many of these infections or at least delay their onset. Medications targeted against HIV infection to keep the immune system strong can help protect against these infections for some time. Unfortunately, none of these medications cures HIV.

> HIV infects cells of the immune system called CD4 cells. The CD4 cell count at any given time determines the types of infections to which a person is vulnerable.

As noted above, although women make up a relatively small percentage of those infected with HIV and those with AIDS in the United States, they are one of the fastest-growing groups among the newly infected. Most often these are women who are at some risk for HIV, such as those who use injection drugs and share works, or who have a sexual partner who is an injection drug user. Women often have a poorer prognosis than men, possibly because of inadequate access to health care.

Until recently, research into HIV and its clinical manifestations focused on men, but we are now beginning to have a better idea of how

HIV affects women. The treatment regimens for HIV are currently the same for women as for men, but there are differences between women and men with HIV infection. Women with HIV infection are more likely to have such AIDS-defining illnesses as candida (yeast) in the throat, recurrent bacterial pneumonia, and progressive multifocal leukencephalopathy. Men, on the other hand, are more likely to have such illnesses as Kaposi's sarcoma, oral hairy leukoplakia, *Pneumocystis carinii* pneumonia, and prolonged herpes outbreaks.

Women with HIV infection and AIDS are also at higher risk for gynecological problems. Infected women acquire cervical cancer more often than women without HIV, and the course of the cancer can be much more aggressive. Therefore, women with HIV infection and AIDS should be screened for cervical cancer more closely (every six months initially, then, if normal, yearly thereafter) (see "The Pap Smear" in the section on genital warts). The treatment of cervical cancer is the same for both groups. Frequent yeast infections can be a sign of HIV infection in otherwise healthy women, but the connection is by no means automatic (see the section on fungal infections). In addition, women infected with HIV are more likely to have problems with their periods and to experience early menopause.

The following is a list of symptoms that may be caused by HIV infection but may also result from other causes. See your health care provider if you have any of these symptoms:

—Unexplained weight loss
—Unexplained loss of appetite
—Swollen glands
—Fever that is not going away
—Cough or shortness of breath
—Sores or rashes that aren't healing
—Persistent diarrhea
—Persistent yeast infections or genital symptoms
—Changes in memory
—Persistent headaches
—Weakness of the arms or legs

HOW IS HIV TRANSMITTED?

Infection takes place in three ways—sexual transmission, exchange of blood or other body fluid, and exchange of fluids from mother to child—and these are discussed in detail below. At this time no vaccine is available to prevent people from becoming infected with HIV, and studies of various vaccines have been disappointing. The virus mutates (that is, its surface proteins change) quickly. Because vaccines are usually directed against surface proteins in an effort to kill the virus, such subtle but important changes in the virus over time mean that a vaccine that may be effective at one time may not be effective a short while later. Research is in progress to find an effective vaccine.

It is important to remember that even if a person with HIV is being treated with medication, there is still a risk of passing the infection through unprotected sex to an uninfected partner. The ways in which HIV can be transmitted are outlined below. HIV *cannot* be transmitted by hugging, coughing or sneezing, sharing dishes or toilet seats, or working with someone who is HIV positive. There is no need to sterilize household surfaces touched by someone with HIV, for example, as the virus does not last long outside the body. However, if an item such as a razor or toothbrush is contaminated with blood, transmission could occur.

Sexual Transmission

HIV can be transmitted through unprotected genital and anal sex, and oral sex as well. How much of a risk of transmission any given sexual exposure carries depends on what type of contact it is (see Chapter 5 for a description of safer and unsafe sexual practices) and how infectious a partner is. People with HIV are particularly infectious when they are newly infected (and this may even be before a blood test registers as positive) and later in their illness, when they have AIDS. It is at these times that the largest quantities of virus are circulating. *However, it is possible to transmit the virus through an unprotected sexual contact regardless of the stage of illness.*

A person can become infected from a single sexual contact with an infected partner. Blood, semen, vaginal secretions, and breast milk have high amounts of virus. Saliva, urine, and tears also contain HIV, but in lower quantities, and are not sufficient to transmit HIV unless blood is present. Women are at higher risk than men of becoming HIV infected if exposed through sexual activity, possibly because they have more mucosal tissue in the genital area, which is more vulnerable to infection through small breaks or tears. Some people, however, have repeated exposures to infected partners and either do not become infected at all or become infected only after a period of time. Recent studies have shown that a particular gene may offer protection against becoming infected with HIV; however, at this point there is no way that a person can be tested for this gene in the course of routine medical screening, and no one should assume that he or she is somehow immune.

On the other hand, a person who discovers that a previous or current partner is infected with HIV should not assume that he or she, too, is infected and therefore abandon safer sex practices. *Testing is the only way to know whether or not an individual is infected.* Similarly, if one partner in a relationship is tested for HIV, the results reveal nothing about the other partner's HIV status. People often assume that if they have been together for a while with a person who is tested and is found to be HIV negative, then they are also HIV negative and don't need to be tested. This is not true. *Both partners must be tested six or more months after any other sexual contacts or exposure to risk factors, must be found to be HIV negative, and must remain mutually monogamous and free of other risk factors to know that they are free of HIV.*

People who have genital ulcer diseases, such as herpes, are more vulnerable to becoming infected with HIV, since breaks in the skin (even if they are not noticeable) make transmission of the virus easier. Having other sexually transmitted diseases, such as gonorrhea, can also facilitate transmission of HIV. Thus efforts to control the spread of other sexually transmitted infections can also help prevent the spread of HIV, and routine testing for STDs can provide information to help protect against becoming infected with HIV. It is very important to be tested for other STDs as a part of routine health care and not to assume that an HIV test is a complete screen for infections. A person who puts himself or herself at risk of acquiring other STDs puts himself or herself at risk for acquiring HIV infection.

> HIV infection is not the only sexually transmitted infection, and having other STDs may increase the chance of spreading and acquiring HIV infection.

Women who use oral contraceptives (the pill) as their birth control method and do not use a barrier method to protect against STD transmission may also be at slightly higher risk of acquiring HIV in-fection. This is because in many women oral contraceptives cause changes in the cervix that make the inner columnar cells more visi-ble (a process called *ectopy*), and it is these cells that are most vul-nerable to infection (by HIV as well as the agents responsible for other STDs) during unprotected sex. However, it is not recommended that women stop using birth control pills; rather, they should be cautious (as should everyone) about risk factors for acquiring HIV.

Most birth control methods—such as progesterone shots or im-plants, intrauterine devices, birth control pills, and sterilization—do not offer any protection against STDs, and some (as just noted for the pill) may actually increase the risk if condoms aren't used as well.

Exchange of Blood or Other Body Fluids

HIV can be transmitted by blood and other body fluids in the follow-ing ways:

—Through a transfusion with infected blood or an infected blood product
—Through a stick with a needle that has infected blood on it
—Through a splash of infected body fluids onto a mucous membrane or a break in the skin
—Through exchanging needles or other works for injection drug use

Today the risk in the United States of becoming infected with HIV through a transfusion of a unit of blood or a blood product is approxi-mately 1 in 450,000 to 1 in 660,000. Those who received blood or blood products before 1985 (the year in which screening of blood and blood products for HIV became mandatory) are at greater risk for hav-ing been infected, particularly if they received multiple transfusions between 1978 and 1985. All blood and blood products are screened for HIV with the same tests that are used to test people for the virus. Be-cause there is a possibility that the person who donated a given unit of blood was newly infected with HIV and that older blood tests would not yet show a positive re-sult, newer tests are also per-formed that can detect HIV ear-lier. Advances in screening of

The risk of acquiring HIV infection from a blood transfusion since 1985 has been between 1 in 450,000 and 1 in 660,000.

donated blood may decrease this risk even further in the future. Blood transfusions in other countries may pose a higher risk, depending on when the particular country initiated screening of its blood supply and which tests are used to test donated blood.

Health care workers are at risk through contact with potentially infected patients and their body fluids. Other people are sometimes also inadvertently exposed to body fluids or needle-stick injuries. The risk of infection in this way depends on how much virus is present in the fluid or on the object (is the infected person encountered late or early in the infection, or during the middle period?) and how long the object has sat around after being used. It also depends on what type of injury a person sustains (was it a small scratch or a deep wound that went into the muscle?). A person who is stuck with a needle containing blood from an infected person runs about a 0.3 percent risk of becoming infected with HIV.

> Health care workers who are stuck with a needle containing HIV-infected blood run about a 0.3 percent risk of becoming infected. This risk is decreased when medications commonly used to treat HIV infection are started soon after infection.

Wearing gloves when coming into contact with potentially infected body fluids decreases the likelihood of becoming infected. Wearing two sets of gloves (a practice referred to as double gloving) decreases the risk from a needle-stick injury by about 50 percent compared with using just one set of gloves. This risk is reduced even further with the use of antiviral drugs immediately after exposure (see the discussion of treatment).

There is no evidence of transmission from infected health care workers to their patients, except for the widely publicized incident of an infected dentist who was found to have infected five of his patients during the 1980s. Exactly how this transmission occurred is not clear. A study of 15,000 patients of 32 HIV-infected physicians found that none of them had been infected by their providers.

Drug users who share injection drug works have a high risk of becoming infected with HIV. In "shooting galleries," where persons often share injection drug equipment and may exchange sex for drugs, one study found that a large percentage of the equipment was contaminated with HIV. Using household bleach to sterilize the equipment for at least five minutes (and washing it with water afterwards) may decrease the risk of infection but does not eliminate it. The use of sterile needles, sometimes available through a needle exchange program, decreases the risk of HIV infection through injection drug use.

Exchange of Fluids from Mother to Child

An infected mother can transmit HIV to her child through the placenta when the baby is in the womb, by exposure to vaginal secretions at birth, or through breast milk by breastfeeding. Most children who are born to infected mothers acquire the infection while in the womb or at delivery, but breastfeeding is discouraged if the mother is HIV positive.

Eighty-five percent of women who are HIV positive are of childbearing age, and between 1 and 2 percent of pregnant women in urban settings in the United States are HIV positive. Because testing is not mandatory, many women do not know they are infected and that their children are at risk.

> **A potential consequence of the increase in the number of infected women is an increase in the number of children infected in the womb or during childbirth.**

While in the womb, a baby receives antibodies from the mother through the placenta. Infants born to mothers who are HIV positive almost always have antibody to HIV when they are born, whether or not they are infected. These antibodies from the mother can stay in the baby's circulation for up to eighteen months. For this reason, tests are performed to determine if the infant has the virus and not just the antibody. These include tests to detect the genetic material of the virus (the polymerase chain reaction, or PCR, test and the branched HIV-DNA amplification test, also known as the *viral load test*) and tests that identify one of the proteins or antigens found on the surface of the virus (the p24 antigen), as well as culturing for HIV. (These tests are described below.) If a child is at risk for infection, testing should be performed periodically from birth until the child reaches one year of age. A child who continues to test positive at one year is most likely truly infected.

An infant born to an untreated mother who is HIV positive has a 15–25 percent risk of being born infected, with a higher risk if the mother is at an advanced stage in her illness. An additional 12–14 percent of infants are infected through breast milk. If the mother has a large amount of circulating virus (which can be the case briefly during the initial infection and for a longer period later in the course of her illness), then an infant runs a 30 percent or greater chance of being infected. Babies born prematurely also seem to have a higher risk of infection, and the use of fetal scalp monitors also makes transmission of HIV easier when the mother is infected. (These devices use tiny electrodes placed on the infant's head while in the womb to monitor the infant's condition; the tiny cuts they create in the scalp can facilitate the transmission of HIV and herpes virus from the mother to the infant.) Trauma to the scalp from forceps may also facilitate transmission. Having a cesarean delivery may decrease the risk of transmission of HIV to a child.

The current recommendations to decrease the risk of transmission from mother to infant include (1) the mother taking antiretroviral medication (such as AZT or nevirapine) during the pregnancy, (2) elective cesarean delivery at thirty-eight weeks of pregnancy, and (3) not breastfeeding. These interventions can decrease the risk of transmission to approximately 2 percent.

> The risk of an HIV-positive woman transmitting the infection to her unborn child is significantly decreased with the use of antiretrovirals during the pregnancy.

Because intervention with medication during the pregnancy may significantly decrease the chance that a baby will become infected, it is very important for a woman who is pregnant or who is thinking about becoming pregnant to know her HIV status. Testing is not mandatory, however, and the decision remains each woman's alone.

TESTING FOR HIV

Deciding to be tested for HIV may be a difficult step. Even for those who believe they are at low risk, the process can be nerve wracking. A person must be emotionally ready to be tested, because obviously the test results may be life altering. A person who is going to be tested should consider how she or he will react if the results are positive or if they are negative. Anyone considering having an HIV test should consider these questions:

—Do you want to bring someone with you when you get your
results?

—Before you are tested, do you want to tell a friend or sexual
partner that you are going to be tested?

—Do you have someone to talk with after you are tested?

—If you test negative, what will you do in the future to lower
your risk of becoming infected?

If you test positive, the person who gives you your results should
be able to offer referral to a clinic that cares for persons infected with
HIV (if the facility where you are tested does not provide that care) and
also, if you wish, refer you to services for psychological support. This
clinic can also provide screening for other sexually transmitted and
nonsexually transmitted infections, as well as information about
safer sex and how to prevent transmission to others. It is also a good
idea to have the test repeated if a positive result is obtained, especially
if you are at low risk for infection, on the chance that there was an er-
ror at the laboratory.

The emotional reactions to a positive diagnosis are varied and often intense. Many people are stunned, confused, angry. If you find out
you're HIV positive, talk with your health care provider or a counselor, a trusted friend, or family member. Take time to adjust to the
diagnosis, and seek information before you make any major life decisions.

Many (but not all) states require an HIV-positive result to be reported to the state health department. This information cannot be
given to anyone else (such as insurance companies), and health care
providers cannot divulge your information to anyone else without
your permission.

Who should be tested? Sexually active adults who have had unprotected sexual contact in the past should consider being tested, even
if they feel and look fine, since, as we have seen, most people who are
infected would not otherwise know it. People who have been infected
with another STD should also be tested for HIV, since they may be at
greater risk for the infection. Those who have had a blood or blood
product transfusion before 1985 in the United States should consider
being tested, especially if they received blood or blood product transfusions between 1978 and 1985, which was when the epidemic began
in this country. And if a person has such unexplained symptoms as

fever, weight loss, and lymph node swelling, then HIV should be considered as a possible diagnosis and testing should be performed. Women who are considering a pregnancy or are pregnant may benefit from testing. Injection drug users who have shared needles or works should also be tested. Some people may decide not to be tested because "there's nothing I could do about it anyway," but there are in fact good reasons to know. First, medications are available that can lengthen the time for which you remain healthy and without evidence of infection, slow the effect of the virus on your immune system, and prevent complications. Second, if you find out you are infected, you can take steps to prevent transmission of HIV to a partner.

Telling a partner you have HIV infection can be extremely difficult. In most states, anonymous partner notification programs are available to contact partners who need to be tested. For those living with HIV and entering into a new relationship, partners need to be told. Your health care provider, or some of the AIDS information resources listed in the appendix of this book, can provide suggestions about how to talk with new partners. A support group for people living with HIV may also help.

Many couples entering into new sexual relationships decide to be tested jointly for HIV. This is a good idea. If both partners are tested for HIV more than six months from their last sexual contact with other partners or exposure to any other risk factor, test negative, and are mutually monogamous, then they can assume that they are negative for HIV. However, if there is continued risk of infection—such as contact with other partners or injection drug use—then couples cannot assume they are safe and should continue to use a barrier method to help protect themselves against infection.

If you intend to be tested for HIV, you should consider the issue of confidentiality. Insurance companies, if they know that you have sought testing for the infection, may label you as "high risk" and deny you insurance coverage or certain benefits in the future—even if you test negative. This consequence has prevented many people from being tested. Others who didn't know about this practice, and who sought testing from a health care provider on their insurance plans, now have the test as part of their permanent records and may be denied insurance coverage in the future. Check in your area for a clinic that performs anonymous testing. To preserve your anonymity, such

a testing center requires only
your first name, or else you are
assigned a number without having to give your name at all.
Most public health clinics provide this service. There is also a
home HIV test that is anony-
mous (discussed below). People who do test positive should refer their
partners for testing; health care providers can help with this.

> If you wish to be tested for HIV, consider having the test done anonymously so that the result does not become part of your permanent medical record.

The following five types of tests are available to test for HIV infection or to monitor the progress of an infected individual.

Antibody Tests

In most clinical settings, testing for HIV involves a test called the EIA,
or enzyme immunoassay, as a first step. This is a test for antibody, or
the body's immune response to infection with either HIV-1 (the most
common source of infection in the United States) or HIV-2. It can be
performed on blood or saliva in a medical setting as well as on blood
through a home testing kit (available in most pharmacies and drug
stores). The testing procedure for samples collected in the home test
is the same as that for samples taken in a clinic. The home testing kits
require a finger stick, to test blood, or a specimen of saliva.

The antibody test is very sensitive. Most infected people (about
95%) will show a positive EIA test about three months after the time
of possible infection. Everyone who is positive should show a positive
test six months after infection, although very rarely a positive result
may take longer to show up. The
risk of a false negative test after
six months from infection is
0.001–0.3 percent, depending on
the number of people infected in
a particular geographic area. People who do not form antibody
may have a rare deficiency in antibody formation, called *agam-
maglobulinemia.*

> Most infected people will show a positive blood test for HIV three months after infection. With rare exceptions, by six months after infection, all those who are infected will show a positive test for HIV.

Test results are generally straightforward—either positive or negative—but occasionally they are not. Some people have an antibody

in their systems that reacts positively to the EIA test but is not an antibody to HIV; nevertheless, the test shows a positive or reactive result. That is why any positive EIA test must be confirmed by another test to make sure it is accurate. Approximately 1 out of every 200 people who are tested has a positive EIA test when he or she is not in fact infected.

The EIA test can also be falsely positive or reactive because of medical conditions in which excess antibody is formed (such as some rheumatologic diseases, like lupus and rheumatoid arthritis), a recent immunization, or a recent viral illness. The body is constantly making antibodies in response to one thing or another, and sometimes such an antibody can "trip" the test positive. On the other hand, some people do not have an obvious risk factor such as these but nevertheless have reactive EIA tests, even though they are not infected with HIV. The EIA test has a sensitivity of 93.4–99.6 percent and a specificity of 99.2–99.8 percent. This means that between 93 and 100 percent of people who are truly positive will test positive and that of those who test negative, 99–100 percent are really not infected. Thus the EIA is a reliable screening test, but it is not 100 percent accurate.

If the EIA is positive, another test, usually the Western blot or an immunofluorescence assay, is done to confirm the result. Through this sequence of testing, most people who test positive are accurately detected as HIV infected.

> Sometimes test results are not clear-cut. Make sure your health care provider explains your results so that you can understand them.

The presence of antibodies to a certain combination of proteins from HIV on the Western blot assay determines whether or not a person is infected. To confirm that an EIA test is positive, antibodies must be seen on a Western blot to at least two of the following three proteins: p24, gp41, and gp120/160. This test may also take six months after a person has been infected to react positive.

Test results can show no antibodies to HIV (a negative result) or enough antibodies to indicate a positive result for HIV. However, there may also be some reactivity on this test but not enough to indicate infection. There are two possible explanations: a person may be newly infected but not yet have formed a full panel of antibody, or a person may not be infected. These partially reactive Western blot results are referred to as *indeterminate*. A repeat test a few months after the first test will help distinguish between the two scenarios. If there is a strong suspicion that a person has a newly acquired HIV infection and the preliminary tests are negative, the health care provider may order a blood test to look for the genetic material of the virus (not a typical screening test). A positive test for the genetic material should be followed up by the standard screening tests to verify that there is, in fact, an infection. If a person is newly infected and shows an indeterminate Western blot result, then eventually he or she should show a true positive result on the test. If the test is reactive for some other reason, then it may show an indeterminate pattern indefinitely or swing back and forth between a negative result and an indeterminate result.

> **The EIA and Western blot tests will detect most people who are infected.**

These results are sometimes confusing, even to health care providers, so make sure you receive an explanation of any test results. Clinics that perform many HIV tests (either STD clinics or health department STD clinics) can help clarify these results if your health care provider has not explained them clearly enough to you.

p24 Antigen Test

As its name suggests, the p24 antigen test is designed to detect a specific protein on the surface of the virus: the p24 antigen. Antigens stimulate a person's immune system to make antibodies, which are also proteins, and help the body to fight off the infection. The p24 antigen test may detect the presence of infection more quickly than the antibody tests discussed previously, and it is currently used by blood banks to detect the virus in those who are infected but have not yet developed antibody. It has a very high sensitivity for detecting HIV early in the course of infection, when the level of circulating virus is very high. It is not, however, recommended as a routine screening test for HIV at this point, because for those persons beyond the initial, acute stage of infection, its sensitivity is not as high as that of the EIA and Western blot assay.

The p24 antigen test is also useful in detecting infection in newborns born to HIV-infected mothers, since these babies may have passively acquired their mothers' antibody to HIV infection and therefore would test positive on the EIA and Western blot assay, whether or not they were truly infected. The presence of the p24 antigen in an infant indicates true infection. Some of the tests designed to detect the genetic material of the virus (described later) may be more accurate than this test for the detection of HIV infection in newborns, and they are now used more commonly for testing newborns.

Culture

Evaluation of the virus through culture is a technique that is not used in routine clinical practice, but mostly in the research setting. HIV is difficult to grow in culture, and the process takes a long time. The tests described above are more sensitive and cheaper.

Testing for the Genetic Material of the Virus

Two types of tests are available to look specifically for the genetic material of the virus: qualitative and quantitative.

The *qualitative test* seeks to detect the presence or absence of HIV but does not indicate how much of the virus is present. It is not performed as often as the quantitative tests, which do tell how much virus is present and are therefore more useful for observing a person who is infected with HIV to determine where he or she is in the course of the illness and how effective treatment is.

The qualitative test has about 97 percent sensitivity and about 98 percent specificity. This means that it detects ninety-seven out of one hundred people who are infected, and that ninety-eight out of one hundred people who test negative truly are not infected. The test is not as accurate as the EIA/Western blot combination, so it is not routinely used for screening purposes. Instead it is employed in a few select situations, such as diagnosing infection in the newborn. This test may also be useful in those cases in which the EIA and Western blot assay are inconclusive for adults and an additional test is necessary.

The *quantitative tests*, or *viral load tests*, are also known as PCR tests. There are several types, all of which look for the genetic material of the virus and then "amplify" it to readable quantities. These tests measure the quantity of virus circulating in the blood. One reason they are not recommended for screening purposes is that it is possible at different stages in the course of a person's infection with HIV to have levels of virus that are undetectable by these assays. Thus a "negative" test does not always exclude infection. Similarly a "positive" test may, rarely, be a false positive.

The quantitative tests are thought to have between 86 percent and greater than 98 percent sensitivity. However, new viral load assays are currently being evaluated, and in the near future more sensitive tests may be available that would be more useful for screening purposes. At this time these tests are about five times more expensive than the EIA and Western blot assay, and this is another factor to consider when deciding on one particular test over another. The quantitative tests are used primarily to follow the course of an HIV-infected person's illness, and they are useful in determining when medications should be initiated or changed (see "Treatment"). They can also clarify inconclusive EIA and Western blot tests and help in identifying infected newborns.

Testing for Damage to the Immune System

The test most commonly used to follow the course of a person's illness is the CD4 or T-helper-cell count. As mentioned earlier, the CD4 cell is a type of cell in the immune system that is attacked and destroyed by HIV; the number of circulating CD4 cells at any given time offers insight into the progression of the illness and information about prognosis and response to therapy. Another type of immune system cell, the CD8 cell or T-suppressor cell, can also be measured, and the ratio of CD4 to CD8 cells can be useful in monitoring the progress of the infection. *These tests are not used to determine if someone has HIV infection.* People with other medical problems can demonstrate a decline in their CD4-cell level for various reasons, and those with HIV can have normal CD4 counts.

> Many tests are available to screen for HIV infection and to assess how a person with HIV infection is doing. Make sure your health care provider explains these tests, and their results, clearly to you.

TREATMENT

There have been many advances in treatment for HIV infection and in our understanding of how the virus works over the past twenty years, but unfortunately no cure is anticipated in the near future. Since 1985, drugs called "nucleoside analogues" have been available to prolong the interval that a person with HIV infection can live without developing AIDS and its related illnesses. These medications have also been shown to delay death from AIDS. These drugs act by binding to RNA and preventing the virus from making DNA.

Newer medications, called *protease inhibitors* and non-nucleoside reverse transcriptase inhibitors (NNRTIs), offer additional hope for people infected with HIV to live longer and healthier lives. In the future these medications may offer an opportunity to treat newly exposed persons and prevent them from becoming infected. This strategy has been employed for persons who were exposed to infection in a health care setting, and it may also be an option for people exposed in other ways.

All of these medications are expensive and have side effects. Their cost poses a serious problem for many people, although several of the manufacturers in the United States have instituted programs to offer these medications at lower cost to those who need them and cannot afford them. Unfortunately, in developing areas of the world, where poverty is a way of life for many and the number of HIV-infected people is escalating rapidly, there is no hope that these medications will be available to most of the people infected with HIV. Therefore the enthusiasm generated by the development of such new medications must be tempered by the realization that the majority of people in the world who are infected with HIV will not be able to use them because of their cost.

When to start treatment and which treatments to start are the topics of much research and discussion. HIV infection should be treated by health care providers and clinics that know the latest guidelines for how and when to prescribe these treatments, because prescribing them incorrectly, or taking medications in the wrong way, can lead to resistance and so limit treatment options in the future. Centers that specialize in HIV treatment also have counsel-

There are many branches in the decision tree for a person living with HIV infection, including such questions as when to start medications and which medications to use. It is essential to have a health care provider who listens and is up to date on treatment advances.

ing services available for people who need help in sorting through the emotions that a diagnosis brings. Studies have shown that the providers who care for larger numbers of patients with HIV infection often offer the best care, because they are more up to date with newer developments in treatment options. If you believe you have recently been infected, your health care provider will most likely offer you treatment right away, or refer you to a specialist for treatment, probably even before confirmatory tests are back. Talk with your health care provider about the benefits and drawbacks of treatment at this stage.

Many people with HIV infection have decided to combine the traditional therapies provided by Western medicine (described in more detail below) with alternative or complementary therapies, such as herbal therapy, acupuncture, dietary changes, and vitamins. Ask your HIV health care provider which of these options have been proven useful and which may be harmful or interact with your medications. An HIV diagnosis can be emotionally devastating, and dealing with the emotional effects can be as important as dealing with the physiological effects. Psychological support from an HIV specialist or primary care provider, or a psychologist, psychiatrist, psychiatric nurse practitioner, or social worker, to name just a few, can be extremely important at the time of diagnosis and later, as one adjusts to life with HIV. Many centers that offer treatment for HIV also provide psychological counseling.

As during any difficult period in one's life, there are always choices. People with HIV infection have control over how they choose to define themselves and how they continue to lead their lives. After dealing with the initial emotional trauma of learning of their HIV-positive status, infected people sometimes develop a much greater understanding of themselves and their lives, often making changes for the better, both physically and emotionally. Many people find that they begin to pursue options they had never thought possible or do things they had always wanted to do. A well-chosen counselor can help with this important transitional period.

It is also important for those infected with HIV to maintain a healthy lifestyle and have routine health maintenance examinations. Preventive dentistry should be followed, and women with HIV infection should have a pelvic examination and Pap smear every six months.

A healthy lifestyle—avoiding smoking, illicit drug use, and alcohol—should be a goal, since these things may harm the immune system. Unsafe sex (that is, without a barrier such as a latex condom) not only puts a partner at risk for acquiring HIV but also puts the HIV-infected person at risk for acquiring other sexually transmitted infections. Having sex after a diagnosis of HIV is a decision that requires open communication between partners and an understanding of the risks of transmission and ways to decrease them. Talk with your health care provider about this, and see Chapter 5, "What is 'Safer Sex'?"

What should a medical examination for a person with HIV consist of? A complete medical history, physical examination, and laboratory evaluation (including a blood chemistry panel and complete blood count) should be performed. A skin test and chest X-ray to check for tuberculosis are also essential. Those determined to be positive must have treatment to prevent a reactivation of the disease, to which they will be more susceptible once infected with HIV, a virus that suppresses the immune system. A test for syphilis—the Venereal Disease Research Laboratory (VDRL) test or rapid plasma reagin (RPR) test—must also be done for the same reason. In addition to a test for syphilis, a screen for all sexually transmitted infections should be performed. See Chapter 3 for a full description of what an STD examination entails.

Testing for toxoplasmosis should also be carried out after the initial HIV diagnosis. As will be discussed later, people who have toxoplasma antibody have a history of infection, even though they may not remember being infected, since infection is frequently symptom free. This puts them at risk for reactivation of toxoplasmosis as their medical condition worsens. Immunization against pneumococcal pneumonia, influenza (yearly, in the fall), and hepatitis A and B for sexually active persons is also recommended.

The health care provider of an infected person will use the CD4 or T-helper-cell count and the viral load test and monitor the person's physical condition to decide on the best time to start or alter the various medications available to treat HIV infection.

There can be significant variation in an individual's CD4 count, even on a daily basis. A "normal" CD4 count is greater than 500; however, if a person without HIV infection experiences a serious illness or stress, this number can temporarily drop below 500. Similarly, most HIV-infected people will have CD4 counts greater than 500 during the early part of their infection. This *daily* variation can sometimes be up to 150 points in HIV-positive individuals, and even more in those who are HIV negative. A CD4 count that is significantly different from the previous count should be rechecked, ideally at the same time of day that the first count was obtained, to determine if the variation is real. In general, people with a CD4 count of less than 500 are more susceptible to infections; this susceptibility increases when the CD4 count falls below 200.

> CD4 counts can vary by up to 150 points in a single day. Before treatment decisions are made, the count should be taken again and consideration given to using a viral load assay to define the course of illness.

The viral load test may be a better indicator of disease progression than the T-helper-cell count, and it may indicate disease progression more quickly. This test can also be used to determine whether or not medication changes have been effective.

> Both the T-helper-cell count and the viral load test are recommended to follow the progression of HIV infection and the response to medications.

For instance, with the initiation of a new medication, one would hope to see a rise in the T-helper-cell count and a decrease in the viral load. It is assumed that when the viral load is low (and therefore the amount of circulating virus is low) disease progression has been slowed. Your health care provider can explain this in more detail.

The T-helper-cell count and viral load are usually checked every three to six months or so, or about three to four weeks after every change in the dose or type of antiretroviral medication or protease inhibitors. It is not recommended that the viral load be checked for up to one month following a viral or bacterial illness or after a vaccination, since these situations can temporarily raise the viral load. In addition, there are some slight differences among the tests, so the same viral load test should always be used for the same person.

All of the drugs used to treat people with HIV infection must be taken exactly as prescribed to decrease the risk of resistance, and all have potentially serious side effects.

Because many of these medications are new, and because clinical trials are currently under way to evaluate how best to use them, the recommendations for their use are frequently changing. Therefore, the following guidelines are just that—guidelines. I will not provide specific dosages, because some of these would probably have changed even before this book is published. The decision as to which medications to use (if any at all) must be arrived at after discussions between the patient and the health care provider.

There are three classes of medications to treat HIV:

1. Nucleoside analogues:
   —Thymidine analogues, such as stavudine (dT4) and zidovudine (AZT)
   —Non-thymidine nucleoside analogues, such as didanosine (ddI), lamivudine (3TC), and zalcitabine (ddC)
2. Non-nucleoside reverse transcriptase inhibitors: nevirapine and delavirdine
3. Protease inhibitors: saquinavir mesylate, indinavir, ritonavir, and nelfinavir

A combination of classes of medications—such as a thymidine nucleoside analogue, a non-thymidine nucleoside analogue, and a protease inhibitor—is the current recommended treatment. A combination of drugs is called "HAART," for "highly active antiretroviral therapy." Use of one drug alone is not recommended, because it is less effective.

If you are taking or planning to take medication, talk with your health care provider about which combination is best for you. You should take the medications as prescribed; taking them incorrectly can increase the chance that the virus will become resistant to the medications. In the near future, combinations of medications in a single pill may make taking these medications for treatment of HIV infection much easier.

The goal of all types of treatment is to decrease the viral load to undetectable levels. If the viral load is greater than 30,000 to 50,000, then medication may be considered even if the T-helper-cell count is stable and a person is feeling well physically. If the T-helper-cell count is decreasing, or a person is experiencing progression of the HIV infection with various opportunistic infections, then medications may be considered even if the viral load is low and stable. In some cases when the viral load is less than 5000–10,000 copies, the HIV-infected person and his or her health care provider may decide that it is best to start treatment. However, the higher the count, the more likely the health care provider is to recommend treatment.

If a person experiences toxicity or intolerable side effects from a medication regimen, then an alternative regimen can be chosen. Many people do experience side effects from these medications, and changes in medication or dose reductions are sometimes needed.

> Many treatment options are currently available for HIV infection, and the treatment plan must be individualized for each person. Treatment guidelines are constantly changing as new research is performed.

Treatment of Opportunistic Infections

In addition to the drug regimens used to treat HIV infection itself, there are medications that can be used to protect a person from what are called *opportunistic infections:* those to which a person with HIV becomes vulnerable once the T-helper-cell count begins to fall. There are many infections for which people with low CD4 counts have increased vulnerability; some of the most common are discussed below. In general, it is important to avoid possible infection by foods, such as uncooked fish, meat, or eggs; to keep any wounds clean; to avoid sharing razors or toothbrushes with others; and to avoid unprotected sex or sharing needles for drug use, which put not only others but the HIV-infected person at risk.

Pneumocystis carinii Pneumonia. Early in the HIV epidemic, *Pneumocystis carinii* pneumonia was the major cause of death among people with AIDS. Now, with the use of medications to prevent infection, it is still common but occurs much less frequently. HIV-infected persons are vulnerable to this type of lung infection if their T-helper-cell counts drop below 200. Several medications have proven effective in the treatment of this infection; of these the antibiotic trimethoprim-sulfamethoxazole is the most effective and best tolerated. Other options—which tend to have more side effects and are not as well tolerated—include oral dapsone and pentamidine in an aerosol (inhaled) form.

Toxoplasmosis. Toxoplasmosis is an infection caused by the parasite *Toxoplasma gondii.* Approximately 80 percent of all adults have been infected with this parasite at some point in their lives, and most healthy people experience no symptoms or problems from this infection. However, in people with AIDS this infection can reactivate and cause problems in the central nervous system, such as encephalitis and pockets of infection in the brain. A blood test can tell whether someone has been infected and therefore is at risk of the *Toxoplasma gondii* infection reactivating as the HIV infection progresses. Trimethoprim-sulfamethoxazole is the medication of choice; alternatives are pyrimethamine and dapsone.

Tuberculosis. Skin testing for tuberculosis will detect whether a person has been exposed to the disease in the past. This test is a particularly good idea for people with HIV, because a reactivation of the tuberculosis can occur as the immune system declines. If a skin test is positive, the medication isoniazid is recommended to kill the bacterium and prevent the disease from occurring.

Mycobacterium avium Complex Infection. When the T-helper-cell count falls below 50, about 30 percent of people with AIDS will develop infection with this organism. Symptoms include fever, night sweats, weight loss, and stomach pain. Three medications that have proven effective in treating this infection are clarithromycin, azithromycin, and rifabutin.

Fungal Infections. Fungal infections are very common among persons with AIDS, and they include cryptococcal meningitis and fungal infections of the esophagus and mouth. Fluconazole has been shown to prevent these infections; however, because it interacts with other medications that are commonly used to treat HIV infection, it is recommended that fluconazole be used only to treat active infections and not to prevent potential infection.

Herpes Simplex Infections. Approximately 70 percent of people who are infected with HIV also have genital herpes. This is a much higher rate than in the rest of the population, where the average infection rate is about 25 percent. It is possible that people may have become infected with herpes through the same sexual risks that exposed them to HIV. In addition, any disease that causes sores or lesions in the genital area puts a person at higher risk of acquiring HIV, since any breaks in the skin, even if microscopic, can facilitate transmission. As with the rest of the population, people with HIV infection may not know they have herpes, because they can be symptom free or only mildly symptomatic and not recognize these symptoms as being from herpes. In general, people with HIV infection and herpes have more frequent and severe herpes outbreaks than those without HIV. The antiviral medications can be used to treat outbreaks when they occur or can be taken every day to prevent an outbreak (see the section on herpes). The use of suppressive acyclovir may also prevent reactivation of the chicken pox virus (in those infected as children) as herpes zoster, or shingles. People with AIDS who are taking suppressive acyclovir also seem to have more prolonged survival times than those who are not, although the reasons for this finding are unclear.

DISCUSSION OF the treatment of the various opportunistic infections that can occur with HIV infection in any further detail is beyond the scope of this book, and you should speak with your health care provider about this subject.

Treatment When Someone Has a Known Exposure to HIV

As discussed earlier, some people, such as health care workers, have the potential to be exposed to HIV in the workplace. Despite being trained to decrease the likelihood of HIV infection through taking so-called *universal precautions* (using barriers to prevent contact with infected body fluids), they can nevertheless be exposed accidentally. Persons who are at the highest risk are those who sustain a needle-stick injury from a large-bore needle that has recently been used on an HIV-positive person and has visible blood on it. A person who is stuck with a needle that has sat around for an unknown length of time has a lower likelihood of becoming infected with HIV, since the virus does not last long outside the body. However, because of the uncertainty, any needle stick or cut with glass or a scalpel that has been in contact with another person's body fluids, any splash of body fluids onto mucosal surfaces, or any splash of fluid onto nonintact skin (such as the site of a skin rash, scratch or scrape, or blister) should be considered a risk.

The risk of acquiring HIV from a fluid that was splashed onto broken skin has been estimated to be 0.3 percent (3 in 1000). The risk of an exposure through a splash onto a mucous membrane is estimated to be less: under 0.1 percent (1 in 1000). As mentioned in the discussion of transmission, the most potentially infectious body fluids are *blood, semen, vaginal fluids, and breast milk.* Fluids from which there is a doubtful risk of transmission are saliva, urine, feces, sweat, tears, and vomit, unless any of these fluids is also mixed with blood. Any other body fluids, such as fluid from the lung or amniotic fluid, could potentially transmit HIV. Fluids from a person known to be HIV-positive are more infectious if they are from someone whose virus is very active, as evidenced by a high viral load assay or a low CD4 count.

If a person has experienced a significant exposure to a body fluid known to present a risk for HIV transmission, then a decision must be made about whether to start medications that may prevent that person from becoming infected. The decision must be reached in consultation with a health care provider and must be based on the information provided by the most current studies.

For people with significant risk of infection, treatment with antiretrovirals following an exposure to blood or other potentially infectious body fluids reduced the likelihood that they would become infected. The sooner medication was started, the more protection was offered. The current recommendation for massive exposure is to start therapy with antiretrovirals within one hour after the exposure and continue for twenty-eight days. If a person had a very-high-risk exposure and the medications were not initiated within this time frame, then in some situations they may be started later. These medications obviously have side effects, and the decision to use them must be an individual one. About one-third of those who have begun taking these medications after exposure discontinue them because of their side effects.

As discussed previously, it is not yet clear whether it makes sense to take these medications if an exposure has occurred other than in a work setting, such as during unprotected sexual contact. Some health care centers are offering this option to persons who have experienced a very-high-risk sexual exposure. However, there is some concern that offering this treatment after an unsafe sexual experience may lead people to engage in riskier sexual practices. This possibility will need to be monitored as time goes on, and studies of post-sexual and post–injection drug use exposure are under way. If the medications are started, and the person who was the source of the body fluid is later found not to be infected with HIV, then the medications can be discontinued.

> Using the antiretroviral medications to prevent infection with HIV after a high-risk exposure is routine after needle-stick injuries in health care settings. Whether this approach is useful for other high-risk exposures, such as those resulting from sexual contacts, remains to be seen.

Whether or not a person opts to use these medications, follow-up blood tests for HIV are recommended at six weeks, three months, and six months after exposure. A person testing negative after six months is considered to be negative for HIV (excluding the exceedingly rare possibility that someone may take longer than six months to convert to positive status). When a person believes that he or she may have been exposed to HIV, it is a good idea to practice safer sex with partners or consider abstaining from sex altogether until testing has shown negative results. This again must be an individual decision, following recommendations made based on the level of risk to which the person has been exposed.

LYMPHOGRANULOMA VENEREUM

incidence: very rare
cause: bacterium (*Chlamydia trachomatis*)
symptoms: lymph node swelling, painful ulcers
treatment: antibiotics

WHAT IS IT?

Lymphogranuloma venereum (LGV) is an infection caused by three types of the bacterium *Chlamydia trachomatis*. Other types of this bacterium cause the more common chlamydia infections, such as urethritis and cervicitis (see the section on chlamydia).

HOW COMMON IS IT?

Although some types of the bacterium *Chlamydia trachomatis* are very common in the United States, the types that cause LGV are not, and fewer than 1000 people are diagnosed with LGV each year in this country.

LGV is common in the developing world, especially in Africa, Asia, and South America, and most people who live in the United States and contract the disease do so when they travel to another part of the world and have unprotected sex with an infected person. Poor people living in urban areas of the United States are also at higher risk. Having multiple sexual partners is a risk factor for acquiring LGV, as it is for other sexually transmitted diseases.

WHAT ARE THE SYMPTOMS?

The symptoms of LGV are very different from the typical chlamydia symptoms of urethritis and cervicitis (see the section on chlamydia). Men are more likely than women to have noticeable symptoms.

Three stages of symptoms can occur with LGV. In the first stage, a small red bump or ulcer occurs in the genital or anal area; it is painless, transient, and usually not noticed. The lesion appears a few days to a few weeks after infection; it can occur on skin outside the genital and anal areas, but it occurs more commonly on the head of the penis or on the cervix or labia. The bump usually heals without a scar.

The second stage (and the most commonly noticed symptom of LGV) consists of lymph node swelling in the groin area. This stage usually occurs within ten days to six months after infection. At this point, the bacterium also enters the bloodstream, and it can cause infection at sites distant from the site of initial infection, such as the liver, lung, and brain. Although the lymph node swelling usually occurs on one side of the groin, it can occur on both sides at the same time. The lymph nodes are usually painful; they may rupture and drain pus, and the person may experience fever.

During this stage, men and women may also experience inflammation and infection of the urethra, which is usually symptom free. Women can also have infection and inflammation of the cervix.

A person who has been infected in the anal area through receiving anal intercourse may develop rectal ulcers with pain and discharge. Even if a person has not received anal intercourse but has an LGV infection in the genital area, it is possible for the infection to spread to the anal and rectal area and cause bleeding and pain with bowel movements.

Those who perform oral sex on infected persons can become infected in the mouth; oral LGV infection causes mouth ulcers and lymph node enlargement in the neck.

If LGV is not treated with antibiotics at the second stage, the symptoms will often resolve on their own, usually over weeks to months, but scarring and chronic genital or anal ulcers can occur later, even after years have passed: this is the third stage of infection. Scarring in the rectum can cause strictures that may be so severe that they block the passage of stool. If inflammation and scarring interfere with the drainage of the lymph nodes in the genital area, significant enlargement of the genital tissues, called *genital elephantiasis,* can occur. Surgical repair of the scarring may be necessary under these circumstances.

> The symptoms of LGV are significant lymph node swelling and genital ulcers, which can lead to scarring if not treated early.

HOW IS LYMPHOGRANULOMA VENEREUM TRANSMITTED?

Lymphogranuloma venereum is transmitted through sexual contact with a person who is infected. The infection can be transmitted through unprotected oral, anal, or genital sexual contact. Condoms decrease the risk of transmission. Pregnant women who are infected do not transmit the infection to the fetus while it is in the womb, but the infant may become infected by transmission as it travels through the birth canal.

> Lymphogranuloma venereum is transmitted through sexual contact or from mother to child at birth.

TESTING FOR LYMPHOGRANULOMA VENEREUM

The first two stages of LGV produce symptoms that are similar to the symptoms of many other diseases (including colitis, proctitis, proctocolitis, Crohn's disease, and ulcerative colitis) as well as other STDs (such as syphilis, herpes, and chancroid). The second stage of LGV can also be confused with tuberculosis and plague, as well as cancers such as Hodgkin's disease. Swollen lymph nodes may also be mistaken for a hernia in the groin area.

The similarities among these diseases make it essential to perform a blood test for the specific strains of *Chlamydia trachomatis* that cause LGV. This test looks for antibodies, or the body's immune response to the infection, and is the method of choice today. In addition, using either the genital ulcer or fluid from the swollen lymph node, the lesions may be tested for the bacterium that causes this infection.

Testing for LGV involves a blood test to detect the body's immune response (antibodies) to the infection.

If a person has lymph node swelling in the groin area, he or she should be tested for other, more common, sexually transmitted infections (such as syphilis and HIV infection), as well as nonsexually transmitted causes of such swelling. Because people with LGV in the United States are likely to be infected with other STDs as well, a complete screening for sexually transmitted infections is recommended whenever the diagnosis of LGV is made. Because LGV causes open sores in the genitals, HIV is transmitted more easily to individuals with LGV.

TREATMENT

Lymphogranuloma venereum is treated with antibiotics. The recommended treatment is doxycycline, or erythromycin if a person can't take doxycycline. Close weekly follow-up by a health care provider is essential until the symptoms have cleared, and antibiotics must be continued until the infection has resolved. Surgical draining of swollen, pus-filled lymph nodes may be necessary.

Scarring is not uncommon, even when the treatment is started early and has been successful. Surgical repair of the scarring may be necessary after the infection has been successfully treated with antibiotics.

Anyone who has had sexual contact with an infected person, usually within the sixty days before that person became symptomatic, must be treated with antibiotics and should be tested for other STDs as well.

MOLLUSCUM CONTAGIOSUM

incidence: common
cause: virus (*Molluscum contagiosum*)
symptoms: painless, dimpled bumps
treatment: topical treatments, but will resolve without treatment

WHAT IS IT?

Molluscum contagiosum (molluscum for short) is a skin infection caused by the virus *Molluscum contagiosum,* which is a member of the poxvirus family. It is usually a relatively benign infection that causes harmless skin lesions and does not become chronic. Molluscum is very common among children, who often have lesions on the face, trunk, or extremities and usually acquire the infection through nonsexual contact. Adults usually acquire the infection in the genital area through sexual contact.

HOW COMMON IT IS?

Since most people do not seek treatment for molluscum and the infection is not reportable to health departments in the United States, it is difficult to estimate how common it is. Molluscum is a commonly seen skin problem in pediatric clinics and STD clinics. It occurs throughout the United States and the world, but it is probably more common in warmer areas.

People who have compromised immune systems, such as those with AIDS, often have extensive lesions on the face and other areas of the body. It is not clear whether the virus is latent on the skin and becomes active when the immune system weakens or whether persons with AIDS are more vulnerable to new infection.

WHAT ARE THE SYMPTOMS?

The *Molluscum contagiosum* virus causes small bumps in the skin that are usually flesh colored but range in color from white to yellow to pink. The lesions do not usually itch or hurt. There may be only a few lesions or there may be many, and individual lesions may grow together to form larger bumps. The bumps have a characteristic "dent" or umbilication in the center, which can be hard to see. If a lesion is lanced with a sterile needle, a white core can be expressed, as when one squeezes a pimple; this core contains the virus particles.

The lesions can become infected, and this makes them difficult to distinguish from lesions resulting from other infections, such as herpes. People with molluscum—and even some health care providers—often confuse the lesions with warts.

The lesions appear between one week and six months after infection, and the interval may occasionally be even longer, up to several years in certain cases. This does not mean that a person has been reinfected: the virus acquired from the initial infection can continue to show skin manifestations for a long time.

> Molluscum lesions take weeks or months to show up after initial infection. They are often confused with warts.

The bumps, when they are sexually transmitted, can appear anywhere in the genital area and sometimes on the upper thighs and lower abdomen. They usually appear on outside skin surfaces rather than on mucosal surfaces. If the bumps are left untreated, they will eventually disappear on their own and heal without scarring, but this may take some time. Lesions can vanish within one week of appearing, or it may take several years (the range is one week to four years). Most lesions resolve on their own within a few months.

People with other skin disorders, such as eczema, may have more difficulty clearing molluscum. Using topical steroids may also delay healing of the molluscum, since the steroids inhibit the body's immune response where they are applied. The use of oral steroids for another medical problem, such as asthma, can delay healing, as can suppression of the immune system as a result of other medical problems, such as AIDS. An evaluation for an underlying immune system problem should be considered in someone with widespread molluscum (that is, lesions all over the body or outside the usual areas of infection). Such widespread lesions can be difficult to treat.

HOW IS MOLLUSCUM CONTAGIOSUM TRANSMITTED?

The virus is transmitted by skin-to-skin contact with a person who is infected, whether or not that person has symptoms. The virus can also be transmitted through the saliva of a person with facial molluscum. It is also believed that the virus can be transmitted through inanimate objects, such as towels. Multiple members of the same family often become infected, either through direct contact or from inanimate objects.

> Some people may be infected and symptom free and still transmit molluscum to others.

In adults, when the lesions are in the genital area, lower abdomen, or upper thighs, the infection has usually (though not always) been transmitted through sexual contact. The risk of molluscum infection increases with the number of sexual partners that a person has. Children with molluscum on the face may develop lesions in the genital area, most likely by transmitting the virus there themselves.

TESTING FOR MOLLUSCUM CONTAGIOSUM

A health care provider who has expertise in diagnosing sexually transmitted infections can usually make the diagnosis of molluscum contagiosum by looking at the bumps. There is no blood test or other test to routinely diagnose this infection. If there is doubt, a lesion can be biopsied to assist in making the diagnosis, but this is rarely necessary because the skin lesions are in most cases easily identified by sight.

One of the treatments for molluscum, freezing the bumps with liquid nitrogen, can help to accentuate the central umbilication that is a classic feature of the lesions. Another way to help make a diagnosis is to lance a large lesion to express the characteristic core of virus, which is hard, white, and waxy in appearance.

Partners should be referred to a health care provider for examination. If no lesions are seen, no treatment is necessary.

TREATMENT

As noted previously, if left untreated, the lesions eventually disappear on their own, but the process may take several months. To speed up this process, there are two treatment options. The first is freezing the lesions with liquid nitrogen—which is also the standard treatment for another sexually transmitted skin infection, genital warts. Another common treatment for warts, topical liquids such as podophyllin (10–25% solution) or trichloroacetic acid (80–90% solution), can be used either alone or in addition to the liquid nitrogen. These treatments basically destroy the virus as well as the skin cells containing the virus.

The second treatment option is to nick the skin of the lesions with a sterile needle and then express the central core of virus. This is easier if the lesions are larger. The lesions tend to be well vascularized, so bleeding can occur with this method. Patients can be taught to perform this procedure themselves.

> Treatment of the molluscum lesions will speed resolution. However, they will disappear on their own if left alone.

Treatment may not be successful in people with such underlying immune system problems as AIDS.

The lesions are usually not red, tender, or filled with pus. If these features are noted, it may be a sign that there is a secondary bacterial infection, most often with the common bacteria found on the skin. Such infections occur in about 40 percent of those with molluscum infection. If a secondary bacterial infection is suspected, antibiotic treatment may be necessary.

MUCOPURULENT CERVICITIS

incidence: common
cause: bacteria (chlamydia, gonorrhea, others), virus (herpes virus), protozoa (trichomonas)
symptoms: discharge, spotting between periods; often none
treatment: directed at the underlying cause

WHAT IS IT?

There are many different types of infection of the cervix. Some, such as those caused by chlamydia and gonorrhea, involve the inner part of the cervix, resulting in an infection called *endocervicitis*. Others, such as trichomonas and yeast infections, involve primarily the outer part of the cervix, resulting in an infection called *ectocervicitis*. Still others, such as those caused by herpes viruses, may involve both the inner and the outer part of the cervix. Sometimes these different infections occur at the same time, and it can be difficult to distinguish them from one another without performing tests.

The term *mucopurulent cervicitis* (MPC) is often used to describe infections of the endocervix, and MPC is used throughout this section as a synonym for *endocervicitis* unless otherwise specified. For more specific information about the types of infection that can cause MPC, see the appropriate sections in this part of the book.

Mucopurulent cervicitis is a term used to describe infection of the cervix by one of several sexually transmitted organisms.

HOW COMMON IS IT?

Infections of the cervix are very common. It is estimated that between four and six million women in the United States are diagnosed with MPC each year and that even more women have undetected infection, but there are no good statistics. Accurate numbers are not available, since cervicitis is not reportable to the health department in every state. MPC seems to be much more common among younger, sexually active women, women who are pregnant, and women who use oral birth control pills and do not use a barrier method to protect against sexually transmitted diseases. Any woman can become infected, however, if she is sexually active with an infected partner.

WHAT ARE THE SYMPTOMS?

Many women with MPC do not have symptoms, and MPC is often discovered only on examination. Some symptoms that a woman may notice are a vaginal discharge, often yellow in color; spotting with blood after intercourse or between periods; pain with intercourse; and burning with urination.

Depending on what is causing the infection of the cervix, there may be other symptoms, such as itching and redness of the labia in trichomonas infection or a sore on the labia from herpes. There can also be pelvic discomfort, although usually this is a symptom that would make a health care provider suspect pelvic inflammatory disease, a complication of cervicitis (see the section on pelvic inflammatory disease).

Sexually transmitted cervical infections can be symptom free or can cause vague symptoms.

HOW IS MUCOPURULENT CERVICITIS TRANSMITTED?

The organisms that cause MPC are transmitted through sexual contact with a partner who is infected. This is generally through genital contact, although it may be possible for women who have sex with women to transmit these organisms through sex toys. Genital rubbing, without penetration, may also be sufficient to transmit herpes virus from one partner to another.

A man or woman performing oral sex on a woman probably does not transmit gonorrhea, chlamydia, or the bacteria that cause nongonococcal urethritis since there is no direct contact with the cervix, although genital herpes infection with the cold sore type of herpes virus (type 1) can occur through oral sex. The use of dental dams or plastic wrap may help prevent such infection.

Condoms, if they are used properly and do not break, effectively prevent transmission of the bacteria that cause cervicitis (such as chlamydia and gonorrhea), as well as such protozoa as trichomonas, through vaginal intercourse. However, herpes simplex virus may be transmitted even with the use of condoms (see the section on herpes). The cervical cap and diaphragm, used with the spermicide nonoxynol-9, also may help prevent such bacterial infections as gonorrhea and chlamydia, but condoms are still the best method of protection.

TESTING FOR MUCOPURULENT CERVICITIS

The symptoms of MPC may be vague, and it may be difficult to diagnose based on history alone. Therefore a pelvic examination is necessary to diagnose MPC. Many women mistakenly believe they are being tested for infections when they have a Pap smear, which is the screen for cervical cancer (see the section on genital warts). A Pap smear may sometimes reveal changes consistent with herpes or trichomonas infection, but the real purpose of a Pap smear is to screen for cervical cancer, and specific tests must be performed to determine the causes of MPC.

Testing for cervicitis involves a gynecological examination.

The diagnosis of MPC is made based on characteristic observations during the examination and under the microscope. On examination, a discharge may be noticed; a sample will be examined under the microscope to help determine if it is coming from the cervix or the vagina. The cervix may show some telltale signs of infection, such as easy bleeding when it is swabbed, emission of pus from the opening (the os), and excessive redness. On examination of the cervical discharge under a microscope, numerous white blood cells can be seen. Occasionally, gonorrheal organisms can be seen under the microscope (as noted, gonorrhea is one cause of MPC). Cultures may be performed for specific bacteria. The health care provider will also determine whether there is infection higher up in the pelvic organs (see the section on pelvic inflammatory disease).

TREATMENT

Treatment of the underlying infection should cure the cervicitis. For bacterial causes, antibiotics (usually chosen to cover gonorrhea and chlamydia) are used. If trichomonas is seen or suspected, or if herpes simplex is suspected, treatment is directed toward these organisms. Through careful examination and testing, your health care provider will be able to decide which medication is best for you. As with all infections discussed in this book, it is important not to self-treat, since the decision about which medications to use is a complicated one, and self-treatment will often make it more difficult in the long run to sort out what is actually happening. For example, if someone starts to have symptoms, begins taking an antibiotic that was prescribed for another type of infection, and then visits a health care provider for evaluation because the medication didn't work, it may be difficult to determine the cause of the initial symptoms. Douching may also mask the symptoms and make diagnosis more difficult.

After you have been seen, diagnosed, and treated for the infection, your health care provider may recommend a follow-up visit to ensure the treatment has worked. If your symptoms get worse during treatment, return to see your health care provider as soon as possible.

Partners of women diagnosed with MPC must also be evaluated and treated, whether or not they have symptoms themselves and whether or not they show evidence of infection on examination. It is important not to resume sexual activity until both you and your partner have been treated.

NONGONOCOCCAL URETHRITIS

incidence: common
cause: bacteria (chlamydia and others), virus (herpes virus), protozoa (trichomonas)

symptoms: burning with urination, discharge; often none
treatment: directed at the underlying cause

WHAT IS IT?

Nongonococcal urethritis (NGU) is an infection of the urethra (the tube that carries urine from the bladder) in men that is sexually transmitted and is not caused by gonorrhea. It can be caused by several organisms, including *Chlamydia trachomatis* (the most common cause), *Ureaplasma urealyticum, Mycoplasma genitalium, Trichomonas vaginalis,* and the herpes virus. (See the sections on chlamydia infection, trichomoniasis, and herpes for more information.) Men who perform anal sex on partners may develop urethral infections from the bacteria that are normally found in stool. *NGU, therefore, is not a specific "bug" but rather a syndrome with several possible causes.* Before many of the specific organisms that cause this infection were identified, it was also known as nonspecific urethritis.

HOW COMMON IS IT?

Nongonococcal urethritis is the most common problem for which men seek help in sexually transmitted disease clinics. It is estimated that four to six million men in the United States are infected with NGU each year. Men of any age can become infected, although NGU is most often diagnosed in younger men (those in their teens to twenties) who are more sexually active and less likely to be following safer sex practices. A man can be infected and not know it.

> **About four to six million men are diagnosed with NGU each year in the United States.**

WHAT ARE THE SYMPTOMS?

About half the time, men who are infected with NGU do not have any symptoms and would not know they were infected unless they were tested. If symptoms do occur, they include painful urination, a discharge from the penis (which may only be noticed as stains in the underwear), or an itchy or ir-

> **Half the men infected with NGU do not have any symptoms.**

ritated feeling in the penis. Sometimes the discharge may be noticed only after urination. There may also be an alteration in the flow of urine, such as a "spray" or two streams, which occurs because of the inflammation in the urethra. Often these symptoms are very mild. They usually take between one and three weeks after infection to show up, but they may take much longer.

Urethritis can, rarely, progress to infection in the prostate or epididymis, and this may be the first indication that infection is present (see the section on epididymitis). Usually NGU does not cause such symptoms as fever, chills, and nausea. If the urethritis is caused by the herpes virus rather than bacteria, there are sometimes lesions on the genital skin. Although the symptoms of urethritis caused by gonorrhea are usually more severe and occur more quickly after infection than those of NGU, this is not always the case.

Women who become infected with the bacteria that cause NGU in men have different symptoms (see the sections on chlamydia, mucopurulent cervicitis and pelvic inflammatory disease).

Men and women can become infected in the throat with the bacteria that cause NGU. Usually they do not experience any symptoms, although occasionally there can be some mild throat irritation. When a man or woman has an NGU bacterial infection in the anal or rectal area, there are often no symptoms; if they do occur, they may include rectal discharge, bleeding, and pain.

HOW IS NONGONOCOCCAL URETHRITIS TRANSMITTED?

Nongonoccal urethritis is transmitted through sexual contact with a partner who is infected: genital (penis to vagina), oral (penis to throat), or anal (penis to rectum). Men who perform anal sex may become infected with stool bacteria in the urethra. Correct use of a condom during sexual contact decreases the risk of transmission of NGU. Condoms should be used for genital, oral, or anal intercourse with a partner who has not been tested, since a person can be infected but have no symptoms. Although many men believe otherwise, there is no evidence that urethritis is caused by allergic reactions, masturbation, too much caffeine,

> NGU can be transmitted through oral, anal, or genital sexual contact with an infected partner. Condoms, if used correctly, help prevent transmission.

too little water, too much alcohol, spicy foods, or too much or too little sex.

TESTING FOR NONGONOCOCCAL URETHRITIS

To test for NGU, a urethral swab may be taken and examined for white blood cells. A small swab is inserted a short distance into the urethra (this may cause momentary discomfort). If examination under a microscope reveals a certain number of white cells ($\geq$5), then the diagnosis of urethritis is made. If a man has urinated within the past four hours, the results may not be accurate, because the urine can wash away the signs of infection and the results would be falsely negative. For the urethral swab test to provide the most accurate results, the man should not urinate (preferably overnight) before this examination.

If the results of the urethral swab test are negative but symptoms persist, the examination is usually repeated after the man has not urinated overnight. Alternatively, the man is instructed not to urinate overnight, and then the first part of the morning stream is examined under the microscope. More than ten white blood cells per field under the microscope, or evidence of white blood cells (a "positive leukocyte esterase test") on a urinalysis of the first-stream urine, are also indicative of infection. Tests should also be done for chlamydia and gonorrhea—these tests may show infection even if the test for NGU does not—and any infection that is found should be treated (see the sections on chlamydia and gonorrhea). Both gonorrhea and chlamydia are reportable to the state health department in most states.

If a partner has been exposed to NGU in the throat or anal area, tests can be performed in these areas for specific organisms such as chlamydia and herpes virus, but not for all the bacterial organisms that can cause NGU, since some of them are difficult to culture.

TREATMENT

The treatment of choice for bacterially caused NGU is antibiotics, most commonly doxycycline or azithromycin. If a person can't take these antibiotics, then erythromycin, ofloxacin, or levofloxacin are recommended. The type of antibiotic chosen for initial treatment is the same for chlamydia as for the other bacterial causes of NGU. If herpes is thought to be the cause of the urethritis, then an antiherpes medication is used (see the section on herpes). If trichomonas is suspected, metronidazole is prescribed. All of these medications have possible side effects and interactions with other medications, and any treatment decision must take these factors into account. Ask your health care provider which medication is best for you.

Partners of a person diagnosed with NGU must also be evaluated and treated, whether or not the partner shows symptoms or evidence of infection on examination. All sexual contacts, generally within the past sixty days, must be treated. It is important not to resume sexual contact with a person until he or she has been completely treated and all symptoms have resolved in both partners.

If evidence of infection persists after treatment, another examination should be performed. If symptoms resolve, no follow-up examination is necessary. The medications are effective in about 95 percent of cases, but recurrence of infection occurs after successful treatment in about 10–20 percent of cases. Taking the medication incorrectly, having sexual contact with a partner who did not receive treatment, or having sex with a new, untested partner can all cause reinfection. If none of these possible explanations applies, a different antibiotic is usually prescribed.

Symptoms may occasionally persist even after several courses of antibiotics and eradication of the organism that caused the NGU. In this situation no further treatment is usually given, and the symptoms usually resolve on their own with time. If you did not take the medication as prescribed, or if you had sex again with an infected partner, you may be given another course of the antibiotic or you may be treated for the more unusual causes of NGU (such as trichomonas). Talk with your health care provider about this.

PELVIC INFLAMMATORY DISEASE

incidence: common
cause: bacteria (chlamydia, gonorrhea, vaginal bacteria)
symptoms pelvic pain, discharge, pain with intercourse, spotting between periods
treatment: antibiotics

WHAT IS IT?

Pelvic inflammatory disease (PID) is an infection of the pelvic organs in women that can involve the uterus (in which case the infection is called *endometritis*), the Fallopian tubes (*salpingitis*), the ovaries (*ovarian abscess*), or the peritoneum (the lining of tissue around the pelvic organs; *pelvic peritonitis*). One, several, or all of these organs can be affected. PID is usually caused by sexually transmitted bacteria such as gonorrhea and chlamydia, but it can be caused by other bacteria as well. It is the most serious infection of the genital area in women.

HOW COMMON IS IT?

It is estimated that about one million women develop PID each year in the United States, but this is likely to be an underestimate since in many parts of the country PID is not reportable to the local health department. Three-quarters of the women infected are younger than twenty-five, but women of any age can be infected.

About 85 percent of cases of PID are caused by sexually transmitted bacteria; a woman who has unprotected genital intercourse with a male partner infected with PID-causing bacteria is at high risk for becoming infected. The sexually transmitted bacteria break down the defenses in the cervix that normally prevent vaginal bacteria from moving up into the pelvic organs; this breakdown allows these bacteria to contribute to the infection.

The other 15 percent of cases of PID are caused by gynecological procedures that mechanically open the cervix and allow the vaginal bacteria to rise into the pelvic organs and cause infection. Women who have an invasive gynecological procedure—such as an abortion, insertion of an intrauterine device (IUD), or hysterosalpingography (an X-ray study to examine the Fallopian tubes and uterus by means of injection of dye into these structures)—are at increased risk for developing PID. In addition, women who use IUDs as a birth control method run a higher risk for developing PID if exposed to sexually transmitted infections. Women who douche are also in the high-risk category, possibly because douching pushes vaginal

> Certain gynecological procedures, the use of an IUD, and douching all may make women more susceptible to PID.

bacteria higher up into the genital tract. Women who have had PID in the past are at increased risk of having it again, because scarring from the infection makes them more vulnerable.

Men, obviously, do not get PID, but they can be infected with the bacteria that cause it.

WHAT ARE THE SYMPTOMS?

The most common symptom of PID is pain in the pelvis and lower abdomen. The pain is usually dull, and it can occur on one side or both sides of the pelvis. Other symptoms—discharge and an odor from the vaginal area, burning with urination, fever, and spotting between periods or after sexual intercourse—may also be present. A woman may notice heavier than usual periods and pain during intercourse. With more severe infection, there can be fever and chills, and nausea and vomiting. In addition, PID can sometimes spread into the abdominal cavity and cause infection around the liver, experienced as pain in the upper right part of the abdomen. This rare condition is known as Fitz-Hugh Curtis syndrome. In other cases there may be no symptoms with PID or symptoms may be very mild, and the infection may go undetected until it is discovered during a pelvic examination.

PID can cause no symptoms, mild symptoms, or severe symptoms.

Symptoms generally occur within a few days to a few months after infection, but they may take longer to show up. With each episode of PID, a woman undergoes a 20 percent reduction in her future fertility and runs a 20 percent risk of being subject to chronic pelvic pain and an increased risk of an ectopic (tubal) pregnancy.

HOW IS PELVIC INFLAMMATORY DISEASE TRANSMITTED?

The bacteria that cause PID are usually transmitted through unprotected sexual contact with an infected person. Two common causes are gonorrhea and chlamydia. Other bacteria that can cause PID either are sexually transmitted (e.g., *Mycoplasma hominis*) or are vaginal bacteria that are not sexually transmitted (e.g., *Gardnerella vaginalis*).

PID is usually caused by sexually transmitted bacteria such as gonorrhea and chlamydia.

Women with multiple sexual partners are at increased risk for PID. A woman who has unprotected sex with an infected partner while she is menstruating is also at higher risk, since at this time of the month the natural defenses of the cervix are less effective. Younger women may be more vulnerable because they are more likely to practice unsafe sex and may have more frequent exposure to partners who are infected with sexually transmitted bacteria.

For women who are sexually active with male partners, condoms can help prevent transmission of PID-causing bacteria if they are used correctly and consistently and if the condom does not break or leak. Cervical caps and diaphragms may also help decrease the risk of infection, but they are not as effective as condoms. Whatever their sexual orientation, women who have had unprotected sexual contacts in the past and who have never been examined for sexually transmitted diseases should be examined and tested for STDs that can cause PID, even if they are symptom free.

TESTING FOR PELVIC INFLAMMATORY DISEASE

Testing for PID requires a pelvic examination and is based on both the examination and symptom history. Evidence of infection may include a yellowish discharge from the cervix, and the cervix may be red and bleed easily when it is swabbed—abnormal signs that indicate cervicitis. With a cervical infection, secretions collected on a swab inserted into the opening of the cervix (the os) are often seen to contain white blood cells when examined under a microscope. Often, white blood cells are seen in an examination of the vaginal secretions. With PID, there is also pain when the cervix is moved by a finger inserted into the vagina (*cervical motion tenderness*). There is usually also pain with pressure over the uterus and ovaries. A woman may experience a fever, and a blood test may reveal an elevated white blood cell count. It is important to note that no single finding on examination or in the history can be used to make the diagnosis of PID. Many health care providers offer treatment if the possibility of PID is high, even if the diagnosis lacks certainty, because the consequences of untreated infection can be devastating.

A surgical procedure called a *laparoscopy* may be performed to help confirm the diagnosis of PID. The procedure is carried out in a hospital, with the woman under anesthesia. A tiny incision is made below the umbilicus (belly button) and a *laparoscope* is inserted into the abdomen to enable the health care provider to look directly at the uterus, Fallopian tubes, and ovaries to see if they are infected. An *ultrasound* study may also be performed, which may show a collection of pus or infected tissue (an abscess) in the ovaries or Fallopian tubes, or other evidence of pelvic organ infection. A biopsy of the uterus is another means of establishing whether an infection is present.

> PID is diagnosed during a pelvic examination; a variety of methods may be used to confirm the diagnosis.

Tests for sexually transmitted bacteria such as gonorrhea and chlamydia are usually performed. These tests may be negative even when PID is present, because many bacteria can cause PID and it is not possible to test routinely for all of them in most clinical settings. During the examination, the health care provider will make sure the woman does not have other conditions—such as pregnancy (particularly an ectopic, or tubal, pregnancy), appendicitis, irritable bowel syndrome, endometriosis, or bladder infection—that could mimic the symptoms of PID.

TREATMENT

The treatment of choice for PID is antibiotics that treat all the potential bacterial causes of the disease. As noted above, health care providers would rather treat a woman for PID if there is *any* chance that she has it, even if the disease cannot be conclusively diagnosed, because the potential consequences of missing the diagnosis are so severe.

Sometimes the bacteria causing PID are not identified, but the treatment is the same whether or not they are identified. And the treatment of PID is the same whether or not it is thought to be sexually transmitted. Most women with PID are treated as outpatients, but about 20 percent must be hospitalized. A woman who has severe pain, or who cannot take oral antibiotics because she is nauseated and vomiting, is pregnant, or doesn't respond to treatment as an outpatient, is usually admitted to the hospital to allow antibiotics to be administered intravenously. Younger women may be hospitalized to make sure they receive their full course of treatment. Furthermore, if there is suspicion of a localized area of infection (an abscess) or if there is any question about the diagnosis, a woman is usually admitted to the hospital. Women who are pregnant and have PID are also usually hospitalized for aggressive treatment of the disease. Irrespective of the circumstances, any decision regarding hospitalization must be discussed with one's health care provider.

Some of the medications used to treat PID for women admitted to the hospital are an intravenous antibiotic (cefotetan or cefoxitin) plus doxycycline; other options are available for women who cannot take these antibiotics. If a woman shows improvement in a few days, the intravenous medication can be switched to pills, to finish out the two-week course. An outpatient treatment regimen would use levofloxacin or ofloxacin, with or without metronidazole, depending on the patient and geographic location. Other options exist as well.

About seventy-two hours after outpatient treatment has begun, a follow-up visit is usually scheduled; if things have improved, another follow-up visit is scheduled after treatment. If her condition is not improving, the woman may be admitted to the hospital so that intravenous antibiotics can be administered. Any woman with PID must abstain from sex during treatment. Even if the cause of the infection is suspected to be a nonsexually transmitted organism, any sexual partner within the past two months must be treated as a contact, regardless of whether or not he has symptoms or shows evidence of infection on examination. Further follow-up visits after treatment has been completed are essential to make sure the treatment was effective. If you have an IUD and are diagnosed with PID, your health care provider may recommend that the IUD be removed. Talk with your health care provider about this.

A single episode of PID changes the anatomy of the pelvic organs, so that a woman is at higher risk for developing PID again if she is infected with these bacteria. Thus it is especially important that she protect herself from becoming reinfected in the future.

Very rarely, and only in cases of severe infection, a hysterectomy (removal of the pelvic organs) must be performed to eliminate the infection. Fortunately most women respond well to the antibiotics, although the complications, such as scarring, can sometimes still occur, especially if the woman delayed seeking treatment.

PROCTOCOLITIS, PROCTITIS, AND ENTERITIS

incidence: common
cause: bacteria, viruses, protozoa; varies depending on the location of the infection
symptoms: rectal pain, discharge, diarrhea
treatment: directed at the underlying cause

WHAT ARE THEY?

Proctocolitis, proctitis, and enteritis are intestinal syndromes caused by infection with bacteria, viruses, or protozoa that can be transmitted sexually as well as by nonsexual means. *Proctocolitis* is an infection and inflammation of the rectum and the colon. It is usually caused by shigella, salmonella, campylobacter, *Entamoeba histolytica*, or lymphogranuloma venereum (LGV) infections. *Proctitis* is an infection and inflammation of the rectum, lower than in proctocolitis; it is usually caused by gonorrhea, chlamydia, herpes, syphilis, or LGV, and is usually a result of receiving anal intercourse. *Enteritis* is an infection and inflammation of the small intestine, which is usually caused by giardia. In persons with HIV infection, enteritis may also be caused by cytomegalovirus *Mycobacterium avium* complex, cryptosporidium, isospora, and salmonella infections.

> Many organisms that are sexually transmitted can cause intestinal infections. Different types of STDs affect different areas of the gastrointestinal system.

HOW COMMON ARE THEY?

Some of these infections, such as chlamydia, gonorrhea, herpes, LGV, and syphilis, can be transmitted only through sexual contact. Women who have a gonorrhea or chlamydia infection of the cervix can develop proctitis when infected secretions travel to the anal area. Many of the other infections are most common among men and women who engage in anal intercourse or in oral-anal contact, a practice called *rimming*. But remember, some of these infections are not sexually transmitted, and are very common among travelers, who acquire them by eating improperly prepared food. We do not have reliable information about how many of the people who are diagnosed with these infections each year have acquired them through sexual contact, but we do know that in the era of HIV the practice of safer sex among men who have sex with other men has led to a decrease in the prevalence of the infections in this group.

WHAT ARE THE SYMPTOMS?

Whether or not the organisms that cause proctocolitis, proctitis, and enteritis are acquired sexually, the symptoms are usually those of a gastrointestinal illness. How much time elapses between initial infection and the appearance of symptoms depends on which infection is present. Although abdominal pain and rectal discharge are common, the specific symptoms depend on which area of the gastrointestinal tract is involved.

The symptoms of proctitis include pain in the anal area, a mucous discharge from the anal area, constipation, and feeling an urgent need to have a bowel movement without being able to do so, despite straining. Blood may be noticed in the stool or when wiping after a bowel movement. If the proctitis is caused by herpes or syphilis, then lesions may be present. In men, infections such as chlamydia and gonorrhea usually produce far fewer symptoms when they are present in the rectum than when they are present in the urethra.

The symptoms of proctocolitis are generally the same as for proctitis, with the addition of diarrhea and abdominal pain. Less often, proctitis and proctocolitis are symptom free.

The symptoms of enteritis include diarrhea and cramping or pain in the abdominal area, often in the lower left abdomen. Nausea and bloating often accompany these symptoms. The diarrhea may be bloody, depending on which organism has caused the infection, and there may also be a mucous rectal discharge. Other possible symptoms include fever, chills, and malaise (a generalized sense of not feeling well). Significant weight loss can result if food is not absorbed well because of inflammation in the bowel.

HOW ARE PROCTOCOLITIS, PROCTITIS, AND ENTERITIS TRANSMITTED?

Proctitis is transmitted sexually primarily when a man or woman receives penile penetration in the anal area and, in women, when genital infection affects this area. Enteritis is transmitted sexually when a person ingests fecal material, either through oral-anal sex or through oral-genital sex when the anal-genital area has been contaminated by fecal material. Not all enteritis is sexually transmitted. A person can become infected with the nonsexually transmitted organisms that cause enteritis by eating improperly prepared food that is contaminated with fecal material. Proctocolitis can be acquired by oral-anal and oral-genital sex.

A man who performs anal intercourse can become infected (and usually remains symptom free) and then infect others by performing anal intercourse on them. Some people who receive anal intercourse practice rectal douching; these infections can be transmitted if the equipment for rectal douching is shared. Douching can also cause injury to rectal tissues, making transmission of sexually transmitted infections more likely. People who are infected with certain diseases, such as herpes, through genital-genital sexual contact may experience outbreaks in the anal area (see the section on herpes), but only rarely inside the rectum.

If condoms are used correctly during anal intercourse and if they do not break or leak, they will help provide protection against proctitis and proctocolitis. Oral-anal contact should be avoided if a person's infection status is not known. Dental dams or plastic wrap may provide some protection against these infections for those who practice oral-anal intercourse, but they should not be relied on completely. Only tiny amounts of the bacteria *Shigella*, for example, are required to cause infection. As noted previously, even symptom-free persons who are infected can transmit these infections. To prevent nonsexual transmission, proper food handling techniques, hand washing, and efforts to avoid contamination of water and food products are essential.

TESTING FOR PROCTOCOLITIS, PROCTITIS, AND ENTERITIS

The first step in testing for these infections is examination by a health care provider. If you have symptoms in the anal or rectal area, and if your sexual practices have involved either anal intercourse or oral-anal contact, tell your health care provider. This is important, because the range of possible diagnoses for these symptoms is greater for a person who has participated in these sexual practices. Raising this issue may be awkward for you, and even your provider may feel too embarrassed to ask you (or not even think to ask), but being open about this part of your history will help you receive the correct diagnosis and appropriate care.

Testing usually involves culturing lesions, culturing stool, and looking into the colon with special instruments to examine the infected areas.

For proctitis, a visual examination of the anal area and of the mucosal area of the rectum is necessary. The latter can be performed by *anoscopy* (which involves inserting a small plastic or metal scope into the anal area to allow the health care provider to see the internal tissue) or *sigmoidoscopy,* which involves looking farther into the colon with a flexible tube.

If areas farther up in the colon may be involved (as in proctocolitis), then a more comprehensive test, a *colonoscopy,* may be done. In this test, the health care provider (usually a gastroenterologist) looks at the entire colon through a longer flexible tube. No matter which procedure is performed, a swab is used to take a sample of material that is then examined for white blood cells under the microscope; cultures can be performed for gonorrhea and chlamydia, which are two of the most common causes of proctitis. Sometimes a biopsy of the rectal tissue may be taken to make a diagnosis; this painless procedure is performed during the sigmoidoscopy or colonoscopy.

Samples of stool or any rectal discharge may be examined under the microscope for white blood cells. The stool may also be examined for evidence of protozoan and bacterial infections. Any sores are tested for herpes and syphilis; if no sores are present, then blood tests for these two infections may be carried out, and these may be repeated in several months (see the sections on herpes and syphilis).

To diagnose enteritis, a stool sample is examined under the microscope for white blood cells and cultures are performed for the parasites and bacteria that can cause the disorder. The most common organism known to cause enteritis through sexual transmission is *Giardia lamblia,* a parasite. Several stool samples are usually taken to evaluate for this pathogen. Bacteria such as salmonella, shigella, and campylobacter can also cause enteritis and can be sexually transmitted. In persons infected with HIV, many more infectious organisms can cause enteritis, and special tests must be performed for them.

TREATMENT

Treatment of these infections is directed at the underlying cause. For proctitis caused by bacterial infection with gonorrhea and chlamydia, the treatment is ceftriaxone and doxycycline. Treatment is usually started before the culture results return from the laboratory and is based on what is seen on examination. The treatments for chlamydia, gonorrhea, herpes, LGV, and syphilis are described in the respective sections in this part of the book.

The treatments for the bacterial causes of enteritis, such as salmonella and shigella and campylobacter infections, are antibiotics. Giardia infections are usually treated with metronidazole.

If it is thought the illness was sexually transmitted, sexual contacts must be examined, tested, and treated. For some organisms that cause enteritis, such as giardia and shigella, evaluation of nonsexual household contacts (parents, spouses, children, and siblings) is also recommended, since these infections are fairly easy to transmit nonsexually as well, especially through improper food handling.

> **Treatment for these infections involves eliminating the organism responsible. Several organisms may be involved.**

PUBIC LICE

incidence: common
cause: lice (*Phthirus pubic*)
symptoms: genital itching, nits on pubic hair
treatment: topical creams

WHAT IS IT?

Pubic lice or crabs are caused by a tiny parasite called *Phthirus pubis* that is usually transmitted through sexual contact. Other types of lice, such as head lice and body lice, are usually not sexually transmitted. Pubic lice are called crabs because of their crab-like appearance under the microscope.

HOW COMMON IS IT?

Because nonprescription treatments for this infection are available and because this is not an infection that is required to be reported to local health departments, there is no way to know exactly how many people are infected. However, it is estimated that as many as three million people a year may have pubic lice. Most of those infected are in their teens and twenties, although anyone of any age can become infected.

WHAT ARE THE SYMPTOMS?

Infected persons usually notice the nits (eggs) of the lice at the base of follicles in the pubic hair. The hair on the thighs or trunk, the hair of a beard or mustache, eyelash or eyebrow hair, and (rarely) the hair on the scalp may also be infected. Nits look like tiny white specks on the hair follicles. Multiple nits are usually attached to a single hair follicle. Finding the adult lice is much harder because the adults are only about a millimeter in length. Itching may or may not be present. Sometimes people notice tiny, rust-colored spots on their underwear, the result of bleeding from those places where the lice are feeding on the skin. Symptoms may take from a few days to a month to appear after a person becomes infected.

> **Pubic lice do not always cause itching.**

HOW ARE PUBIC LICE TRANSMITTED?

Infection usually occurs through skin-to-skin contact with an infected person, often through sexual contact. Coming into contact with the bedding or clothing of a person who is infected can also cause infection. Pubic lice do not survive off the body (such as in clothing or bedding) for more than a day or two.

> **Lice can be transmitted through sexual contact with an infected person or through contact with an infected person's bedding or clothing.**

TESTING FOR PUBIC LICE

A health care provider can usually diagnose pubic lice by examining the affected areas; in addition, the nits and lice can be examined under the microscope.

TREATMENT

Pubic lice are treated with topical creams, permethrin rinse cream, or pyrethrins with piperonyl butoxide. Some of these medications are available without a prescription. Second-line choices are malathion lotion (which has an odor) or a pill called ivermectin. Ask your health care provider about medication dosing. Ivermectin should be avoided for women who are pregnant or breastfeeding and for small children. In the past, a topical application of the medication lindane was recommended, but this drug can be toxic (it can cause seizures and a serious blood disorder called "aplastic anemia"), so it is no longer a first-line treatment.

The medications are applied to all infected areas (excluding the eyelashes), left on for a brief period (usually four to ten minutes, depending on the medication used), and then washed off. Retreatment may be necessary if symptoms last more than a week after the first treatment. After treatment, the nits on the hair can be removed with a fine-toothed comb.

> **There are several inexpensive medications to treat pubic lice, some of which are available without a prescription. Lice are easy to treat and do not cause permanent damage.**

Lice infestation of the eyelashes is treated by applying a heavy layer of petroleum jelly to the eyelashes twice a day for about ten days. This kills the nits by smothering them. Standard lice treatments can be harmful to the eyes and therefore should not be applied to the eyelashes.

Bedding and clothing that have been in contact with an infected person within the last seventy-two hours must also be treated, either by washing them in hot water and drying them on the hot cycle of the dryer, by dry cleaning, or by keeping them away from contact with people for at least seventy-two hours, after which time the lice will have died.

Treatment of all sexual partners within the past month is recommended, even if they have no symptoms. It is important to abstain from sex while you are being treated. Treatment of furniture and pets is not required. People who have not had intimate contact with the infected person, or who have not slept in the person's bedding or worn his or her clothing, do not need to be treated.

SCABIES

incidence: common
cause: mite (*Sarcopetes scabei*)
symptoms: bumps and burrows on the skin that itch, especially at night
treatment: topical creams

WHAT IS IT?

Scabies is a very contagious skin infection caused by the mite *Sarcopetes scabei,* a parasite that lives in and on the skin. Scabies can be sexually transmitted.

HOW COMMON IS IT?

It is not known how many people are diagnosed with scabies each year, but the infection is common.

WHAT ARE THE SYMPTOMS?

When a person is infected with scabies, the adult female mites burrow into the skin and lay eggs, which hatch in about ten days. The body's immune response to the mites causes itching and a rash, usually two to four weeks after first infection. In a person who has had scabies in the past, however, the symptoms may start within a day after reinfection, because the immune system "remembers" the previous infection and can mount a quicker response.

The scabies rash is a series of tiny, wavy lines (the burrows) and dots or tiny bumps that may look like little blisters. Bigger bumps or small nodules can also occur, especially in the groin area and in the armpits. The rash generally occurs in adults in the genital area, around the waist (belt line), in the armpits, on the wrists, on the hands (primarily on the webs between the fingers), in the crooks of the arms, on the elbows, on the buttocks, and on the ankles and feet. Other regions of the body may also show symptoms, although the palms and soles, upper back, neck, face, and scalp are usually not affected in adults.

> An itchy rash on the genitals and wrists and in the webs of the fingers is typical of scabies.

Most people who have a scabies infection develop the rash on the hands and wrists, and this is usually the first place where symptoms are seen. The itching is usually worse at night and after a shower. There is also a variant of the infection called "Norwegian scabies," which consists of a similar distribution of the rash but with much more scaling over the rash.

Children often have less characteristic rashes, making scabies in a child more difficult to diagnose. They can have rashes on the scalp, palms, and soles, and they often also have secondary bacterial infection, which may make some of the bumps look like tiny pimples.

If a person is either taking oral steroids for a medical condition such as asthma or using a topical steroid cream on the rash, then the lesions may be harder to recognize. Steroids suppress the immune system, and since the symptoms of scabies result primarily from the body's immune response to the infection, they may be somewhat lessened.

HOW IS SCABIES TRANSMITTED?

Transmission occurs through skin-to-skin contact with an infected person, either sexual or nonsexual, or through contact with bedding or clothing that has been in contact with an infected person. The infection is usually not transmitted through casual contact, for example in a workplace.

In adults, scabies is usually transmitted by sexual contact with an infected partner, but intercourse is not necessary to transmit scabies sexually. Children transmit scabies to one another through close physical contact. Multiple members of the same family frequently become infected, often through contact with the clothing or bedding of an infected person. Outbreaks sometimes occur in hospitals and nursing homes.

There is another type of scabies mite that can be transmitted from animals to humans, particularly from dogs. Outbreaks are not uncommon among entire families in which there is an infected dog. This scabies mite is different from the human scabies mite but can still cause infection in humans, as well as symptoms similar to those previously described. The human scabies mite does not infect animals, however, and the animal scabies mite cannot be transmitted from one person to another. The infection caused by the animal scabies mite resolves on its own without treatment.

TESTING FOR SCABIES

Scabies is usually not difficult to diagnose when the rash and symptoms are typical, although the rash may be confused with other skin problems that cause rashes. For this reason it is useful to perform a test to help with the diagnosis. Scrapings of the lesions may show evidence of the burrowing mites or the feces of the mites under the microscope.

TREATMENT

Scabies is treated by applying permethrin cream from the neck down at night and washing it off in the morning (after eight to fourteen hours). This procedure kills the mites. An alternative is a pill called ivermectin, which is taken twice, at the time of diagnosis and then two weeks later; ivermectin should be avoided for women who are pregnant or breastfeeding and for small children. Lindane lotion or cream is an alternative, but it is not recommended as first-line treatment because it can cause seizures and a serious blood disorder called "aplastic anemia." Lindane should be avoided in people with an extensive rash from scabies or other skin problems, since this increases the likelihood of seizures. Also, some resistance of scabies to lindane has been reported. Sexual partners and close household contacts should also be treated, even if they do not have symptoms. People who do not have body contact or share clothing or bedding with the infected person do not need to be treated.

> There are several topical creams to treat scabies, which are easy to use and inexpensive.

The itching may persist for a week or two after treatment. Medications that relieve itching, such as diphenhydramine, are available without prescription. If new skin rashes are seen after treatment, then the treatment may not have been successful and another application may be necessary. Frequent reapplication of the medications can be irritating to the skin, however, and it may cause a rash that can be misinterpreted as being caused by persistent scabies. If the symptoms persist longer than a few weeks after treatment, then a return visit to a health care provider is a good idea.

The nodules that sometimes occur with scabies may take longer to disappear than the rash and itching—sometimes several months. Injection of steroids into the lesions or the use of a topical steroid cream for a short period of time may help to speed resolution. These treatments can be administered by your health care provider.

Just as important as treatment with medication is treatment of clothes and bedding that have been in contact with an infected person within the last seventy-two hours. They should be laundered in hot water and dried on a hot cycle, dry cleaned, or kept out of contact for more than seventy-two hours, after which time the mites will have died of starvation. Furniture and pets do not need to be treated.

Norwegian scabies (also called "crusted scabies") is much more difficult to treat and may require more than one treatment. It is more common among people with a compromised immune system, such as people with cancer or HIV. Lindane should be avoided for treatment of this type of scabies because, given the extensive skin rash, it could cause toxicity. A dermatologist or infectious disease specialist should be consulted to help with the treatment of Norwegian scabies.

SYPHILIS

incidence: common
cause: bacterium (*Treponema pallidum*)
symptoms: painless ulcer with primary syphilis; rash, lymph node swelling, and hair loss with secondary syphilis; heart and neurological problems in later stages
treatment: antibiotics

WHAT IS IT?

Syphilis is an infection caused by the bacterium *Treponema pallidum*, which can be transmitted through sexual contact or from mother to child during pregnancy. This bacterium can infect many different organ systems and cause a full range of symptoms. Although antibiotics effectively treat syphilis, the disease is still a major health problem, and epidemics of syphilis still occur in some areas of the United States.

HOW COMMON IS IT?

More than 50,000 people are diagnosed with syphilis each year in the United States. The number of people infected with syphilis in this country reached a peak in the late 1940s, but with the discovery of penicillin, which was the first successful treatment for syphilis, the number began declining. In the late 1970s and early 1980s there was a resurgence of the disease in men who had sex with other men. However, with increased awareness of HIV and the importance of safer sex practices among this group, heterosexuals became the primary reservoir for infection. More recently there has again been a resurgence in men who have sex with other men.

As the incidence of syphilis among heterosexuals rises, however, more infected children are being born to mothers with syphilis. Infection of a newborn can cause devastating, lifelong problems. Syphilis screening is routine for women who obtain prenatal care in the United States. But many women for various reasons do not seek health care during pregnancy, or are excluded from it, and sexually transmitted diseases, including syphilis, are therefore not detected.

Recently there have been epidemics of syphilis in certain areas of the country, particularly in the South and coastal urban areas, despite an overall decline in the past few years in the number of people infected. In other areas of the world, such as Africa and Southeast Asia, the rates of infection are much higher. People infected with syphilis in the United States are more often those who are poor, those who use drugs, and those who engage in sex in exchange for drugs and therefore do not have access to, or seek, medical care. Syphilis is more common in HIV-positive people than in non-HIV-positive populations; a person with syphilis lesions is more susceptible to becoming infected with HIV, because open sores in the skin make transmission more likely.

WHAT ARE THE SYMPTOMS?

The symptoms of syphilis are numerous and varied. Many organ systems can be affected. People who have compromised immune systems, such as those with AIDS, may have a more aggressive course of infection and less typical symptoms.

Syphilis is divided into early and late stages of infection. Early infection is further subdivided into primary syphilis, secondary syphilis, and early latent syphilis. Late infection is also subdivided, into late latent syphilis, tertiary syphilis, and neurosyphilis. How long the infection has been present and the nature of the symptoms determine the stage of infection, what type of treatment is necessary, and how long it must be administered.

After infection with syphilis, symptoms of *primary syphilis* can take between ten and ninety days to appear, with the average interval being around three weeks. The first symptom is an ulcer, called a *chancre*, which is usually painless. There is usually only one chancre, which occurs at the site where infection took place. This can be on any area of the skin or on any mucous membrane. Rarely, the lesion is slightly painful, especially if there is a secondary infection with skin bacteria. (Other STDs that can cause similar symptoms are herpes, chancroid, and granuloma inguinale; see "Testing for Syphilis" below for a discussion of how the diagnosis of syphilis is confirmed.)

A swab taken from the chancre is usually seen to contain the syphilis-causing bacterium, *Treponema pallidum*, when examined under the microscope. There is usually a nonpainful swelling of the lymph nodes in the area of the infection. Often the infected person does not realize that he or she is infected, especially since a painless lesion is easy to miss, particularly if it is in the vagina or on the cervix for a woman or in the urethra for a man. The lesion usually disappears on its own after a few weeks without treatment.

If a person is not diagnosed and treated at this point, symptoms of *secondary syphilis* can appear several months later. This stage occurs when the syphilis-causing bacterium enters the bloodstream from the lesion. It can "seed" any organ and cause a variety of symptoms:

—A red, flat, nonitching rash over the whole body, including the palms and soles
— Swelling of the lymph nodes throughout the body
— Fever
— Sore throat
— Joint aches
— Headaches
— Patchy hair loss
— Wart-like lesions in the genital area that are not warts but manifestations of secondary syphilis

There can also be painless lesions on the mucous membranes and neurological changes, among other symptoms. People with secondary syphilis may also feel like they have the flu, and in fact these symptoms are so vague

> Syphilis is called the "great mimic" because its symptoms can imitate those of other diseases.

that they can easily be mistaken for other medical problems. All of these symptoms will eventually resolve without causing further problems, but this does not mean that the infection has gone away.

During both the primary and secondary stages of syphilis, a person is very infectious to partners. As can be imagined, both phases of the infection are often missed, either because the initial lesion is not noticed or because the symptoms are thought to have another cause, since they are so vague. In addition, since both of these phases are transient, people may think the problem has gone away when the symptoms resolve, but this is not the case. People with infection persisting beyond this point can live for many years, often decades, without experiencing further symptoms. Infection may be detected only through routine blood testing, and it is then called *latent syphilis*. People are still potentially infectious during this time, especially soon after resolution of the secondary syphilis stage.

The syphilis-causing bacterium can cause destruction of internal organs, a stage known as *tertiary syphilis* or *late syphilis*. This stage is rarely seen today, since the discovery of antibiotics has made syphilis so treatable, but virtually any organ system—such as the bones, liver, eyes, skin, and heart—can be damaged. If infection progresses to the brain, it is called *neurosyphilis*. In these stages the infection can be life threatening.

Infected newborns may have no symptoms, or the symptoms may be severe enough to cause brain damage and death. At birth, a child who is infected may not have a positive blood test, because the disease may take several weeks to show up on blood tests; for this reason, children born to high-risk mothers must have follow-up tests performed a few weeks after birth. Symptoms in infected newborns include brain damage, bone deformities, dental malformations, hearing loss, and rash. Women who are pregnant and are infected with syphilis have a higher risk of miscarriage: only 20 percent of women with syphilis will carry a fetus to term and deliver a normal, healthy baby. In the United States and in many other parts of the world, testing for syphilis is a routine part of prenatal health care.

HOW IS SYPHILIS TRANSMITTED?

Syphilis is transmitted through sexual or other intimate contact with an infected person, or from mother to unborn child. The chancres or sores of primary syphilis and the rashes and skin lesions of secondary syphilis are very infectious, so people with syphilis are most infectious during the primary and secondary stages of the infection, although the disease can be transmitted during certain later stages as well. The blood, semen, and vaginal secretions of an infected person may also be infectious.

> **Syphilis can be transmitted through sexual or other intimate contact, or from mother to child.**

Not only oral, anal, or genital sexual contact but even touching infected areas can result in transmission. People can transmit syphilis even if they are not symptomatic. Common routes through which the bacterium may enter the person being infected include breaks in the skin (which may be so tiny that they are invisible to the naked eye) or contact with mucous membranes.

TESTING FOR SYPHILIS

There are two ways in which syphilis is routinely diagnosed: (1) microscopic identification of the bacterium *Treponema pallidum* from swabs taken from the lesions and (2) identification of the body's immune response to the infection through blood tests. Lesions that are moist, such as the chancres or skin lesions seen in secondary syphilis, can be swabbed and examined under a special microscope for the syphilis-causing bacterium. However, most clinics do not have the ability to perform this test or do not have clinicians who are expert at looking for the syphilis-causing bacterium in this way.

> **Testing for syphilis involves either examining swabs taken from lesions for the syphilis-causing bacterium or performing blood tests to detect the body's immune response to the disease.**

The syphilis blood tests are designed to detect antibodies, which are proteins that the body makes in response to syphilis infection. The most common of these tests are the VDRL (Venereal Disease Research Laboratory) and RPR (rapid plasma reagin) tests. An infected person may take up to three months after infection to show a positive test result, although most people do so within a few weeks of infection. These tests first show up as positive during primary syphilis, and they will remain positive (usually reaching a peak during secondary syphilis) unless a person receives treatment. If a person is successfully treated for syphilis, the tests will usually return to normal about twelve months after treatment. Thus, these two tests can be used to determine whether or not a given treatment for syphilis is effective.

A small percentage of the population (1–2%) will test positive on the VDRL and RPR tests even though they are not infected with syphilis. These false positive results are more common in pregnant women and in those who have an underlying medical problem (such as lupus) or another infection (such as tuberculosis).

If a person tests positive, then standard practice calls for a second test to be performed to determine whether he or she is really infected with syphilis. This second test, called the treponemal antibody test or fluorescent treponemal antibody absorbed test (FTA-ABS), is very specific for syphilis and detects different antibodies than the tests described earlier. This test occasionally also shows a positive result for a person who is not infected with syphilis, but this is rare. Once a person has a positive FTA-ABS test due to infection with syphilis, this test usually does not revert to normal (although the likelihood of doing so is higher if syphilis is treated in the primary stage), even after successful treatment; it is therefore not a good test for monitoring whether or not treatment has been successful.

These tests can also be performed on body fluids other than blood, such as fluid from the spinal canal to determine whether the infection is affecting the neurological system (neurosyphilis).

If all the tests for syphilis are negative and the disease is still suspected, a blood test is usually repeated at about three months from the suspected date of infection; as already noted, it may take up to three months after infection to show a positive blood test. These tests are complex and require interpretation by a health care provider.

Partners of people diagnosed with syphilis should seek testing and treatment from their health care provider. People who have had sex with an infected person within ninety days of that person being diagnosed (regardless of the stage) should be treated, whether or not they have symptoms. Long-term partners of people with syphilis that is diagnosed in the late stages should be evaluated and treated, with treatment depending on the stage of their syphilis infection. People diagnosed with syphilis should be tested for other STDs as well, including

HIV. Infants with syphilis are tested in the same way as adults. Syphilis is reportable to the health department in most states, and there are anonymous partner notification programs so that persons who may have been infected can be called in for treatment.

TREATMENT

The best treatment for syphilis is still one of the oldest antibiotics: penicillin. For the treatment of syphilis, penicillin must be given as an injection, not as an oral dose. The dosage and duration of treatment depend on the stage of the infection. For primary, secondary, and early latent syphilis, a single dose of penicillin usually eliminates the infection. Some people develop fever, chills, muscle aches, headache, and a worsening of the chancre or rash about eight hours after the shot; this reaction, called the *Jarisch-Herxheimer reaction*, is probably due to the rapid killing of the bacteria. It is temporary, usually resolving within twenty-four hours, and it does not lead to permanent problems. It is not an allergic reaction to penicillin. It usually occurs in people who have early infection with syphilis.

For a person who has late latent syphilis or syphilis of unknown duration, injections are given weekly for three consecutive weeks. A person who develops neurosyphilis must be hospitalized and receive intravenous penicillin for ten to fourteen days.

To determine whether treatment has been successful, follow-up visits for a VDRL or RPR test are essential. If the treatment was successful, then the test result will be lower than it was previously. If treatment has not been successful, this may be because the infection has involved the nervous system or the person has been reinfected. As already indicated, neurosyphilis is treatable but requires a longer course of therapy as well as hospitalization for the administration of intravenous antibiotics.

> Follow-up is essential to ensure that the infection is being treated successfully. The VDRL and RPR blood tests are used for this purpose. A health care provider will recommend a schedule of follow-up visits based on the specific stage of infection.

People who are allergic to penicillin can be treated with other medications, such as doxycycline and tetracycline, if they have primary or secondary syphilis. However, for pregnant women the only recommended regimen is penicillin. The treatment may not be as effective in people infected with HIV as in those not infected, and for this reason close monitoring and follow-up testing are essential in HIV-positive persons. An HIV specialist should be consulted in these cases.

TRICHOMONIASIS

incidence: very common
cause: protozoa (*Trichomonas vaginalis*)
symptoms: genital itching, redness, discharge; often none in men
treatment: antibiotics

WHAT IS IT?

Trichomoniasis ("trich") is an infection caused by a protozoan organism called *Trichomonas vaginalis*. It is a common sexually transmitted infection.

HOW COMMON IS IT?

Trichomoniasis is probably the most common sexually transmitted infection in the world. Each year, about five million women are diagnosed with the infection in the United States alone. A similar number of men are probably infected, but the statistics are available only for women, since it is they who usually have symptoms and seek health care.

> **Approximately three million women are infected with trichomoniasis each year in the United States.**

Who is at highest risk? People are more likely to be infected if they have unprotected sex with multiple partners. The more sexual partners a person has, the higher the likelihood that he or she will become infected with trichomonas. In one study, trichomonas infection was found in about 5 percent of women on routine gynecological visits, in about 13–25 percent of women attending sexually transmitted disease clinics, and in 50–75 percent of prostitutes.

WHAT ARE THE SYMPTOMS?

Trichomonas infections occur exclusively in the genital area. They do not occur in the mouth or anal area. In women, the symptoms of trichomoniasis include a yellow-green, frothy discharge in the vagina; vaginal and labial itching, irritation, and redness; and a fishy odor from the vagina. Because of the irritation, intercourse may be painful. Lymph node swelling in the groin may also occur. Some women have only a discharge, without all the other symptoms of irritation. Some experience burning with urination, because they have an infection in the urethra as well as in the vagina. Others experience pain in the abdomen, although we don't know why, because the infection is located exclusively in the vagina and not higher up.

Women who have trichomoniasis usually have symptoms, although about 5 percent of infected women are symptom free. Symptoms usually show up about a week or two after infection but may take longer. Approximately one-third of women who are infected and do not initially have symptoms will develop symptoms within six months or so after infection. Why some women develop symptoms and others don't is not clear.

Recently a link has been established between trichomonas infection and problems in pregnancy. Pregnant women with trichomoniasis have a higher incidence of premature rupture of membranes and premature delivery of the infant. Vaginal infection with trichomonas can also be passed to the newborn during delivery, causing either genital or lung infection in the child.

Trichomonas infection can cause premature delivery and premature rupture of membranes as well as infection in the newborn.

Men usually do not experience any symptoms of trichomonas infection, although a few men have symptoms of urethritis (urethral infection), such as burning with urination, discharge, or simply a sensation of irritation in the penis. (See the section on nongonococcal urethritis.) If left untreated, trichomonas has been shown to cause scarring (called strictures) in the urethra, which may impair the flow of urine.

HOW IS IT TRANSMITTED?

Trichomonas infection is acquired through sexual contact with a partner who is infected, most often through heterosexual (vagina-penis) contact, but women who have sex with other women can transfer the infection through the use of sex toys. The throat and the anal or rectal area are not sites of infection, so the infection is not transmitted through oral sex or anal intercourse. Although trichomonas can exist for several hours in body fluids outside the body, and therefore the possibility exists that transmission may take place by nonsexual means, there are no documented cases of transmission by toilet seats or towels. Once genital secretions dry, they are not infectious to others.

> Trichomoniasis is transmitted through sexual contact and from an infected mother to her newborn child during delivery.

Having unprotected vaginal intercourse with a partner who is infected can transmit trichomoniasis, even if the infected partner does not have any symptoms. Using condoms correctly and consistently helps prevent transmission.

> Condoms, if used correctly, help prevent transmission of trichomonas infection.

For women who have sex with other women, vaginal fluid exchange can lead to infection. Testing prior to sexual contact, the use of condoms on sex toys for each partner, or not sharing sex toys at all can decrease the risk of infection.

TESTING FOR TRICHOMONIASIS

For women, a pelvic examination is necessary to test for trichomonas infection, both to detect the signs of the infection and to gather samples for examination. Often, there is redness of the labia and vagina, and frothy, bad-smelling yellow-green discharge in the vagina. The discharge has a higher pH than the normal, more acidic, vaginal secretions. The outer part of the cervix (ectocervix) may be red and irritated, with tiny red dots; these are small hemorrhages, and the condition is called "strawberry cervix."

When the discharge is examined under the microscope, the individual trichomonas organisms can be seen. Often, bacterial vaginosis occurs with trichomoniasis, and this can be seen under the microscope as well. The protozoans move in a characteristic way that is apparent under the microscope, so microscopic examination is the oldest and still the most common method to evaluate for trichomonas infection; it may miss infection in about 30–40 percent of cases, however.

> Diagnosis can usually be made in women by examining vaginal secretions. Cultures may be necessary to make the diagnosis.

There are also tests that can detect trichomonas in vaginal secretions by looking for the genetic material of the trichomonas organism, and these tests can be done in the health care provider's office. If there is still concern, the health care provider may send a specimen of vaginal secretion for culture, which is the most sensitive test available.

Trichomoniasis is harder to diagnose in men than in women. Cultures can be taken from the urethra, urine, or semen to make the diagnosis, although this approach may not reveal trichomonas, even in men who have the infection. The only evidence may be white blood cells from a urethral swab test seen under the microscope (see the section on nongonococcal urethritis). Trichomonas infection is estimated to cause between 2 and 5 percent of cases of nongonococcal urethritis in men in the United States. Men most often seek treatment for trichomonas infection because their partners have been diagnosed with trichomoniasis rather than as a result of symptoms they have noticed in themselves.

TREATMENT

Two medications have been found to be effective for treating trichomoniasis in men and women, and both can be taken as a single dose by mouth: metronidazole and tinidazole. Although metronidazole is also available as a cream, *only the pill form is effective for trichomoniasis.* The cream form does not treat the infection in the urethra and genital glands; therefore, even though the symptoms disappear, recurrence is common.

> Oral antibiotics are about 95 percent effective in treating trichomoniasis.

If symptoms persist after treatment, a follow-up examination is recommended, since no treatment is 100 percent effective and infection may persist. The sexual contacts over the past two months of anyone who has been diagnosed with trichomonas infection must also be treated.

When these medications do not work, an additional course of antibiotics is necessary. Sometimes trichomonas can be difficult to eradicate, and the health care provider may refer a patient to a specialist. Those being treated for trichomoniasis should not have sexual contact until they and their partners have been treated, have taken all their medication, and have achieved complete resolution of their symptoms.

A word about metronidazole and tinidazole and their side effects: these medications should not be taken with alcohol, since the combination can cause violent nausea and vomiting. Furthermore, you should not drink alcohol for twenty-four hours after stopping the metronidazole or for seventy-two hours after stopping the tinidazole.

Trichomonas infection can pose a risk to the unborn child, as noted above. However, there is a debate on whether or not treatment of the infection during pregnancy helps decrease this risk. Tinidazole is not recommended for use in pregnancy; the evidence suggests that metronidazole may be safe. Pregnant women should discuss the risks and benefits of treatment with their health care provider.

A P P E N D I X

R E S O U R C E S

ADDITIONAL INFORMATION ON STDs AND HIV/AIDS

AIDS Hotline
www.aidshotline.org
Provides information on AIDS and STDs and on state AIDS hotlines.

American Social Health Association
www.ashastd.org
National STI Hotline: 919-361-8488, Monday through Friday,
9:00 A.M. to 6:00 P.M. EST
Call hotline to ask questions about STIs.
For prerecorded information on STIs and testing: 919-361-4848

Centers for Disease Control and Prevention
www.cdc.gov/std
STD Hotline and HIV/AIDS Hotline: 1-800-232-4636
Traveler's Health Hotline: 1-877-394-8747

Herpes
Herpes Resource Center (American Social Health Association)
www.ashastd.org
Provides up-to-date information on herpes blood testing,
location of herpes support groups, online chat room on herpes,
and excellent literature about herpes and other STDs.

Home Access Health Corporation

www.homeaccess.com

Provides information on the company's FDA-approved at-home testing kit for HIV (also an at-home testing kit for hepatitis C).

HPV

National HPV and Cervical Cancer Prevention Resource Center

www.ashastd.org

Provides up-to-date information on HPV and cervical cancer screening, location of HPV support groups, online chat room on HPV, and excellent literature about HPV and other STDs.

Planned Parenthood

www.plannedparenthood.org

To find a Planned Parenthood Health Center in your area, call 1-800-230-PLAN

Recurrent Laryngeal Papillomatosis Foundation

www.rrpf.org

Provides regional contact information.

Abortion: The loss of a pregnancy; an abortion can be spontaneous (a miscarriage) or induced.

Abstinence: The act of voluntarily doing without something, such as sex.

Acquired immunodeficiency syndrome (AIDS): A condition caused by the human immunodeficiency virus (HIV), in which the immune system is damaged and a person becomes susceptible to various infections and malignancies.

Analingus: Oral-anal sexual contact; also known as rimming.

Anoscopy: A procedure in which a scope is used to look into the anus, to examine the mucous membranes and help diagnose infection.

Antibiotic: A medicine used to treat a bacterial infection.

Antibody: A protein produced by the immune system to help fight off infection; antibodies are made in response to antigens.

Antifungal: A medicine used to treat a fungal infection.

Antigen: A protein on the surface of an organism that stimulates an immune response (the production of antibodies).

Antiretroviral: A medicine used to treat a retroviral infection, such as that caused by HIV.

Antiviral: A medicine used to treat a viral infection, such as herpes.

Aphthous ulcer: A small, painful ulcer inside the mouth, which is not caused by herpes.

Arthritis: Inflammation of a joint or joints: one of the symptoms of Reiter's syndrome.

Asymptomatic: Without symptoms.

Autoinoculation: Infection of oneself.

Bacterium: A microscopic single-celled organism; some bacteria (such as gonorrhea and chlamydia) can cause infection whereas others (such as *Lactobacillus* in the vagina of a woman) do not cause disease and are important for the health of humans.

Barrier method: A method of birth control and STD protection that provides an impenetrable barrier (such as a latex condom) between sexual partners.

Benign: Not serious.

Bisexual: Describing a person who has sex with partners of the same sex and of the opposite sex.

Carrier: A person who has an infection and can pass that infection to others, but who may be symptom free him- or herself, such as a carrier of hepatitis B.

Celibacy: The state of abstaining from sexual intercourse.

Cervicitis: Inflammation and/or infection of the cervix.

Chancre: A painless ulcer seen in primary syphilis.

Chronic: Lasting a long time.

Colonoscopy: A procedure that consists of inserting a flexible tube into the rectum to visualize the entire colon.

Conjunctivitis: Irritation and inflammation of the conjunctiva, which is the mucous membrane covering the inner surface of the eyelids.

Culture: A laboratory test in which an organism is grown to help diagnose the cause of an infection.

Cunnilingus: Oral-genital sexual contact on a female.

Discharge: In this book an abnormal fluid produced from an opening, such as the cervix, rectal area, or penis.

Douching: Application of a stream of fluid (douche) to wash an area (such as the vagina or rectum); douching is not recommended because it can promote infection.

Dysplasia: The appearance of abnormal cells; a precursor to cancer.

Dysuria: Burning with urination.

Ectopic pregnancy: A pregnancy in which the fertilized egg implants outside the uterus, such as in a Fallopian tube; some sexually transmitted infections, such as chlamydia, increase the likelihood of an ectopic pregnancy; also known as a *tubal pregnancy*.

Elephantiasis: The enlargement of parts of the body and hardening of the skin on those parts; elephantiasis can occur if blood or lymph drainage from the area is impaired, such as from scarring.

Endometriosis: The implanting of endometrial tissue (the lining of the uterus) in areas outside the uterus.

Endometrium: The lining of the uterus.

Epididymitis: Infection and inflammation of the epididymis, a structure that sits above each testicle in the scrotum.

Episodic: In this book, describing a symptom that comes and goes.

Fellatio: Oral-genital contact on a man.

Fungus: Yeast; an organism that lives off other organisms.

Groin: The area between the top of the leg and the lower abdomen.

Herpes simplex virus (HSV): The virus that causes herpes; there are two types, herpes simplex 1 and herpes simplex 2.

Heterosexual: A person who has sex with partners of the opposite sex.

Homosexual: A person who has sex with partners of the same sex.

Human immunodeficiency virus (HIV): The virus that causes acquired immunodeficiency syndrome (AIDS).

Human papillomavirus (HPV): The virus that causes genital warts.

Immune system: The complex system with which the body fights off disease.

Immunocompromised: Describing a person whose immune system is not functioning properly, thus making him or her more vulnerable to disease.

Infertility: The inability to have children.

Inflammation: Redness, swelling, and warmth in a tissue of the body, which can result from infection or injury.

Injection drug users: People who inject drugs into their bodies.

Intercourse: Sexual coupling; the term is usually interpreted to include oral, genital, or anal sex.

Intrauterine device (IUD): A device that is inserted into the uterus for contraception.

Intravenous: Occurring in the veins.

Jaundice: Yellowing of the skin and eyes, as may be seen with hepatitis.

Lesion: In this book, any kind of abnormality on the skin, such as redness, a bump, or a break in the skin.

Lymph node: A part of the immune system; lymph nodes are made up of small groups of cells of the immune system located in clusters around the body, such as in the armpits or in the groin; they can enlarge as a result of infection or malignancy.

Malignancy: A disease state in which cells of the body grow in an unregulated manner and can spread to other areas of the body (metastasize).

Menstruation: A period; the flow of blood from the uterus, which occurs monthly in most women if no fertilized egg implants in the uterus, as the endometrium is shed.

Mucopurulent: Characterized by a combination of mucus and pus, as in mucopurulent cervicitis.

Mucopurulent cervicitis (MPC): A sexually transmitted infection of the cervix.

Mucous membranes: The thin, delicate, mucus-secreting linings of various anatomical structures, such as the genitals, mouth, and eyes.

Nongonococcal urethritis (NGU): A sexually transmitted urethral infection that is not gonorrhea; it is also known as nonspecific urethritis (NSU).

Organism: An individual animal, plant, bacterium, or protozoan.

Outercourse: Sexual contact (such as sensual massage) that does not include the exchange of body fluids.

Pap smear: A procedure in which the cells of the cervix are examined to look for cancerous changes; a screen for cervical cancer.

Papule: A bump.

Pathogen: Anything that causes disease.

Pelvic inflammatory disease (PID): An infection of the uterus, Fallopian tubes, and/or ovaries in women.

Prodrome: A set of symptoms indicating the onset of disease (e.g., in herpes, tingling or itching in the genital area may indicate a herpes outbreak is about to occur).

Prophylactic: Anything used to prevent the acquisition of a disease; a prophylactic can be a medicine or a device (such as a condom).

Protozoan: A microscopic organism, such as trichomonas.

Pus: A collection of white blood cells and dead cells at the site of an inflammation.

Rash: An eruption of spots, splotches, or patches on the skin.

Reiter's syndrome: A disorder of the immune system that can follow infection with chlamydia as well as other infections; Reiter's syndrome is characterized by urethritis, arthritis, and conjunctivitis, as well as other symptoms.

Retrovirus: A specific type of virus: HIV is a retrovirus.

Rimming: Analingus; oral-anal sexual contact.

Safer sex: A set of practices that help reduce the risk of STD transmission between partners.

Screen: To test for evidence of an infection or condition.

Semen: The milky fluid ejaculated during an orgasm in a man; it contains fluids from the prostate, seminal vesicles, and testicles as well as sperm.

Sensitivity: A measure of how often a test will detect a person who is truly infected; for example, a test that has a 99 percent sensitivity will detect 99 out of 100 people who have the infection.

Sexually transmitted disease (STD): A disease that is transmitted through sexual contact; often also called a *sexually transmitted infection (STI)*. (Formerly called *venereal disease*.)

Sigmoidoscopy: A procedure that consists of inserting a small flexible tube into the rectum to visualize the lower colon.

Specificity: A measure of how specific a test is; for example, on a test that has a 99 percent specificity, 99 people out of 100 who do not have the disease will test negative (in other words, one person will have a false positive result).

Speculum: A plastic or metal device used to look inside the vagina of a woman during a pelvic examination.

Spermicide: A substance that kills sperm.

Torsion of the testicle: A medical emergency in which the blood vessels to the testicle are twisted; torsion can lead to the death of the testicle if not repaired quickly.

Tubal pregnancy: A pregnancy in which the fertilized egg implants in a Fallopian tube or another area outside the uterus; some sexually transmitted infections, such as chlamydia, increase the likelihood of a tubal pregnancy; also known as an *ectopic pregnancy.*

Ulcer: An open sore.

Urethritis: Inflammation of the urethra, often caused by infection.

Virus: A microscopic agent that can cause infection but can survive only in connection with living cells; examples are the herpes simplex virus and the human papillomavirus.

White blood cells: Cells in the body that are part of the immune system and that help the body to fight infection; when they collect at the site of an inflammation, along with dead cells, they are known as *pus.*

R E F E R E N C E S

PART I

Ament, L. A., and Whalen, E. Sexually transmitted diseases in pregnancy: diagnosis, impact, and intervention. *J Obstet Gynecol Neonatal Nurs* 25:657, 1996.

Bailey, J. V., et al. Sexually transmitted infections in women who have sex with women. *Sex Transm Infect* 80:244, 2004.

Berger, B. J., et al. Bacterial vaginosis in lesbians: a sexually transmitted disease. *Clin Infect Dis* 21:1402, 1995.

Centers for Disease Control. *HIV Infection and AIDS: Are You at Risk?* [consumer pamphlet]. Atlanta: Department of Health and Human Services, 1994.

Centers for Disease Control. Increases in fluoroquinolone-resistant Neisseria gonorrhoeae among men who have sex with men—United States, 2003, and revised recommendations for gonorrhea treatment, 2004.

Centers for Disease Control. *Sexually Transmitted Disease Surveillance, 2004.* Atlanta: Department of Health and Human Services, National Center for HIV, STD, and TB Prevention, 2005.

Centers for Disease Control. Sexually transmitted diseases treatment guidelines, 2002. *MMWR* 51(RR-6), 2002.

Centers for Disease Control. Sexually transmitted diseases treatment guidelines, 2006. *MMWR* 55(RR-11), 2006.

Chesson, W., et al. The estimated direct medical cost of sexually transmitted diseases among American youth, 2000. *Perspect Sex Reprod Health* 36:11, 2004.

Chu, S. Y., et al. Epidemiology of reported cases of AIDS in lesbians: United States 1980–1989. *Am J Public Health* 80:1380, 1990.

Condoms, Contraceptives and STDs: Does Your Birth Control Method Protect You from Sexually Transmitted Disease? [consumer pamphlet]. Research Triangle Park, N.C.: American Social Health Association, 1994.

Condoms in the Prevention of Sexually Transmitted Diseases: The Proceedings of a Conference. Research Triangle Park, N.C.: American Social Health Association, 1997.

Diamant, A. L., et al. Lesbians' sexual history with men: implications for taking a sexual history. *Arch Intern Med* 159:2730, 1999.

Drew, W. L., et al. Evaluation of the virus permeability of a new condom for women. *Sex Transm Dis* 17:110, 1990.

Ferris, D., et al. A neglected lesbian health concern: cervical neoplasia. *J. Fam Pract* 43:581, 1996.

Fethers, K., et al. Sexually transmitted infections and risk behaviours in women who have sex with women. *Sex Transm Infect* 76:345, 2000.

Finding the Words: How to Communicate about Sexual Health [consumer pamphlet]. Research Triangle Park, N.C.: American Social Health Association, 1994.

Handsfield, H. H. *Color Atlas and Synopsis of Sexually Transmitted Diseases,* 2nd ed. New York: McGraw-Hill, 2000.

Holmes, K. K., ed. *Sexually Transmitted Diseases,* 3rd ed. New York: McGraw-Hill, 2006.

Holmes, K. K., et al. Effectiveness of condoms in preventing sexually transmitted infections. *Bull World Health Organ* 82:454, 2004.

How reliable are condoms? Reprint from *Consumer Reports.* Yonkers, N.Y.: Consumers Union of the United States.

How to Use a Condom [consumer pamphlet]. Eatontown, N.J.: Ansell Inc., Medical Products Division.

Long, G. E., and Rickman, L. S. Infectious complications of tattoos. *Clin Infect Dis* 18:610, 1994.

Marrazzo, J. M., et al. Characterization of vaginal flora and bacterial vaginosis in women who have sex with women. *J Infect Dis* 185:1307, 2002.

Marrazzo, J. M., et al. Papanicolaou test screening and prevalence of genital human papillomavirus among women who have sex with women. *Am J Public Health* 91:947, 2001.

Marx, R., et al. Crack, sex and STDs. *Sex Transm Dis* 18:92, 1991.

Ness, R. B., et al. Condom use and the risk of recurrent pelvic inflammatory disease, chronic pelvic pain, or infertility following an episode of pelvic inflammatory disease. *Am J Public Health* 94:1327, 2004.

Richardson, B. A. Nonoxynol-9 as a vaginal microbicide for prevention of sexually transmitted infections. *JAMA* 287:1171, 2002.

STD News [quarterly newsletter published by the American Social Health Association, Research Triangle Park, N.C.], 1995–1998.

Stine, K. Lesbians and STDs. Lecture given at the Reproductive Health 1997 Conference, Portland, Oregon, March 1997.

Wechsler, H., et al. Health and behavioral consequences of binge drinking in college: a national survey of students at 140 campuses. *JAMA* 272:1672, 1994.

Wendel, P. J., and Wendel Jr., G. D. Sexually transmitted diseases in pregnancy. *Semin Perinatol* 17:443, 1993.

Wilkinson, D., et al. Nonoxynol-9 spermicide for prevention of vaginally acquired HIV and other sexually transmitted infections: systematic review and meta-analysis of randomised controlled trials including more than 5000 women. *Lancet* 2:613, 2002.

Winks, K., and Semans, A. *The Good Vibrations Guide to Sex*. Pittsburgh: Cleis Press, 1994.

PART II

The following references providing information about specific sexually transmitted diseases were used as general references in this part of the book.

Centers for Disease Control. Sexually transmitted diseases treatment guidelines, 2006. *MMWR* 55(RR-11), 2006.

Handsfield, H. H. *Color Atlas and Synopsis of Sexually Transmitted Diseases*, 2nd ed. New York: McGraw-Hill, 2000.

Holmes, K. K., ed. *Sexually Transmitted Diseases*, 3rd ed. New York: McGraw-Hill, 2006.

Bacterial Vaginosis

Berger, B. J., et al. Bacterial vaginosis in lesbians: a sexually transmitted disease. *Clin Infect Dis* 21:1402, 1995.

Berman, S. M., et al. Low birth weight, prematurity, and postpartum endometritis: association with prenatal cervical *Mycoplasma hominis* and *Chlamydia trachomatis* infection. *JAMA* 257:1189, 1987.

Burtin, P., et al. Safety of metronidazole in pregnancy: a meta-analysis. *Am J Obstet Gynecol* 172:525, 1995.

Caro-Paton, T., et al. Is metronidazole teratogenic? A meta-analysis. *Br J Clin Pharmacol* 44:179, 1997.

Eschenbach, D. A., et al. Diagnosis and clinical manifestation of bacterial vaginosis. *Am J Obstet Gynecol* 158:819, 1988.

Hauth, J. C., et al. Reduced incidence of preterm delivery with metronidazole and erythromycin in women with bacterial vaginosis. *N Engl J Med* 333:1732, 1995.

Hay, P., et al. Oral clindamycin prevents spontaneous preterm birth and mid trimester miscarriage in pregnant women with bacterial vaginosis. *Int J STD AIDS* 12(suppl 2): 70, 2001.

Hill, L.V.H., et al. Prevalence of lower genital tract infections in pregnancy. *Sex Transm Dis* 15:5, 1988.

Hillier, S. L., et al. Association between bacterial vaginosis and preterm delivery of a low-birth-weight infant. *N Engl J Med* 333:1737, 1995.

Holst, E., et al. Bacterial vaginosis: microbiological and clinical findings. *Eur J. Clin Microbiol* 6:536, 1987.

Jackson, P., et al. Single dose metronidazole prophylaxis in gynaecological surgery. *N Z Med J* 89:243, 1979.

Joesoef, M. R., et al. Intravaginal clindamycin treatment for bacterial vaginosis: effects on preterm delivery and low birth weight. *Am J Obstet Gynecol* 173:1527, 1995.

Kurki, T., et al. Bacterial vaginosis in early pregnancy and pregnancy outcomes. *Obstet Gynecol* 80:173, 1992.

Larrson, P. G., et al. Incidence of pelvic inflammatory disease after first trimester legal abortion in women with bacterial vaginosis after treatment with metronidazole: a double blind, randomized study. *Am J Obstet Gynecol* 166:100, 1992.

McGregor, J. A., et al., Bacterial vaginosis is associated with prematurity and vaginal fluid mucinase and sialidase: results of a controlled trial of topical clindamycin cream. *Am J Obstet Gynecol* 170:1048, 1994.

Morales, W. J., et al. Effect of metronidazole in patients with preterm birth in the preceding pregnancy and bacterial vaginosis: a placebo-controlled, double-blind study. *Am J Obstet Gynecol* 171:345, 1994.

Piper, J. M., et al. Prenatal use of metronidazole and birth defects: no association. *Obstet Gynecol* 82:348, 1993.

Vejtorp, M., et al. Bacterial vaginosis: a double blind randomized trial of the effect of treatment of the sexual partner. *Br J Obstet Gynaecol* 95:920, 1988.

Vermeulen, G. M., and Bruinse, H. W. Prophylactic administration of clindamycin 2% vaginal cream to reduce the incidence of spontaneous preterm birth in women with an increased recurrence risk: a randomised placebo-controlled double-blind trial. *Br J Obstet Gynaecol* 106:652, 1999.

Chancroid

Becker, T. M., et al. *Haemophilus ducreyi* infection in South Florida: a rare disease on the rise? *South Med J* 80:182, 1987.

Blackmore, C. A., et al. An outbreak of chancroid in Orange County, California: descriptive epidemiology and disease-control measures. *J Infect Dis* 151:840, 1985.

Bowmer, M. I., et al. Single-dose ceftriaxone for chancroid. *Antimicrob Agents Chemother* 31:67, 1987.

Boyd, A. S. Clinical efficacy of antimicrobial therapy in *Haemophilus ducreyi* infections. *Arch Dermatol* 125:1399, 1989.

Diaz-Mitoma, F., et al. Etiology of non-vesicular genital ulcers in Winnipeg. *Sex Transm Dis* 14:33, 1987.

Dickerson, M. C., et al. The causal role for genital ulcer disease as a risk factor for transmission of human immunodeficiency virus: an application of the Bradford Hill criteria. *Sex Transm Dis* 23:429, 1996.

Dylewski, J., et al. Laboratory diagnosis of *Haemophilus ducreyi*: sensitivity of culture media. *Diagn Microbiol Infect Dis* 4:241, 1986.

Fast, M. W., et al. Antimicrobial therapy of chancroid: an evaluation of five treatment regimens correlated with in vitro sensitivity. *Sex Transm Dis* 10:1, 1983.

Greenblatt, R. M., et al. Genital ulceration as a risk factor for human immunodeficiency virus infection *AIDS* 2:47, 1988.

Hammond, G. W., et al. Clinical, epidemiological, laboratory and therapeutic features of an urban outbreak of chancroid in North America. *Rev Infect Dis* 2:867, 1980.

Hansen, E. J., and Loftus, T. A. Monoclonal antibodies reactive with all strains of *Haemophilus ducreyi*. *Infect Immunol* 44:196, 1984.

Jones, C. C., et al. Cultural diagnosis of chancroid. *Arch Dermatol* 127: 1823, 1991.

Kunimoto, D. Y., et al. Urethral infection with *Haemophilus ducreyi* in men. *Sex Transm Dis* 15:37, 1988.

Martin, D. H., and DiCarlo, R. P. Recent changes in the epidemiology of genital ulcer disease in the United States: the crack cocaine connection. *Sex Transm Dis* 21(suppl 2):576, 1994.

Marx, R., et al. Crack, sex and STD's. *Sex Transm Dis* 18:92, 1991.

Museyi, K., et al. Use of an enzyme immunoassay to detect serum IgG antibodies to *Haemophilus ducreyi*. *J Infect Dis* 157:1039, 1988.

Plummer, F. A., et al. Antimicrobial therapy of chancroid: effectiveness of erythromycin. *J Infect Dis* 148:726, 1983.

Plummer, F. A., et al. Clinical and microbiologic studies of genital ulcers in Kenyan women. *Sex Transm Dis* 12:193, 1985.

Plummer, F. A., et al. Epidemiology of chancroid and *Haemophilus ducreyi* in Nairobi. *Lancet* 2:1293, 1983.

Sturm, A. W., and Zanen, H. C. Characteristics of *Haemophilus ducreyi* in culture. *J Clin Microbiol* 19:672, 1984.

Chlamydia Infection

Brunham, R. C., et al. Etiology and outcome of acute pelvic inflammatory disease. *J Infect Dis* 158:510, 1988.

Cates, W. Jr., and Wasserheit, J. N. Genital chlamydia infections: epidemiology and reproductive sequelae. *Am J Obstet Gynecol* 164:1771, 1991.

Centers for Disease Control. Screening tests to detect *Chlamydia trachomatis* and *Neisseria gonorrhoeae* infections, 2002. *MMWR* 51(RR-15), 2002.

Gravett, M. G., et al. Independent associations of bacterial vaginosis and chlamydia infections with adverse pregnancy outcome. *JAMA* 256:1899, 1986.

Hammersclag, M. R. *Chlamydia trachomatis* in children. *Pediatr Ann* 23:349, 1994.

Harrison, H. R., et al. Cervical *Chlamydia trachomatis* and mycoplasmal infections in pregnancy: epidemiology and outcomes. *JAMA* 250: 1721, 1983.

Harrison, H. R., et al. Cervical *Chlamydia trachomatis* infection in university women: relationship to history, contraception, ectopy and cervicitis. *Am J Obstet Gynecol* 153:244, 1985.

Kousa, M., et al. Frequent association of chlamydial infection with Reiter's syndrome. *Sex Transm Dis* 5:57, 1978.

LeBar, W. D. Keeping up with new technology: new approaches to diagnose chlamydia infection. *Clin Chem* 42:809, 1996.

Paavonen, J., et al. Prevalence and manifestations of endometritis among women with cervicitis. *Am J Obstet Gynecol* 152:280, 1985.

Schacter, J. Immunodiagnosis of sexually transmitted disease. *Yale J Biol Med* 58:443, 1985.

Stamm, W. E., et al. Asymptomatic *Chlamydia trachomatis* urethritis in men. *Sex Transm Dis* 13:163, 1986.

Stamm, W. E., et al. *Chlamydia trachomatis* urethral infections in men: prevalence, risk factors, and clinical manifestations. *Ann Intern Med* 100:47, 1984.

Weber, J. T., and Johnson, R. E. New treatments for chlamydia genital infections. *Clin Infect Dis* 20(suppl 1):566, 1995.

Weinstock, S., et al. *Chlamydia trachomatis* infection in women: a need for universal screening in high prevalence populations? *Am J Epidemiol* 135:41, 1992.

Donovanosis

Bowden, F. J., et al. Pilot study of azithromycin in the treatment of genital donovanosis. *Genitourin Med* 72:17, 1996.

De Boer, A., et al. Cytologic identification of Donovan bodies in granuloma inguinale. *Acta Cytol* 28:126, 1984.

Hoosen, A. A., et al. Granuloma inguinale in association with pregnancy and HIV infection. *Int J Gynecol Obstet* 53:133, 1996.

Mitchell, K. M., et al. Donovanosis in Western Australia. *Genitourin Med* 62:191, 1986.

O'Farrell, N. Global eradication of donovanosis: an opportunity for limiting the spread of HIV infection. *Genitourin Med* 71:27, 1995.

Rosen, T., et al. Granuloma inguinale. *J Am Acad Dermatol* 11:433, 1984.

Schneider, J., et al. Extragenital donovanosis: three cases from Western Australia. *Genitourin Med* 62:196, 1986.

Epididymitis

Barnes, R. C., et al. Urinary tract infections in sexually active homosexual men. *Lancet* 1:171, 1986.

Berger, R. E., et al. Etiology and manifestations of epididymitis in young men: correlations with sexual orientation. *J Infect Dis* 155:1341, 1987.

Docimo, S. G., et al. *Candida epididymitis:* newly recognized opportunistic epididymal infection. *Urology* 41:280, 1993.

Gisalson, T., et al. Acute epididymitis in boys: a five-year retrospective study. *J Urol* 124:533, 1980.

Krieger, J. N. New sexually transmitted diseases guidelines. *J Urol* 154:209, 1995.

Melekos, M. D., and Asbach, H. W. Epididymitis: aspects concerning etiology and treatment. *J Urol* 138:83, 1987.

Mulcahy, F. M., et al. Prevalence of chlamydial infection in acute epididymo-orchitis. *Genitourin Med* 63:16, 1987.

Perri, A. J., et al. The Doppler stethoscope and the diagnosis of the acute scrotum. *J Urol* 116:598, 1976.

Fungal (Yeast) Infections

Berg, A. O., et al. Establishing the cause of symptoms in women in a family practice. *JAMA* 251:620, 1984.

Bergman, J. J., et al. Clinical comparison of microscopic and culture techniques in the diagnosis of *Candida vaginitis*. *J Family Pract* 18:549, 1984.

Centers for Disease Control. Non-reported sexually transmitted diseases. *MMWR* 28:61, 1979.

Davidson, F., and Oates, J. K. The pill does not cause "thrush." *Br J Obstet Gynecol* 92:1265, 1985.

Fleury, F. J. Adult vaginitis. *Clin Obstet Gynecol* 24:407, 1981.

Fleury, F. J. Recurrent candida vulvovaginitis. *Chemotherapy* 28(suppl): 48, 1982.

Goode, M. A. Infectious vaginitis: selecting therapy and preventing recurrence. *Postgrad Med* 96:85, 1994.

Horowitz, B. J., et al. *Candida tropicalis* vulvovaginitis. *Obstet Gynecol* 66:229, 1985.

Loendersloot, E. W., et al. Efficacy and tolerability of single dose versus six-day treatment of candidal vulvovaginitis with vaginal tablets of clotrimazole. *Am J Obstet Gynecol* 152:953, 1985.

Multicenter Study Group. Treatment of vaginal candidiasis with a single oral dose of fluconazole. *Eur J Clin Microbiol Infect Dis* 7:364, 1988.

Reef, S. E., et al. Treatment options for vulvovaginal candidiasis, 1993. *Clin Infect Dis* 20(suppl 1):S80, 1995.

Sobel, J. D. Recurrent vulvovaginal candidiasis: a prospective study of the efficacy of maintenance ketoconazole therapy. *N Engl J Med* 315:1455, 1986.

Sobel, J. D., and Chaim, W. Treatment of *Torulopsis glabrata* vaginitis: retrospective review of boric acid therapy. *Clin Infect Dis* 24:649, 1997.

White, D. Effective management of vaginal thrush. *Practitioner* 239:612, 1995.

Genital Warts

Association of Reproductive Health Professionals. *Human Papillomavirus (HPV) and Cervical Cancer, Clinical Proceedings.* Association of Reproductive Health Specialists, March 2001, 13–17.

Bailey, J. V., et al. Lesbians and cervical screening. *Br J Gen Pract* 50:481, 2000.

Bleeker, M.C.G., et al. Condom use promotes regression of human papillomavirus-associated penile lesions in male sexual partners of women with cervical intraepithelial neoplasia. *Int J Cancer* 107:804, 2003.

Campion, M. J., and Singer, A. Vulval intraepithelial neoplasia: clinical review. *Genitourin Med* 63:147, 1987.

Carr, G., and William, D. C. Anal warts in a population of gay men in New York City. *Sex Transm Dis* 4:56, 1977.

Castle, P., et al. Hormonal contraceptive use, pregnancy and parity, and the risk of cervical intraepithelial neoplasia 3 among oncogenic HPV DNA-positive women with equivocal or mildly abnormal cytology. *Int J Cancer* 117:1007, 2005.

Chamberlain, M. J., et al. Toxic effect of podophyllin in pregnancy. *Br Med J* 3:391, 1972.

Chiao, E. Y., et al. Screening HIV-infected individuals for anal cancer precursor lesions: a systematic review. *Clin Infect Dis* 43:223, 2006.

Daling, J. R., et al. Risk factors for condyloma acuminatum in women. *Sex Transm Dis* 13:16, 1986.

de Benedicts, T. J. Intraurethral condyloma acuminatum: management and a review of the literature. *J Urol* 118:767, 1977.

Derkay, C. S. Task force on recurrent respiratory papillomatosis: a preliminary report. *Arch Otolaryngol Head Neck Surg* 121:1386, 1995.

Dilner, J., et al. *Chlamydia trachomatis* infection and persistence of human papillomavirus. *Int J Cancer* 116:110, 2005.

Dinh, T. V., et al. Papanicolaou smears of atypical glandular cells of undetermined significance: histological correlations and suggestions for management. *J Lower Genital Tract Dis* 3(2):73, 1999.

Ferris, D., et al. A neglected lesbian health concern: cervical neoplasia. *J Fam Pract* 43:581, 1996.

Frisch, M., et al. Sexually transmitted infection as a cause of anal cancer. *N Engl J Med* 337:1350, 1997.

Goldie, S., et al. Anal cancer in HIV infection: to screen or not to screen? *AIDS Clin Care* 16(7):53, 2004.

Harris, T. G., et al. Incidence of cervical squamous intraepithelial lesions associated with HIV serostatus, CD4 cell counts, and human papillomavirus test results *JAMA* 293:1471, 2005.

Hogenwoning, C.J.A., et al. Condom use promotes regression of cervical intraepithelial neoplasia and clearance of human papillomavirus: a randomized clinical trial. *Int J Cancer* 107:811, 2003.

HPV in Perspective: A Patient Guide [consumer pamphlet]. Research Triangle Park, N.C.: American Social Health Association, 2003.

HPV News [newsletter published by the American Social Health Association, Research Triangle Park, N.C.], 1992–2006.

Judson, F. N. Condyloma acuminatum of the oral cavity: a case report. *Sex Transm Dis* 8:218, 1981.

Kamb, M. L. Cervical cancer screening of women attending sexually transmitted disease clinics. *Clin Infect Dis* 20(suppl 1):S98, 1995.

Kaufman, R. H., et al. Relevance of human papillomavirus screening in the management of cervical intraepithelial neoplasia. *Am J Obstet Gynecol* 176 (1 part 1): 87, 1997.

Koutsky, L. Epidemiology of genital HPV infection. *Am J Med* 102(5A):3, 1997.

Lutzner, M. A., et al. Different papilloma viruses as the causes of oral warts. *Arch Dermatol* 118:393, 1982.

Manhart, L. E., and Koutsky, L. A. Do condoms prevent genital HPV infection, external genital warts, or cervical neoplasia? A meta-analysis. *Sexually Transm Dis* 29:725, 2002.

Manos, M. M., et al. Identifying women with cervical neoplasia: using human papillomavirus DNA testing for equivocal Papanicolaou results. *JAMA* 281:1605, 1999.

McNeil, C. HPV vaccine treatment trials proliferate, diversify. *J Natl Cancer Inst* 89:280, 1997.

Moscicki, A., et al. Regression of low-grade squamous intra-epithelial lesions in young women. *Lancet* 364:1678, 2004.

Munoz, N., and Bosch, F. X. The causal link between HPV and cervical cancer and its implications for the prevention of cervical cancer. *Bull Pan Am Health Org* 30:362, 1996.

National Cancer Institute Workshop. The 1988 Bethesda System for reporting cervical/vaginal cytological diagnoses. *JAMA* 262:931, 1989.

Oriel, J. D. Anal warts and anal coitus. *Br J Vener Dis* 47:373, 1971.

Oriel, J. D. Natural history of genital warts. *Br J Vener Dis* 47:1, 1971.

Parkin, D. M., et al. Estimates of the worldwide incidence of 18 major cancers in 1995. *Int J Cancer* 54:594, 1995.

A Patient Guide: HPV in Perspective [consumer pamphlet]. Research Triangle Park, N.C.: American Social Health Association, 1995.

Samoff, E., et al. Association of *Chlamydia trachomatis* with persistence of high-risk types of human papillomavirus in a cohort of female adolescents. *Am J Epidemiol* 162:668, 2005.

Sand, P. K., et al. Evaluation of male consorts of women with genital human papillomavirus infection. *Obstet Gynecol* 68:679, 1996.

Saslow, D., et al. American Cancer Society guideline for the early detection of cervical neoplasia and cancer. *CA Cancer J Clin* 52:342, 2002.

Schelct, N. F., et al. Variants of human papillomaviruses 16 and 18 and their natural history in human immunodeficiency virus-positive women. *J Gen Virol* 86(pt 10):2709, 2005.

Schiffman, M., et al. HPV DNA testing in cervical cancer screening: results from women in a high-risk province of Costa Rica. *JAMA* 283:87, 2000.

Schneider, A., et al. Screening for cervical intraepithelial neoplasm grade 2/3: validity of cytologic study, cervicography and human papillomavirus detection. *Am J Obstet Gynecol* 174:1534, 1996.

Schneider, V., et al. Immunosuppression as a high-risk factor in the development of condyloma acuminatum and squamous neoplasia of the cervix. *Acta Cytol* 27:220, 1983.

Shah, K., et al. Rarity of cesarean delivery of juvenile onset respiratory papillomatosis. *Obstet Gynecol* 68:795, 1986.

Silverberg, M. J., et al. Condyloma in pregnancy is strongly predictive of juvenile-onset recurrent respiratory papillomatosis. *Obstet Gynecol* 101:645, 2003.

Slater, G. E., et al. Podophyllin poisoning: systemic toxicity following cutaneous application. *Obstet Gynecol* 52:94, 1978.

Solomon, D., et al. The 2001 Bethesda System: terminology for reporting results of cervical cytology. *JAMA* 287:2114, 2002.

Strickler, H. D., et al. A multifaceted study of human papillomavirus and prostate carcinoma. *Cancer* 82:1118, 1998.

Strickler, H. D., et al. Natural history and possible reactivation of human papillomavirus in human immunodeficiency virus–positive women. *J Natl Cancer Inst* 97:577, 2005.

Tay, S.-K., and Tay, K.-J. Passive cigarette smoking is a risk factor in cervical neoplasia. *Gynecol Oncol* 93:116, 2004.

Trimble, C., et al. Active and passive cigarette smoking and the risk of cervical neoplasia. *Obstet Gynecol* 105:174, 2005.

Winer, R., et al. Consistent condom use from time of first vaginal intercourse and the risk of genital human papillomavirus infection in young women. *N Engl J Med* 354:2645, 2006.

Winer, R., et al. The effect of consistent condom use on the risk of genital HPV infection among newly sexually active young women. Abstract no. MP-120. 16th Biennial Meeting of the International Society for Sexually Transmitted Diseases Research, Seattle, July 11, 2005.

Wright, T. C., Jr., et al. 2001 consensus guidelines for the management of women with cervical cytological abnormalities. *JAMA* 287:2120, 2002.

Gonorrhea

Bignell, C. Antibiotic treatment of gonorrhea: clinical evidence for choice. *Genitourin Med* 72:315, 1996.

Centers for Disease Control. Increases in fluoroquinolone-resistant *Neisseria gonorrhoeae*—Hawaii and California, 2001. *MMWR* 52:1041, 2002.

Centers for Disease Control. Increases in fluoroquinolone-resistant *Neisseria gonorrhoeae* among men who have sex with men—United States, 2003, and revised recommendations for gonorrhea treatment, 2004. *MMWR* 53:335, 2004.

Centers for Disease Control. Screening tests to detect *Chlamydia trachomatis* and *Neisseria gonorrhoeae* infections, 2002. *MMWR* 51(RR-15), 2002.

Centers for Disease Control. *Sexually Transmitted Disease Surveillance 2004 Supplement: Gonococcal Isolate Surveillance Project (GISP) Annual Report, 2004.* Atlanta: Department of Health and Human Services, National Center for HIV, STD, and TB Prevention, 2005.

Ellen, J. M., et al. The link between the use of crack cocaine and the sexually transmitted diseases of a clinic population: a comparison of adolescents and adults. *Sex Transm Dis* 23:511, 1996.

Louv, W. C., et al. Oral contraceptive use and the risk of chlamydia and gonorrhea infections. *Am J Obstet Gynecol* 160:396, 1989.

Moran, J. S. Treating uncomplicated *Neisseria gonorrhea* infections: is the anatomic site of infection important? *Sex Transm Dis* 22:39, 1995.

Rice, J. R., et al. Gonorrhea in the United States 1975–84: is the giant only sleeping? *Sex Transm Dis* 14:83, 1987.

Ross, J. D. Systemic gonococcal infection. *Genitourin Med* 72:404, 1996.

Sherrard, J., and Barlow, D. Gonorrhea in men: clinical and diagnostic aspects. *Genitourin Med* 72:422, 1996.

Tapsall, J. W. What management is there for gonorrhea in the post-quinolone era? *Sex Transm Dis* 33:8, 2006.

Tice, R. W., and Rodriguez, V. L. Pharyngeal gonorrhea. *JAMA* 246:2717, 1981.

Hepatitis A

Bresee, J. S., et al. Hepatitis C virus infection associated with administration of intravenous immune globulin. *JAMA* 276:1563, 1996.

Centers for Disease Control. Prevention of hepatitis A through active or passive immunization: recommendations of the Advisory Committee on Immunization Practices. *MMWR* 45(RR-15), 1996.

Centers for Disease Control. Prevention of hepatitis A through active or passive immunizations: recommendations of the Advisory Committee on Immunization Practices (ACIP). *MMWR* 55(RR-7), 2006.

Centers for Disease Control. Summary of notifiable diseases, United States 1995. *MMWR* 44, 1996.

Corey, L., and Holmes, K. K. Sexual transmission of hepatitis A in homosexual men: incidence and mechanism. *N Engl J Med* 302:435, 1980.

Coulepis, A. G., et al. Detection of hepatitis A virus in the feces of patients with naturally acquired infections. *J Infect Dis* 141:151, 1980.

Coutinho, R. A., et al. Prevalence and incidence of hepatitis A among male homosexuals. *Br Med J (Clin Res)* 287:1743, 1983.

Feinstone, S. M., et al. Hepatitis A: detection by immune electron microscopy of a viruslike antigen associated with acute illness. *Science* 182:1026, 1973.

Innis, B. L., et al. Protection against hepatitis A by an inactivated vaccine. *JAMA* 271:28, 1994.

Lednar, W. M., et al. Frequency of illness associated with epidemic hepatitis A virus infection in adults. *Am J Epidemiol* 122:226, 1985.

Lemon, S. M. The natural history of hepatitis A: the potential for transmission by transfusion of blood or blood products. *Vox Sang* 67(suppl 4):19, 1994.

Lemon, S. M. Type A viral hepatitis: new developments in an old disease. *N Engl J Med* 313:1059, 1985.

McCaustland, K. A., et al. Survival of hepatitis A virus in feces after drying and storage for 1 month. *J Clin Microbiol* 16:957, 1982.

McFarlane, E. S., et al. Antibodies to hepatitis A antigen in relation to the number of lifetime sexual partners in patients attending an STD clinic. *Br J Vener Dis* 57:58, 1981.

Moyer, L., et al. Prevention of hepatitis A virus infection. *Am Fam Phys* 54:107, 1996.

Seef, L. B., and Hoofnagle, J. H. Immunoprophylaxis of viral hepatitis. *Gastroenterology* 77:161, 1979.

Wasley, A., et al. Incidence of hepatitis A in the United States in the era of vaccination. *JAMA* 294:194, 2005.

Werzberger, A., et al. A controlled trial of a formalin-inactivated hepatitis A vaccine in healthy children. *N Engl J Med* 327:453, 1992.

Hepatitis B

Aach, R. D., and Kahn, R. A. Post-transfusion hepatitis: current perspectives. *Ann Intern Med* 92:539, 1980.

Alter, M. J., et al. The changing epidemiology of hepatitis B in the United States: need for alternative vaccination strategies. *JAMA* 263:1218, 1990.

Centers for Disease Control. Changing patterns of groups at high risk for hepatitis B in the United States. *MMWR* 37:429, 1988.

Centers for Disease Control. A comprehensive immunization strategy to eliminate transmission of hepatitis B virus infection in the United States. Recommendations of the Advisory Committee on Immunization Practices (ACIP). Part 1: immunization of infants, children, and adolescents. *MMWR* 54(RR-16), 2005.

Centers for Disease Control. A comprehensive immunization strategy to eliminate transmission of hepatitis B virus infection in the United States. Recommendations of the Advisory Committee on Immunization Practices (ACIP). Part 2: immunization of adults. *MMWR* 2006 (in press).

Dietzman, D. E., et al. Hepatitis B surface antigen (HBsAg) and antibody to HBsAg: prevalence in homosexual and heterosexual men. *JAMA* 238:2625, 1977.

Eddy, D. M. *A Manual for Assessing Health Practices and Designing Practice Guidelines.* Philadelphia: American College of Physicians, 1996.

Heathcote, J., et al. Role of hepatitis B antigen carriers in nonparenteral transmission of the hepatitis B virus. *Lancet* 2:370, 1974.

Hentzner, B., et al. Viral hepatitis in a venereal clinic population. *Scand J Infect Dis* 12:245, 1980.

Hollinger, F. B. Comprehensive control (or elimination) of hepatitis B virus transmission in the United States. *Gut* 38:24S, 1966.

Hoofnagle, J. H., and DiBisceglie, A. M. The treatment of chronic viral hepatitis. *N Engl J Med* 336:347, 1997.

Hoofnagle, J. H., et al. Serologic responses in hepatitis. In: Vyas, G. N., et al., eds. *Viral Hepatitis.* Philadelphia: Franklin Institute Press, 1978, 219.

Katkov, W. N. Hepatitis vaccines. *Med Clin N Am* 80:1189, 1996.

Kim, W. R., et al. Rising burden of hepatitis B in the United States: should the other virus be forgotten? [abstract]. *Hepatology* 36:222A, 2002.

Krugman, S., et al. Viral hepatitis, type B: studies on natural history and prevention re-examined. *N Engl J Med* 300:101, 1979.

Lim, K. S., et al. Role of sexual and non-sexual practices in the transmission of hepatitis B. *Br J Vener Dis* 53:190, 1977.

Lok, A.S.E., and McMahon, B. J. AASLD Practice Guidelines: Chronic hepatitis B. www.aasld.org/netFORUMAASLD/eweb/docs/chronic hep—B.pdf.

MacCallum, F. O. Homologous serum jaundice. *Lancet* 2:691, 1947.

Maynard, J. E. Hepatitis B: global importance and need for control. *Vaccine* 8(suppl):S18, 1990.

Okada, K., et al. E antigen and anti-e in the serum of asymptomatic carrier mothers as indicators of positive and negative transmission of hepatitis B virus to their infants. *N Engl J Med* 294:746, 1976.

Perrillo, R. P. Interferon in the management of chronic hepatitis B. *Dig Dis Sci* 38:577, 1993.

Perrillo, R. P., et al. Hepatitis B e antigen, DNA polymerase activity, and infection of household contacts with hepatitis B virus. *Gastroenterology* 76:1319, 1979.

Pons, J. A. Role of liver transplantation in viral hepatitis. *J Hepatol* 21(suppl 1):146, 1995.

Stevens, C. E., et al. Vertical transmission of hepatitis B antigen in Taiwan. *N Engl J Med* 292:771, 1975.

Szmuness, W., et al. On the role of sexual behavior in the spread of hepatitis B infection. *Ann Intern Med* 83:489, 1975.

Szmuness, W., et al. Passive-active immunization against hepatitis B: immunogenicity studies in adult Americans. *Lancet* 1:575, 1981.

Willson, R. A. Clinical review: extrahepatic manifestations of chronic viral hepatitis. *Am J Gastroenterol* 92:4, 1997.

Wong, K. H., et al. Effect of alpha-interferon treatment in patients with hepatitis B e antigen–positive chronic hepatitis B. *Ann Intern Med* 122:662, 1995.

Wood, A.J.J. The treatment of chronic viral hepatitis. *N Engl J Med* 336: 347, 1997.

Hepatitis C

Aizaki, H., et al. Mother to child transmission of hepatitis C virus variant with an insertional mutation in its hypervariable region. *J Hepatol* 25:608, 1996.

Akahane, Y., et al. Hepatitis C virus infection in spouses of patients with type C chronic liver disease. *Ann Intern Med* 120:748, 1994.

Alary, M., et al. Lack of evidence of sexual transmission of hepatitis C virus in a prospective cohort study of men who have sex with men. *Am J Public Health* 95:502, 2005.

Alter, H. J., et al. Detection of antibody to hepatitis C virus in prospectively followed transfusion recipients with acute and chronic non-A, non-B hepatitis. *N Engl J Med* 321:1494, 1989.

Alter, H. J. New kit on the block: evaluation of second-generation assays for detection of antibody to the hepatitis C virus. *Hepatology* 15:350, 1992.

Alter, M. J. Epidemiology of hepatitis C. *Hepatology* 26(suppl 1):S25, 1999.

Alter, M. J. Epidemiology of hepatitis C in the west. *Semin Liver Dis* 15:5, 1995.

Alter, M. J., and Mast, E. E. The epidemiology of viral hepatitis in the United States. *Gastroenterol Clin N Am* 23:437, 1994.

Alter, M. J., et al. The natural history of community-acquired hepatitis C in the United States. *N Engl J Med* 327:1899, 1992.

Alter, M. J., et al. The prevalence of hepatitis C virus infection in the United States, 1988 through 1994. *N Engl J Med* 341:556, 1999.

Alter, M. J., et al. Testing for hepatitis C virus infection should be routine for persons at increased risk for infection. *Ann Intern Med* 141:715, 2004.

Barrera, J. M., et al. Persistent hepatitis C viremia after acute self-limiting posttransfusion hepatitis C. *Hepatology* 21:639, 1995.

Bennett, W. G., et al. Justification of a single 6-month course of interferon (INF) for histologically mild chronic hepatitis C. *Hepatology* 22:A290, 1995.

Bresters, D., et al. Recombinant immunoblot assay reaction patterns and hepatitis C virus RNA in blood donors and non-A, non-B hepatitis patients. *Transfusion* 33:634, 1993.

Bresters, D., et al. Sexual transmission of hepatitis C virus. *Lancet* 342: 210, 1993.

Bruno, S., et al. Hepatitis C virus genotypes and risk of hepatocellular carcinoma in cirrhosis: a prospective study. *Hepatology* 25:754, 1997.

Calogero, C., et al. Interferon as treatment for acute hepatitis C: a meta-analysis. *Dig Dis Sci* 41:1248, 1996.

Camma, C., et al. Interferon as treatment for acute hepatitis C: a meta-analysis. *Dig Dis Sci* 41:1248, 1996.

Centers for Disease Control. Guidelines for laboratory testing and result reporting of antibody to hepatitis C virus. *MMWR* 52(RR-3), 2003.

Centers for Disease Control. *Hepatitis Surveillance Report No. 60.* Atlanta: Department of Health and Human Services, Public Health Service, 2005.

Centers for Disease Control. Recommendations for prevention and control of hepatitis C virus (HCV) infection and HCV-related chronic disease. *MMWR* 47(RR-19), 1998.

Cerny, A., and Chisari, F. V. Pathogenesis of chronic hepatitis C: immunological features of hepatic injury and viral persistence. *Hepatology* 30:595, 1999.

Chu, C. M., et al. Fulminant hepatic failure in acute hepatitis C: increased risk in chronic carriers of hepatitis B virus. *Gut* 45:613, 1999.

Conroy-Cautilena, C., et al. Routes of infection, viremia and liver disease in blood donors found to have hepatitis C virus infection. *N Engl J Med* 334:1691, 1996.

Diago, M. Intrafamily transmission of hepatitis C virus: sexual and nonsexual contacts. *J Hepatol* 25:125, 1996.

Diamond, C., et al. Viral hepatitis among young men who have sex with men: prevalence of infection, risk behaviors and vaccination. *Sex Transm Dis* 30:425, 2003.

Dienstag, J. L. The natural history of chronic hepatitis C and what we should do about it. *Gastroenterology* 112:651, 1997.

Dienstag, J. L. Sexual and perinatal transmission of hepatitis C. *Hepatology* 26(suppl 1):S66, 1997.

Diepolder, H. M., et al. Possible mechanism involving T-lymphocyte response to non-structural protein 3 in viral clearance in acute hepatitis C virus infection. *Lancet* 346:1006, 1995.

Dusheiko, G. M. Treatment and prevention of chronic viral hepatitis. *Pharmacol Ther* 65:47, 1995.

Farci, P., et al. Lack of protective immunity against reinfection with hepatitis C virus. *Science* 258:135, 1992.

Farci, P., et al. A long-term study of hepatitis C virus replication in non-A, non-B hepatitis. *N Engl J Med* 325:98, 1991.

Fattovich, G., et al. Morbidity and mortality in compensated cirrhosis type C: a retrospective follow-up study of 384 patients. *Gastroenterology* 112:463, 1997.

Garfein, R. S., et al. Viral infections in short-term injection drug users: the prevalence of the hepatitis C, hepatitis B, human immunodeficiency, and human T-lymphotropic viruses. *Am J Public Health* 86: 655 1996.

Gerlach, J. T., et al. Acute hepatitis C: high rate of both spontaneous and treatment-induced viral clearance. *Gastroenterology* 125:80, 2003.

Gretch, D. R. Diagnostic tests for hepatitis C. *Hepatology* 26:43S, 1997.

Gretch, D. R., et al. Use of aminotransferase, hepatitis C antibody, and hepatitis C polymerase chain reaction RNA assays to establish the diagnosis of hepatitis C virus infection in a diagnostic virology laboratory. *J Clin Microbiol* 30:2145, 1992.

Gummer, S. C., and Chopra, S. Hepatitis C: a multifaceted disease. Review of extrahepatic manifestation. *Ann Intern Med* 123:615, 1995.

Gursoy, M., et al. Interferon therapy in haemodialysis patients with acute hepatitis C virus infection and factors that predict response to treatment. *J Viral Hepat* 8:70, 2001.

Hammer, G. P., et al. Low incidence and prevalence of hepatitis C virus infection among sexually active nonintravenous drug-using adults, San Francisco, 1997–2000. *Sex Transm Dis* 30:919, 2003.

Hanley, J. P., et al. Development of anti-interferon antibodies and breakthrough hepatitis during treatment for hepatitis C virus infection in haemophiliacs. *Br J Haematol* 94:551, 1996.

Herion, D., and Hoofnagle, J. H. The interferon sensitivity determining region: all hepatitis C virus isolates are not the same. *Hepatology* 25: 769, 1997.

Hezode, C., et al. Daily cannabis smoking as a risk factor for progression of fibrosis in chronic hepatitis C. *Hepatology* 42:63, 2005.

Hoofnagle, J. H. Hepatitis C: the clinical spectrum of disease. *Hepatology* 26:15S, 1997.

Hoofnagle, J. H. Therapy for acute hepatitis C. *N Engl J Med* 345:1495, 2001.

Hoofnagle, J. H., et al. Fulminant hepatic failure: summary of a workshop. *Hepatology* 21:240, 1995.

Hu, K. Q., and Tong, M. J. The long-term outcomes of patients with compensated hepatitis C virus–related cirrhosis and history of parenteral exposure in the United States. *Hepatology* 29:1311, 1999.

Iwarson, S., et al. Hepatitis C: natural history of a unique infection. *Clin Infect Dis* 20:1361, 1995.

Jaeckel, E., et al. Treatment of acute hepatitis C with interferon alfa-2b. *N Engl J Med* 345:1452, 2001.

Kenny-Walsh, E. Clinical outcomes after hepatitis C infection from contaminated anti-D immune globulin. Irish Hepatology Research Group. *N Engl J Med* 340:1228, 1999.

Koff, R. S., and Dienstag, J. L. Extrahepatic manifestations of hepatitis C and the association with alcoholic liver disease. *Semin Liver Dis* 15: 101, 1995.

Lampertico, P., et al. A multicenter randomized controlled trial of recombinant interferon–alpha 2b in patients with acute transfusion-associated hepatitis C. *Hepatology* 19:19, 1994.

Lau, J. Y., et al. Hepatitis C virus infection in kidney transplant recipients. *Hepatology* 18:1027, 1993.

Lin, H. H., et al. Absence of infection in breast-fed infants born to hepatitis C virus infected mothers. *J Pediatr* 126:589, 1995.

Lissen, E., et al. Hepatitis C virus infection among sexually promiscuous groups and the heterosexual partners of hepatitis C virus infected index cases. *Eur J Clin Microbiol Infect Dis* 12:827, 1993.

Lok, A. S., and Gunaratnam, N. T. Diagnosis of hepatitis C. *Hepatology* 26:48S, 1997.

Mathurin, P., et al. Slow progression rate of fibrosis in hepatitis C virus patients with persistently normal alanine transaminase activity. *Hepatology* 27:868, 1998.

Mazzaro, C., et al. Hepatitis C virus and non-Hodgkin's lymphomas. *Br J Haematology* 94:544, 1996.

Merican, I., et al. Clinical, biochemical and histological features in 102 patients with chronic hepatitis C virus infection. *Q J Med* 86:119, 1993.

Missale, G., et al. Different clinical behaviors of acute hepatitis C virus infection are associated with different vigor of the anti-viral cell-mediated immune response. *J Clin Invest* 98:706, 1996.

Murphy, E. L., et al. Risk factors for hepatitis C virus infection in United States blood donors. *Hepatology* 31:756, 2000.

Nguyen, T., et al. Fluctuations in viral load (HCV RNA) are relatively insignificant in untreated patients with chronic HCV infection. *J Viral Hepat* 3:75, 1996.

NIH Consensus Development Program. *Management of Hepatitis C: 2002.* National Institutes of Health Consensus Conference Statement, June 10–12, 2002. http://consensus.nih.gov/cons/116/091202116cdc _statement.htm.

Nikolaeva, L. I., et al. Virus-specific antibody titres in different phases of hepatitis C virus infection. *J Viral Hepat* 9:429, 2002.

Nishiguchi, S., et al. Randomized trial of effects of interferon-alpha on incidence of hepatocellular carcinoma in chronic active hepatitis C with cirrhosis. *Lancet* 346:1051, 1995.

Ohto, H., et al. Transmission of hepatitis C virus from mothers to infants. *N Engl J Med* 330:744, 1994.

Oshita, M., et al. Increased serum hepatitis C virus RNA levels among alcoholic patients with chronic hepatitis C. *Hepatology* 20:1115, 1994.

Ostapowicz, G., et al. Role of alcohol in the progression of liver disease caused by hepatitis C virus infection. *Hepatology* 27:1730, 1998.

Pawlotsky, J. M., et al. What strategy should be used for diagnosis of hepatitis C virus infection in clinical laboratories? *Hepatology* 27:1700, 1998.

Pereira, B. J., and Levey, A. S. Hepatitis C virus infection in dialysis and renal transplantation. *Kidney Int* 51:981, 1997.

Pessione, F., et al. Effect of alcohol consumption on serum hepatitis C virus RNA and histological lesions in chronic hepatitis C. *Hepatology* 27:1717, 1998.

Poynard, T., et al. Interferon for acute hepatitis C. *Cochrane Database Syst Rev* CD000369, 2002.

Poynard, T., et al. Natural history of liver fibrosis progression in patients with chronic hepatitis C. The OBSVIRC, METAVIR, CLINICIR, and DOSVIRC Groups. *Lancet* 349:825, 1997.

Puoti, C., et al. Clinical histological and virological features of hepatitis C virus carriers with persistently normal or abnormal alanine transaminase levels. *Hepatology* 26:1393, 1997.

Quin, J. W. Interferon therapy for acute hepatitis C viral infection—a review by meta-analysis. *Aust N Z J Med* 27:611, 1997.

Rocca, P., et al. Early treatment of acute hepatitis C with interferon alpha-2b or interferon alpha-2b plus ribavirin: study of sixteen patients. *Gastroenterol Clin Biol* 27:294, 2003.

Roy, K. M., et al. Hepatitis C virus among self declared non-injecting sexual partners of injecting drug users. *J Med Virol* 74:62, 2004.

Rubin, R. A. Chronic hepatitis C: advances in diagnostic testing and therapy. *Arch Intern Med* 154:387, 1994.

Santantonio, T., et al. Natural course of acute hepatitis C: a long-term prospective study. *Dig Liver Dis* 35:104, 2003.

Seeff, L. B. Natural history of hepatitis C. *Hepatology* 26:21S, 1997.

Soffredini, R., et al. Increased detection of antibody to hepatitis C virus in renal transplant patients by third-generation assays. *Am J Kidney Dis* 28:437, 1996.

Sterling, R. D., et al. A comparison of the spectrum of chronic hepatitis C virus between Caucasians and African Americans. *Clin Gastroenterol Hepatol* 2:469, 2004.

Strader, D. B., et al. Diagnosis, management, and treatment of hepatitis C. *Hepatology* 39:1147, 2004.

Takahashi, M., et al. Natural course of chronic hepatitis C. *Am J Gastroenterol* 88:240, 1993.

Thomas, D., et al. Sexual transmission of hepatitis C among patients attending Baltimore sexually transmitted disease clinics: an analysis of 309 sexual partnerships. *J Infect Dis* 171:769, 1995.

Tong, M. J., et al. Clinical outcomes after transfusion-associated hepatitis C. *N Engl J Med* 332:1463, 1995.

Tremolada, F., et al. Antibody to hepatitis C virus in post-transfusion hepatitis. *Ann Intern Med* 114:277, 1991.

van der Poel, C. L., et al. Hepatitis C virus six years on. *Lancet* 344:1475, 1994.

Villano, S. A., et al. Persistence of viremia and the importance of long-term follow-up after acute hepatitis C infection. *Hepatology* 29:908, 1999.

Vogel, W., et al. High-dose interferon-alpha2b treatment prevents chronicity in acute hepatitis C: a pilot study. *Dig Dis Sci* 41:81S, 1996.

Vogt, M., et al. Prevalence and clinical outcome of hepatitis C infection in children who underwent cardiac surgery before the implementation of blood-donor screening. *N Engl J Med* 341:866, 1999.

Wawrzynowicz-Syczewska, M., et al. Natural history of acute symptomatic hepatitis type C. *Infection* 32:138, 2004.

What is the risk of acquiring hepatitis C for health care workers and what are the recommendations for prophylaxis and follow-up after occupational exposure to hepatitis C virus? *Am J Infect Control* 24:411, 1996.

Wiese, M., et al. Outcome in a hepatitis C (genotype 1b) single source outbreak in Germany—a 25 year multicenter study. *J Hepatol* 43:590, 2005.

Willson, R. A. Extrahepatic manifestations of chronic viral hepatitis. *Am J Gastroenterol* 92:3, 1997.

Wood, A.J.J. The treatment of chronic viral hepatitis. *N Engl J Med* 336:347, 1997.

Yano, M., et al. The long term pathological evolution of chronic hepatitis C. *Hepatology* 23:1334, 1996.

Zeuzem, S. [Standard treatment of acute and chronic hepatitis C] (in German). *Z Gastroenterol* 42:714, 2004.

Herpes

Aoki, F. Y., et al. Single-day, patient-initiated famciclovir therapy for recurrent genital herpes: a randomized, double-blind, placebo-controlled trial. *Clin Infect Dis* 42:8, 2006.

Bernstein, D. I., et al. Safety and immunogenicity of glycoprotein D—adjuvant genital herpes vaccine. *Clin Infect Dis* 40:1271, 2005; epub March 24, 2005.

Bodsworth, N. J., et al. Valaciclovir versus acyclovir in patient-initiated treatment of genital herpes: a randomized, double-blind clinical trial. *Genitourin Med* 73:110, 1997.

Boggess, K. A., et al. Herpes simplex virus 2 detection by culture and polymerase chain reaction and relationship to genital symptoms and cervical antibody status during the third trimester of pregnancy. *Am J Obstet Gynecol* 176:443, 1997.

Brocklehurst, P., et al. A randomized placebo controlled trial of suppressive acyclovir late in pregnancy in women with recurrent genital herpes infection. *Br J Obstet Gynaecol* 105:275, 1998.

Brown, Z. A., et al. Effects on infants of first episode genital herpes during pregnancy. *N Engl J Med* 317:1247, 1987.

Brown, Z. A., et al. Genital herpes in pregnancy: risk factors associated with recurrences and asymptomatic shedding. *Am J Obstet Gynecol* 153:24, 1985.

Brown, Z. A., et al. Effect of serologic status and cesarean delivery on transmission rates of herpes simplex virus from mother to infant. *JAMA* 289:203, 2003.

Caplan, L. R., et al. Urinary retention probably secondary to herpes genitalis. *N Engl J Med* 197:920, 1977.

Cherpes, T. L., et al. Cunnilingus and vaginal intercourse are risk factors for herpes simplex virus type 1 acquisition in women. *Sex Transm Dis* 32:84, 2005.

Chosidow, O., et al. Famciclovir vs. aciclovir in immunocompetent patients with recurrent genital herpes infections: a parallel-groups, randomized, double-blind clinical trial. *Br J Dermatol* 14:818, 2001.

Corey, L., and Handsfield, H. H. Genital herpes and public health: addressing a global problem. *JAMA* 283:791, 2000.

Corey, L., et al. Once-daily valacyclovir to reduce the risk of transmission of genital herpes. *N Engl J Med* 350:11, 2004.

Diaz-Mitoma, F., et al. Oral famciclovir for the suppression of recurrent genital herpes: a randomized controlled trial. *JAMA* 280:887, 1998.

Dicerson, M. C., et al. The causal role for genital ulcer disease as a risk factor for transmission of human immunodeficiency virus: an application of the Bradford Hill criteria. *Sex Transm Dis* 23:429, 1996.

Douglas, J. M., et al. A double-blind placebo-controlled trial of the effect of chronic oral acyclovir on sperm production in men with frequently recurrent genital herpes. *J Infect Dis* 157:588, 1988.

Fife, K. H., et al. Valaciclovir versus acyclovir in the treatment of first-episode genital herpes infection: results of an international, multicenter, double-blind, randomized clinical trial. The Valaciclovir International Herpes Simplex Virus Study Group. *Sex Transmit Dis* 24: 481, 1997.

Gilbert, L., et al. Patient and partner perceptions about preventing genital herpes transmission. *Herpes* 12:60, 2005.

Goldmeier, D., et al. Urinary retention and intestinal obstruction associated with anorectal herpes simplex virus infection. *Br J Med* 1:425, 1975.

Hoffman, I. F., and Schmitz, J. L. Genital ulcer disease: management in the HIV era. *Postgrad Med* 98:67, 1995.

Holmberg, S. B., et al. Prior HSV type 2 infection as a risk factor for HIV infection. *JAMA* 258:1048, 1988.

Kaufman, R. H., et al. Clinical features of herpes genitalis. *Cancer Res* 33:1446, 1973.

Koutsky, L. A., et al. A controlled trial of a human papillomavirus type 16 vaccine. *N Engl J Med* 347:1645, 2002.

Lafferty, W. E., et al. Herpes simplex type I as the cause of genital herpes: impact on surveillance and prevention. *J Infect Dis* 181:1454, 2000.

Lafferty, W. E., et al. Recurrences after oral and genital herpes simplex virus infection: influence of anatomic site and viral type. *N Engl J Med* 316:1444, 1987.

Leone, P. A., et al. Valacyclovir for episodic treatment of genital herpes: a shorter 3-day treatment course compared with 5-day treatment. *Clin Infect Dis* 34:958, 2002.

Loveless, M., et al. Treatment of first episode genital herpes with famciclovir. In: *Programs and Abstracts of the 35th Interscience Conference on Antimicrobial Agents and Chemotherapy*. San Francisco, 1995.

McGrath, B. J., and Newman, C. L. Genital herpes simplex infections in patients with the acquired immunodeficiency syndrome. *Pharmacotherapy* 14:529, 1994.

Mertz, G. J., et al. Frequency of acquisition of first episode genital infection with herpes simplex virus from symptomatic and asymptomatic source contacts. *Sex Transm Dis* 12:33, 1985.

Mertz, G. J., et al. Oral famciclovir for suppression of recurrent genital herpes simplex virus infection in women: a multicenter, double-blind, placebo-controlled trial. *Arch Intern Med* 157:343, 1997.

Mertz, G. J., et al. Transmission of genital herpes in couples with one symptomatic and one asymptomatic partner: a prospective study. *J Infect Dis* 157:1169, 1988.

NIH Consensus Development Program. *Management of Hepatitis C: 2002*. National Institutes of Health Consensus Conference Statement, June 10–12, 2002. http://consensus.nih.gov/cons/116/091202116cdc —statement.htm.

Patel, R., et al. Valaciclovir for the suppression of recurrent genital HSV infection: a placebo controlled study of once-daily therapy. *Genitourin Med* 73:105, 1997.

Perry, C. M., and Wagstaff, A. J. Famciclovir: a review of its pharmacological properties and therapeutic efficacy in herpesvirus infections. *Drugs* 50:396, 1995.

Reeves, W. C., et al. Risk of recurrence after first episodes of genital herpes: relation to HSV type and antibody response. *N Engl J Med* 305:315, 1981.

Reiff-Eldridge, R. A., et al. Monitoring pregnancy outcomes after prenatal drug exposure through prospective pregnancy registries: a pharmaceutical company commitment. *Am J Obstet Gynecol* 182:159, 2000.

Reitano, M., et al. Valaciclovir for the suppression of recurrent genital herpes simplex virus infection: a large-scale dose range-finding study. *J Infect Dis* 178:603, 1998.

Riehle, R. A., and Williams, J. J. Transient neuropathic bladder following herpes simplex genitalis. *J Urol* 122:263, 1979.

Roberts, C. M., et al. Increasing proportion of herpes simplex virus type 1 as a cause of genital herpes infection in college students. *Sex Transm Dis* 30:801, 2003.

Romanowski, B., et al. Patients' preference of valacyclovir once-daily suppressive therapy versus twice-daily episodic therapy for recurrent genital herpes: a randomized study. Valtrex HS230017 Study Group. *Sex Transm Dis* 30:226, 2003.

Rooney, J. J., et al. Acquisition of genital herpes from an asymptomatic sexual partner. *N Engl J Med* 314:1561, 1986.

Rosenthal, S. L., et al. The psychosocial impact of serological diagnosis of asymptomatic herpes simplex virus type 2 infection. *Sex Transm Infect* 82:154, 2006.

Ross, C.A.C., and Stevenson, J. Herpes simplex meningoencephalitis. *Lancet* 2:682, 1961.

Sacks, S. L., et al. Patient-initiated, twice-daily oral famciclovir for early recurrent genital herpes: a randomized, double-blind multicenter trial. *JAMA* 276:44, 1996.

Scott, L. L., et al. Acyclovir suppression to prevent cesarean section after first-episode genital herpes. *Obstet Gynecol* 87:69, 1996.

Scott, L. L., et al. Acyclovir suppression to prevent recurrent genital herpes at delivery. *Infect Dis Obstet Gynecol* 10:71, 2002.

Scoular, A. Using the evidence base on genital herpes: optimising the use of diagnostic tests and information provision. *Sex Transm Infect* 78: 160, 2002.

Sheffield, J. S., et al. Acyclovir prophylaxis to prevent herpes simplex virus recurrence at delivery: a systematic review. *Obstet Gynecol* 102: 1396, 2003.

Song, B., et al. HSV type specific serology in sexual health clinics: use, benefits, and who gets tested. *Sex Transm Infect* 80:113, 2004.

Spruance, S., et al. A large-scale, placebo-controlled, dose-ranging trial of peroral valacyclovir for episodic treatment of recurrent herpes genitalis. The Valaciclovir HSV Study Group. *Arch Intern Med* 156:1729, 1996.

Stagno, S., and Whitley, R. J. Herpes infections of pregnancy, II: herpes simplex virus and varicella zoster infection. *N Engl J Med* 313:1327, 1985.

Stamm, W. E., et al. Association between genital ulcer disease and acquisition of HIV infection in homosexual men. *JAMA* 260:1429, 1988.

Stanberry, L. R., et al. Glycoprotein-D—adjuvant vaccine to prevent genital herpes. *N Engl J Med* 347:1652, 2002.

Stenzel, Poore, M., et al. Herpes simplex in genital secretions. *Sex Transm Dis* 14:17, 1987.

Stone, K. M., et al. Pregnancy outcomes following systemic prenatal acyclovir exposure: conclusions from the International Acyclovir Pregnancy Registry, 1984–1999. *Birth Defects Res Part A Clin Mol Teratol* 70:201, 2004.

Sullivan-Bolyai, J., et al. Neonatal herpes simplex virus infection in King County, Washington: increasing incidence and expanding epidemiologic correlates. *JAMA* 250:3059, 1983.

Wald, A. New therapies and prevention strategies for genital herpes. *Clin Infect Dis* 28(suppl.):S4, 1999.

Wald, A., et al. Comparative efficacy of famciclovir and valacyclovir for suppression of recurrent genital herpes and viral shedding. *Sex Transm Dis* 33:529, 2006.

Wald, A., et al. Effect of condoms on reducing the transmission of herpes simplex virus type 2 from men to women. *JAMA* 285:3100, 2001.

Wald, A., et al. Reactivation of genital herpes simplex virus type 2 infection in asymptomatic seropositive persons. *N Engl J Med* 342:844, 2000.

Wald, A., et al. The relationship between condom use and herpes simplex virus acquisition. *Ann Intern Med* 143:707, 2005.

Wald, A., et al. Two-day regimen of acyclovir for treatment of recurrent genital herpes simplex virus type 2 infection. *Clin Infect Dis* 34:944, 2002.

Watts, D. H., et al. A double-blind, randomized, placebo-controlled trial of acyclovir in late pregnancy for the reduction of herpes simplex virus shedding and cesarean delivery. *Am J Obstet Gynecol* 188:836, 2003.

Whittington, W. L., et al. Use of a glycoprotein G–based type-specific assay to detect antibodies to herpes simplex virus type 2 among persons attending sexually transmitted disease clinics. *Sex Transm Dis* 28:99, 2001.

Zimet, G. D., et al. Factors predicting the acceptance of herpes simplex virus type 2 antibody testing among adolescents and young adults. *Sex Transm Dis* 31:665, 2004.

HIV Infection and AIDS

Aberg, J. A., et al. Primary care guidelines for the management of persons infected with human immunodeficiency virus: recommendations of the HIV Medicine Association of the Infectious Diseases Society of America. *Clin Infect Dis* 39:609, 2004.

Blanche, S., et al. A prospective study of infants born to women seropositive for human immunodeficiency virus type 1. *N Engl J Med* 320:1643, 1989.

Carpenter, C. J., et al. Antiretroviral therapy in adults: updated recommendation of the International AIDS Society–USA Panel. *JAMA* 283:381, 2002.

Carpenter, C.C.J., et al. Antiretroviral therapy for HIV infection in 1996: recommendations of an international panel. *JAMA* 273:146, 1996.

Case-control study of HIV seroconversion in health care workers after percutaneous exposure from HIV-infected blood: France, United Kingdom and the United States, January 1988–August 1994. *MMWR* 44:929, 1995.

Centers for Disease Control. 1993 Revised classification system for HIV infection and expanded surveillance case definition for AIDS among adolescents and adults. *MMWR* 41(R-17), 1992.

Centers for Disease Control. *Recommendations for the Use of Antiretroviral Drugs in Pregnant HIV-1 Infected Women for Maternal Health and Interventions to Reduce Perinatal HIV-1 Transmission in the United States.* Atlanta: Department of Health and Human Services, 2002.

Centers for Disease Control. Recommendations of the U.S. Public Health Service Task Force on the use of zidovudine to reduce perinatal transmission of the human immunodeficiency virus. *MMWR* 43(RR-11), 1994.

Centers for Disease Control. Revised guidelines for HIV counseling, testing, and referral and revised recommendations for HIV screening of pregnant women. *MMWR* 50(RR-19):13, 2001.

Centers for Disease Control. Testing for antibodies to human immunodeficiency virus type 2 in the United States. *MMWR* 2006 (in press).

Centers for Disease Control. Update: acquired immunodeficiency syndrome: United States 1994. *MMWR* 44:64, 1995.

Centers for Disease Control. Update: AIDS among women: United States 1994. *MMWR* 44:81, 1995.

Centers for Disease Control. Update: Provisional public health recommendations for chemoprophylaxis after occupational exposure to HIV. *MMWR* 45:468, 1996.

Coffin, J. M. HIV population dynamics in vivo: implications for genetic variation, pathogenesis and therapy. *Science* 267:483, 1995.

Condoms, Contraceptives and STDs: Does Your Birth Control Method Protect You from Sexually Transmitted Disease? [consumer pamphlet]. Research Triangle Park, N.C.: American Social Health Association, 1994.

Corey, L., and Holmes, K. K. Therapy for human immunodeficiency virus infection: what have we learned? *N Engl J Med* 335:1142, 1996.

DeGruttola, V., et al. Infectiousness of HIV between male homosexual partners. *J Clin Epidemiol* 42:849, 1989.

DeVincenzi, I. A longitudinal study of human immunodeficiency virus transmission by heterosexual partners. *N Engl J Med* 331:341, 1994.

Dickover, R. E., et al. Identification of levels of maternal HIV-1 RNA associated with risk of perinatal transmission: effect of maternal zidovudine treatment on viral load. *JAMA* 275:599, 1996.

Fowler, M. G., et al. Update on perinatal HIV transmission. *Pediatr Clin North Am* 47:241, 2000.

Frank, A. P., et al. Anonymous HIV testing using home collection and telemedicine counseling. *Arch Intern Med* 157:309, 1997.

Gerberding, J. L. Management of occupational exposures to blood-borne viruses. *N Engl J Med* 332:444, 1995.

Hammer, S. M., et al. A trial comparing nucleoside monotherapy with combination therapy in HIV-infected adults with CD4 cell counts from 200 to 500 per cubic millimeter. *N Engl J Med* 335:1081, 1997.

Ho, D. D., et al. Rapid turnover of plasma virions and CD4 lymphocytes in HIV-1 infection. *Nature* 373:123, 1995.

Janssen, R. S., et al. The serostatus approach to fighting the HIV epidemic: prevention strategies for infected individuals. *Am J Public Health* 91:1019, 2001.

Katz, M. H., and Gerberding, J. L. Postexposure treatment of people exposed to the human immunodeficiency virus through sexual contact or injection-drug use. *N Engl J Med* 336:1097, 1997.

Katzenstein, D. A., et al. The relation of virologic and immunologic markers to clinical outcomes after nucleoside therapy in HIV-infected adults with 200 to 500 CD4 cells per cubic millimeter. *N Engl J Med* 335:1091, 1997.

Lackritz, E. M., et al. Estimated risk of transmission of the human immunodeficiency virus by screened blood in the United States. *N Engl J Med* 333:1721, 1995.

Melnick, S. L., et al. Survival and disease progression according to gender of patients with HIV infection. *JAMA* 272:1915, 1994.

Morse, S. A. *Atlas of Sexually Transmitted Diseases and AIDS*, 2nd ed. London: Mosby-Wolfe, 1996.

Peterman, T. A., et al. Risk of human immunodeficiency virus transmission from heterosexual adults with transfusion-associated infections. *JAMA* 259:55, 1988.

Pilcher, C. D., et al. Sexual transmission during the incubation period of primary HIV infection. *JAMA* 286:1713, 2001.

Puro, V., et al. Zidovudine prophylaxis after accidental exposure to HIV: the Italian experience. *AIDS* 6:963, 1992.

Sande, M. A. *The Medical Management of AIDS*, 5th ed. Philadelphia: Saunders, 1997.

Saravolatz, L. D., et al. Zidovudine alone or in combination with didanosine or zalcitabine in HIV-infected patients with the acquired immunodeficiency syndrome or fewer than 200 CD4 cells per cubic millimeter. *N Engl J Med* 335:1115, 1996.

Sperling, R. S., et al. A survey of zidovudine use in pregnant women with human immunodeficiency virus infection. *N Engl J Med* 326:857, 1992.

Stockman, J. K., et al. HIV prevention fatigue among high-risk populations in San Francisco. *JAIDS J Acquir Immune Defic Syndr* 35:432, 2004.

Stryker, J., and Coates, T. J. Home access HIV testing: what took so long? *Arch Intern Med* 157:261, 1997.

Tokars, J. I., et al. Surveillance of HIV infection and zidovudine use among health care workers after occupational exposure to HIV-infected blood. *Ann Intern Med* 118:913, 1993.

U.S. Department of Health and Human Service. *Guidelines for the Use of Antiretroviral Agents in HIV-Infected Adults and Adolescents.* Washington, D.C.: Department of Health and Human Services, 2006. http://AIDSinfo.nih.gov.

Wiley, J. A., et al. Heterogeneity in the probability of HIV transmission per sexual contact: the case of male-to-female transmission in penile-vaginal intercourse. *Stat Med* 8:93, 1989.

Wood, A.J.J. Management of occupational exposure to blood-borne pathogens. *N Engl J Med* 332:444, 1995.

Yeni, P. G., et al. Treatment for adult HIV infection, 2004 recommendations of the International AIDS Society–USA Panel. *JAMA* 292:25, 2004.

Lymphogranuloma Venereum

Dan, M., et al. A case of lymphogranuloma venereum of 20 years duration: isolation of *Chlamydia trachomatis* from perianal lesions. *Br J Vener Dis* 56:344, 1980.

Goens, J. L., et al. Mucocutaneous manifestations of chancroid, lymphogranuloma venereum and granuloma inguinale. *Am Fam Phys* 49: 415, 1994.

Mauff, A. C., et al. Problems in the diagnosis of lymphogranuloma venereum. *S Afr Med J* 63:55, 1983.

Munday, P. E., and Taylor-Robinson, D. Chlamydia infection in proctitis and Crohn's disease. *Br Med Bull* 39:155, 1983.

Quinn, T. C., et al. *Chlamydia trachomatis* proctitis. *N Engl J Med* 305: 195, 1981.

Schacter, J. Confirmatory serodiagnosis of lymphogranuloma venereum proctitis may yield false-positive results due to other chlamydial infections of the rectum. *Sex Transm Dis* 8:26, 1981.

Schacter, J., and Osoba, A. O. Lymphogranuloma venereum. *Br Med Bull* 39:151, 1983.

Molluscum Contagiosum

Dennis, J., et al. Molluscum contagiosum, another sexually transmitted disease: its impact on the clinical virology laboratory. *J Infect Dis* 151:376, 1985.

Katzman, M., et al. Molluscum contagiosum and the acquired immunodeficiency syndrome: clinical and immunological details of two cases. *Br J Dermatol* 116:131, 1987.

Ordoukhanian, E., and Lane, A. T. Warts and molluscum contagiosum: beware of treatments worse than the disease. *Postgrad Med* 101:223, 1997.

Mucopurulent Cervicitis

Brunham, E., et al. Mucopurulent cervicitis: the ignored counterpart of urethritis in the male. *N Engl J Med* 311:1, 1984.

Handsfield, H. H., et al. Criteria for selective screening for *Chlamydia trachomatis* infection on women attending family planning clinics. *JAMA* 255:1730, 1986.

Harrison, H. R., et al. Cervical *Chlamydia trachomatis* infection in university women: relationship to history, contraception, ectopy and cervicitis. *Am J Obstet Gynecol* 153:244, 1985.

Manhart, L. E., et al. Mucopurulent cervicitis and *Mycoplasma genitalium*. *J Infect Dis* 187:650, 2004; erratum, 190:866, 2004.

Marrazzo, J. M., et al. Predicting chlamydial and gonococcal cervical infection: implications for management of cervicitis. *Obstet Gynecol* 100:579, 2002.

Marrazzo, J. M., et al. Risk factors for cervicitis among women with bacterial vaginosis. *J Infect Dis* 193:617, 2006.

Paavonen, J., et al. Colposcopic manifestations of cervical and vaginal infections. *Obstet Gynecol Surv* 43:373, 1988.

Paavonen, J., et al. Etiology of cervical inflammation. *Am J Obstet Gynecol* 154:556, 1986.

Rosenberg, M. J., et al. The contraceptive sponge's protection against *Chlamydia trachomatis* and *Neisseria gonorrhea*. *Sex Transm Dis* 14:147, 1987.

Stamm, W. E., et al. Effect of *Neisseria gonorrhea* treatment regimens on simultaneous infection with *Chlamydia trachomatis*. *N Engl J Med* 310:545, 1984.

Nongonococcal Urethritis

Barnes, R. C., et al. Urinary tract infection in sexually active homosexual men. *Lancet* 1:171, 1986.

Fontaine, E. A., et al. Anaerobes in men with urethritis. *Br J Vener Dis* 58:321, 1982.

Holmes, K. K., et al. Etiology of nongonococcal urethritis. *N Engl J Med* 292:1199, 1975.

Krieger, J., et al. Evaluation of chronic urethritis: defining the role for endoscopic procedures. *Arch Intern Med* 148:703, 1988.

Schwebke, J. R., and Hook, E. W., III. High rates of *Trichomonas vaginalis* among men attending a sexually transmitted diseases clinic: implications for screening and urethritis management. *J Infect Dis* 188:465, 2003.

Schwebke, J. R., and Weiss, H. L. Interrelationships of bacterial vaginosis and cervical inflammation. *Sex Transm Dis* 29:59, 2002.

Stimson, J. B., et al. Tetracycline-resistant *Ureaplasma urealyticum*: a cause of persistent nongonococcal urethritis. *Ann Intern Med* 94:192, 1981.

Pelvic Inflammatory Disease

Arredondo, J. L., et al. Oral clindamycin and ciprofloxacin versus intramuscular ceftriaxone and oral doxycycline in the treatment of mild-to-moderate pelvic inflammatory disease in outpatients. *Clin Infect Dis* 24:170, 1997.

Ault, K. A., and Faro, S. Pelvic inflammatory disease: current diagnostic criteria and treatment guidelines. *Postgrad Med* 93:85, 1993.

Bowie, W. R., and Jones, H. Acute PID in outpatients: association with *Chlamydia trachomatis* and *Neisseria gonorrhoeae*. *Ann Intern Med* 95:685, 1981.

Centers for Disease Control. Ectopic pregnancy: United States, 1981–1983. *MMWR* 35:289, 1986.

Cramer, D. W., et al. The relationship of tubal infertility to barrier method and oral contraceptive use. *JAMA* 257:2308, 1987.

Eschenbach, D. A., et al. Acute pelvic inflammatory disease: associations of clinical and laboratory findings with laparoscopic findings. *Obstet Gynecol* 89:184, 1997.

Harrison, H. R. Cervical *Chlamydia trachomatis* infection in university women: relationship to history of contraception, ectopy, and cervicitis. *Am J Obstet Gynecol* 153:244, 1985.

Henry-Suchet, J., et al. Microbiologic study of chronic inflammation associated with tubal factor sterility: role of *Chlamydia trachomatis*. *Fertil Steril* 47:274, 1987.

Hillis, S. D., et al. Delayed care of pelvic inflammatory disease as a risk factor for impaired fertility. *Am J Obstet Gynecol* 168:1503, 1993.

Hillis, S. D., et al. Recurrent chlamydial infections increase the risks of hospitalization for ectopic pregnancy and pelvic inflammatory disease. *Am J Obstet Gynecol* 176(1 part):103, 1997.

Ness, R. B., et al. Bacterial vaginosis and risk of pelvic inflammatory disease. *Obstet Gynecol* 104:761, 2004.

Ness, R. B., et al. Condom use and the risk of recurrent pelvic inflammatory disease, chronic pelvic pain, or infertility following an episode of pelvic inflammatory disease. *Am J Public Health* 94:1327, 2004.

Ness, R. B., et al. Effectiveness of inpatient and outpatient treatment strategies for women with pelvic inflammatory disease: results from the Pelvic Inflammatory Disease Evaluation and Clinical Health (PEACH) randomized trial. *Am J Obstet Gynecol* 186:929, 2002.

Paavonen, J., et al. Prevalence and manifestations of endometritis among women with cervicitis. *Am J Obstet Gynecol* 152:275, 1986.

Puolakkainen, M., et al. Persistence of chlamydial antibodies after pelvic inflammatory disease. *J Clin Microbiol* 23:924, 1986.

Qvigstad, E., et al. Pelvic inflammatory disease associated with *Chlamydia trachomatis* infection after therapeutic abortion. *Br J Vener Dis* 59:189, 1983.

Svensson, L., et al. Ectopic pregnancy and antibodies to *Chlamydia trachomatis*. *Fertil Steril* 44:313, 1985.

Urquhart, J. Effect of the venereal disease epidemic on the incidence of ectopic pregnancy: implications for the evaluation of contraceptives. *Contraception* 19:151, 1979.

Walker, C. K., et al. Anaerobes in pelvic inflammatory disease: implications for the Centers for Disease Control and Prevention's guidelines for treatment of sexually transmitted diseases. *Clin Infect Dis* 28(suppl 1):S29, 1999.

Walker, C. K., et al. Pelvic inflammatory disease: metaanalysis of antimicrobial regimen efficacy. *J Infect Dis* 168:969, 1993.

Westrom, L. Incidence, prevalence and trends of acute pelvic inflammatory disease and its consequences in industrialized countries. *Am J Obstet Gynecol* 138:880, 1980.

Wolner-Hanssen, P., et al. Laparoscopy in women with chlamydial infection and pelvic pain: a comparison of patients with and without salpingitis. *Obstet Gynecol* 61:299, 1983.

Wolner-Hanssen, P., et al. Outpatient treatment of pelvic inflammatory disease with cefoxitin and doxycycline. *Obstet Gynecol* 71:595, 1988.

Proctocolitis, Proctitis, and Enteritis

Bolling, D. R. Prevalence, goals and complications of heterosexual anal intercourse in a gynecological population. *J Reprod Med* 19:120, 1977.

Centers for Disease Control. Amebiasis associated with colonic irrigation: Colorado. *MMWR* 30:101, 1981.

Corey, L., and Holmes, K. K. Sexual transmission of hepatitis A in homosexual men: incidence and mechanism. *N Engl J Med* 302:435, 1980.

Klausner, J. D., et al. Etiology of clinical proctitis among men who have sex with men. *Clin Infect Dis* 38:300, 2004.

Quinn, T. C., et al. The etiology of anorectal infections in homosexual men. *Am J Med* 71:395, 1981.

Rompalo, A. M. Diagnosis and treatment of sexually acquired proctitis and proctocolitis: an update. *Clin Infect Dis* 28(suppl 1):S84, 1999.

Pubic Lice

Sokoloff, F. Identification and management of pediculosis. *Nurse Pract* 19:62, 1994.

Scabies

Molinaro, M. J., et al. Scabies. *Cutis* 56:317, 1995.

Syphilis

Ellen, J. M., et al. The link between the use of crack cocaine and sexually transmitted diseases of a clinic population: a comparison of adolescents with adults. *Sex Transm Dis* 23:511, 1996.

Flores, J. L. Syphilis: a tale of twisted treponemes. *West J Med* 163:552, 1995.

Martin, D. H., and DiCarlo, R. P. Recent changes in the epidemiology of genital ulcer disease in the United States. *Sex Transm Dis* 21(suppl 2):576, 1994.

Ray, J. G. Lues-lues: maternal and fetal considerations of syphilis. *Obstet Gynecol Surv* 50:845, 1995.

Rolfs, R. T., et al. Risk factors for syphilis: cocaine use and prostitution. *Am J Public Health* 80:853, 1990.

Romanowski, B., et al. Serologic response to treatment of infectious syphilis. *Ann Intern Med* 114:1005, 1991.

Stray-Pedersen, B. Cost-benefit analysis of a prenatal prevention program against congenital syphilis. *NIPH Ann* 3:57, 1980.

Trichomoniasis

Kigozi, G. G., et al. Treatment of *Trichomonas* in pregnancy and adverse outcomes of pregnancy: a subanalysis of a randomized trial in Rakai, Uganda. *Am J Obstet Gynecol* 189:1398, 2003.

Klebanoff, M. A., et al. Failure of metronidazole to prevent preterm delivery among pregnant women with asymptomatic *Trichomonas vaginalis* infection. *N Engl J Med* 345:487, 2001.

Kreiger, J. N. Trichomoniasis in men: old issues and new data. *Sex Transm Dis* 22:83, 1995.

Kreiger, J. N. Urologic aspects of trichomoniasis. *Invest Urol* 18:411, 1981.

McLaren, L. C., et al. Isolation of *Trichomonas vaginalis* from the respiratory tract of infants with respiratory disease. *Pediatrics* 71:888, 1983.

Rein, M. F., and Chapel, T. A. Trichomoniasis, candidiasis, and the minor venereal diseases. *Clin Obstet Gynecol* 18:73, 1975.

Schwebke, J. R., and Hook, E. W., III. High rates of *Trichomonas vaginalis* among men attending a sexually transmitted diseases clinic: implications for screening and urethritis management. *J Infect Dis* 188:465, 2003.

Shaio, M. F., et al. Colorimetric one-tube nested polymerase chain reaction for the detection of *Trichomonas vaginalis* in vaginal discharge. *J Clin Microbiol* 35:132, 1997.

Wolner-Hanssen, P., et al. Clinical manifestations of vaginal trichomoniasis. *JAMA* 264:571, 1989.

ABOUT THE AUTHOR

Dr. Lisa Marr completed medical school at the University of Maryland and finished her residency in internal medicine at the University of Pittsburgh. In the mid-1990s Dr. Marr provided patient care, taught medical trainees in the field of STDs, and lectured about STDs to both medical and lay audiences. She was actively involved in research relating to sexually transmitted infections, particularly herpes. She currently lives in Milwaukee, Wisconsin.

DEMCO

APR 1 5 2008